# THE *YOU* YOU'VE NEVER MET

# THE *you* YOU'VE NEVER MET

*How to Stop Experiencing Pain and Chaos
in All of Your Relationships by
Sobering Up, Emotionally Speaking*

DR. ANDREA VITZ

This book details the author's personal experiences with and opinions about her Emotional Sobriety curriculum. The author is not your healthcare provider.

The author and publisher are providing this book and its contents on an "as is" basis and make no representations or warranties of any kind with respect to this book or its contents. The author and publisher disclaim all such representations and warranties, including, for example, warranties of merchantability and healthcare for a particular purpose. In addition, the author and publisher do not represent or warrant that the information accessible via this book is accurate, complete, or current.

The statements made about products and services are not intended to diagnose, treat, cure, or prevent any condition or disease. Please consult with your own physician or healthcare specialist regarding the suggestions and recommendations made in this book.

Except as specifically stated in this book, neither the author nor publisher, nor any authors, contributors, or other representatives will be liable for damages arising out of or in connection with the use of this book.

This is a comprehensive limitation of liability that applies to all damages of any kind, including (without limitation) compensatory, direct, indirect, or consequential damages; loss of data, income, or profit; loss of or damage to property; and claims of third parties.

You understand that this book is not intended as a substitute for consultation with a licensed healthcare practitioner, such as your physician. Before you begin any healthcare program or change your lifestyle in any way, you should consult your physician or another licensed healthcare practitioner to ensure that you are in good health and that the examples contained in this book will not harm you.

This book provides content related to physical and/or mental health issues. As such, use of this book implies your acceptance of this disclaimer.

"The *You* You've Never Met: How to Stop Experiencing Pain and Chaos in All of Your Relationships by Sobering Up, Emotionally Speaking, Rev. Ed."

Copyright © 2021 Dr. Andrea Vitz

All rights reserved. Printed by Ingram Spark in the United States of America. No part of this book may be used or reproduced in any manner whatsoever without written permission except in the case of brief quotations embodied in critical reviews and certain other noncommercial uses permitted by copyright law. For permission requests, write to books@liftedacademy.com, subject line: "Attention: Permissions Coordinator."

ISBN: 978-1-7344090-3-1

*Original Cover Development by Patty Hill*
*Cover and Illustrations by Dustin Eli Brunson*
*Chapter Icon by Mackenzie Clem*
*Cover Photograph by Bambi Cantrell with Hair and Makeup by Tera Kualapa'i Figueroa*

Revised Edition printing 2021.

Vitz, Andrea

Trademark: The *You* You've Never Met

liftedacademy.com/tyynm

For *You*

Shed the secrets burying you.
See the truth about you.
Reveal the lies.

Be so courageous
that you overcome the traumas
you've both endured and inflicted.

Release the shame as well as the anger.
Embrace joy instead of fear.
Experience clarity, not confusion.

No matter who you are,
what's been done to you,
or what you've done.

Be *free*.

# Contents

## You're Here

Chapter 1: An Invitation to Walk With Me ..... 3
Chapter 2: The Me I'd Never Noticed ..... 13
Chapter 3: Ignorant, Not Innocent ..... 19
Chapter 4: Common Misconceptions ..... 28
Chapter 5: Emotional Belligerence ..... 37
Chapter 6: EMSO Training ..... 40

## EMSO FOUNDATIONS: The *You* You've Been Being

Chapter 7: Early-Age Trauma ..... 49
Chapter 8: Trauma-Influenced Self-Beliefs ..... 55
Chapter 9: Trauma Filters ..... 61
Chapter 10: Biochemical Addiction to PANEs ..... 66
Chapter 11: Emotionally-Triggered Behaviors (ETBs) ..... 80
Chapter 12: Intoxicated Identity ..... 89
Chapter 13: Case Studies: Trauma Filters & ETBs ..... 101
Chapter 14: Find My ETBs ..... 105
Chapter 15: What Am I *Actually* Doing? Feeling? And Why? ..... 112
Chapter 16: Anatomy of Emotional Insobriety ..... 145
Chapter 17: Remove (De)Fences ..... 155
Chapter 18: Outgrow Childishness ..... 163
Chapter 19: Escape Jealousy ..... 170
Chapter 20: Free the Self ..... 178
Chapter 21: Release the Critic ..... 188
Chapter 22: Get Real ..... 196
Chapter 23: Remove the Reach ..... 205
Chapter 24: Check Motive! ..... 212
Chapter 25: Case Studies: PANEs & Motives ..... 218

## EMSO INVESTIGATIONS: The *You* You've Never Noticed

Chapter 26: Desire, Intention, Action ... 227
Chapter 27: Readiness for Change ... 234
Chapter 28: R.E.A.Life Investigation ... 242
Chapter 29: A Taste of Freedom ... 281

## EMSO REPAIRS: The *You* You're Revealing

Chapter 30: Choose Freedom ... 289
Chapter 31: Review ... 307
Chapter 32: Reveal ... 314
Chapter 33: Release ... 317
Chapter 34: Repair ... 321
Chapter 35: Merciful Lessons ... 330

## The *You* You've Never Met

Chapter 36: Fighting to Stay the Same ... 339
Chapter 37: Familiar Energy Crisis ... 354
Chapter 38: Choose the Real You ... 375
Chapter 39: You Are Not Alone ... 379
Chapter 40: The *You* You've Never Met ... 383

Afterword: Evolution of Emotional Sobriety ... 387
Author's Notes ... 389
Endnotes ... 391
Glossary of EMSO Terms ... 393
Acknowledgments ... 397
About the Author ... 400

# Foreword

Who are you? A simple question, right? Yet for me, this was a very profound question. Who was I really? Stop and ponder this question for yourself. Do you really know yourself deeply? Do you know why you sometimes have strong emotional reactions with partners, friends, and colleagues that leave you feeling regret and shame?

My personal journey includes an advanced degree in physics and a growing interest in the more profound implications of the quantum world. I regard myself as a citizen of the world, having grown up in South Africa and lived in the UK before settling in California 27 years ago. I'm a curious thinker with an inquiring mind who seeks to develop insight and consciousness on multiple levels.

My career as a successful technology executive had all the makings of a confident and bold man who was talented, innovative, and high-achieving; yet, my sense of self, lack of confidence, and anxiety in the face of conflict stunted my potential and limited my growth.

Decades of searching, reading, and counseling helped me develop some insight into who I was being, and I became more aware of emotional reactions that were unhelpful in relationships with friends, partners, and work colleagues. I recognized my emotional reactions to criticism, my fear of abandonment and failure, and my belief that I simply wasn't good enough lay just beneath the surface. No matter how much I mentally prepared to resist and curtail the hold these emotions had over me, I seemed to experience only partial success. I realized that something in me was causing me to make choices in my life that often yielded painful consequences. I was, however, unable to get to the root cause.

Through reading and personal work, I obtained two important learnings. First is the power and impact of self-image and how it profoundly affects one's life path and success in many areas—work, sports, socially, emotionally, and relationships. Second, I realized that early childhood experiences have a foundational impact on one's emotional tapestry and shape our personality. These two insights remained separate and disconnected for a long time.

I met Dr. Vitz through my gym community and discovered that she had invested many years developing deep insight into the root cause of the emotional challenges so common to all of us. She created the curriculum to develop "emotional sobriety," a term used to describe that state of being where one is no longer controlled by overpowering emotions (not unlike being controlled by a chemical addiction). Her insight has yielded the life-changing insights shared in "The You You've Never Met."

I immediately felt drawn to learn more, as I sensed this work could provide a missing key for my own development and growth. Without hesitation, I purchased my copy of this book and enrolled in her intensive course. The experience was eye-opening. Like many great scientific breakthroughs, a lightbulb turned on as I discovered the deep connection between early childhood experience and adult self-image.

I realized that I had been trying to change my response to emotional triggers by focusing on changing either my behaviors or circumstances instead of looking to the root cause—the self-beliefs. I developed these beliefs in my early childhood as a response to traumatic experiences or what Dr. V. calls our "Trauma-Influenced Self-Beliefs." I realized I'd taken into myself a set of beliefs that were untrue, but nevertheless acted as filters through which I passed all experiences and interactions. Changing these false self-beliefs was the only way to dismantle the filters that repeatedly led me to feel and behave in unhelpful and sometimes destructive ways, sabotaging my own happiness. I cannot overstress how life-changing the insight was when I connected my self-image with my early childhood experiences and the self-beliefs formed during that impressionable time.

I'm entering the next decade of my life with more balance and optimism. I feel much more confident, calm, and rational in situations that were previously emotionally triggering for me. I'm at once taking conflict less personally and taking responsibility for my part in those situations. Reforming self-beliefs unlocks more constructive processing of potentially charged emotional situations.

If you're struggling with relationships at work, home, or with friends, you may find that your emotional responses to triggers seem to be unavoidable and uncontrollable, keeping you in a never-ending cycle of reaction and regret. I recommend this book and training to you and urge you to walk the journey with Dr. Vitz. Allow her to help you identify these imprisoning self-beliefs and behaviors, and begin the work of rediscovering the real you, the original you, the you you were meant to be. Start your healing process and experience the joy and freedom that comes from feeling those emotional triggers ebbing away from your daily life. This is no magic pill; however, let me encourage you as you embark on this life-giving, transformative process. It takes work and time. How much time varies from person to person, but start your new life journey today and notice how your partner, friends, and family also discover the real you, the you you were meant to be, and just how lovable, worthy, and special you truly are.

Larry Robinson
*Chief Product Officer, BrightPlan*

# Preface

I've been called to help people since childhood, which drew me to a profession in healthcare. I became very interested in changing the cause of dis-ease, rather than chasing symptoms, and was thus charmed into the field of chiropractic. I then furthered my quest by becoming a Strength & Rehabilitation Coach. Recognizing that there was a big need for it, inside and outside the fitness world, I became immensely passionate about Emotional Sobriety—or what has now been termed "EMSO"—desirous of delivering the concept to the world in a modern, yet hard-driven, curriculum. I became a Life Coach with an emphasis on Emotional Sobriety to aid in championing that cause. I choose to devote much of my time attempting to fill up the deficit of awareness we face as a society, in that the suffering we consider to be "normal" does not have to be so!

Thus, you're now holding in your hands the revised edition of my first book, which covers the "EMSO Essentials," the first of a three-part curriculum to attain Emotional Sobriety. After teaching this introductory training for some time, I found some of the exercises and direction too advanced for many students. Thus, I decided to move the more progressive work for future books and courses, which have now become the second- and third-tier trainings. By doing so, the intense and profound coursework became simpler to grasp by revising it from its "infancy" to its present, more grown-up state that you're about to read!

Another motivation for this revised edition was to give more "meat" to the discovery and transformation of your secondary addictions. At first, seeming too fast for my students and wanting to work up to it, it became far too important to leave out. Though secondary addictions aren't limited to only drugs and alcohol, the students who've come to me from drug and alcohol recovery are some of the EMSO Training's biggest success stories, which grants this topic the new status as required investigation in addition to our personality addictions.

Everyone is learning at their own pace and ready to receive various lessons and "aha moments" at different times. This may be the perfect time for you to do this work, and it may not be. If you do choose it, even if you find portions of its content intense and even repelling at times, I recommend you see it all the way through. What I'm sharing here is for those interested in massive growth, who are committed to change, and who understand that their life—their behaviors, beliefs, and emotions—is their own responsibility and no one else's. EMSO Training is a difficult undertaking and is completed only by those courageous enough to dive into darkness to see the promise on the other side.

The names of specific individuals used to share real-life experiences in this book have been changed to protect confidentiality, yet we did receive permission to use the specific details. There are levels of trauma which I may never know personally or have yet to encounter in my students. Therefore, some levels of trauma may not be represented in this curriculum. This was written for those with similar challenges shared in its pages, as well as for those whose trauma or particular flavor of suffering seems unique only to you. I'm not a psychotherapist and don't claim to heal any mental health conditions. I don't intend to suggest that this work will cure everyone of their problems, yet I've witnessed people move through their previously insurmountable challenges with this training. They've moved on to enjoy happy and healthy lives, with meaningful and enjoyable family and friend relationships.

Also, some of the words defined throughout this book won't match your previous understanding or the dictionary definition. I've reorganized the meaning of certain words and concepts as they pertain specifically to EMSO, thereby allowing you to understand their essence in greater detail.

Simply put, I'm here to help where I once needed help, and with so many success stories now under my belt, I believe that by putting these ideas into a curriculum—EMSO Training—they're now free to benefit many, many people. I'm here to introduce you to yourself, perhaps in greater detail than you've previously known, and offer you the option for more peace and clarity in your life. This is a gift from me to you from my heart, with the knowledge that came from laboring in love.

Humbly,

Dr. Andrea Vitz

LEVELHEADEDDOC.COM

# YOU'RE HERE
## INTRODUCTION

# 1

# An Invitation to Walk With Me

*Create a future that shines so bright that the past won't recognize you.*

First things first: I'm already yours. I'm already on your side and here with you. Now it's up to you to decide how much of this you're ready to let into your life.

What if I told you that there's a person with greater qualifications to run your life than you? This person is efficient and balanced, and has the answers to your questions. They're poised in their behaviors and have an innate sense of direction to get to wherever they wish to go. They have clarity and resilience in the face of inevitable change. This person knows how to guide you to become even more remarkable, unassailable, and respectable than you already are. They intuitively know how to help correct your flight path when altered. They know how to coach you through tough times.

This exceptional and extraordinary person is the *you* you've never met.

This version of you is waiting to come to the surface. This *you* has been buried under the rubble of who you thought you were supposed to be since you were young. They've been asked to stay "underground" as a means to survive.

Allow me to guide and assist you in ridding the blocks that keep you from knowing and expressing yourself as what I refer to as the "real you."

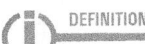

> **REAL YOU:** the innermost *you*, before you experienced any trauma; the original *you* that you were created to be; the *you* that you consciously create; the *you* you've never met.

First, take a moment to listen to yourself. How are you <u>feeling</u> right now? Distracted? Peaceful? Determined? Sad? Are there any sensations in your body? What thoughts are you having? Whatever is here as you begin, welcome it. There's no need to push anything away. This journey we're embarking on together can include all of your emotions, thoughts, and reactions as they appear in you at any moment.

Most of us seem as though we're relatively comfortable with where we are in our lives and relationships. Although our daily lives may not feel particularly fulfilling or even healthy, we have systems and patterns that have become normal for us. Maybe we can't think of a reason to give any time or energy to actively change ourselves or our lives, even if this "norm" is sprinkled with discontent and suffering.

While perhaps there hasn't been enough external pressure to force you to seek change, maybe you're like those of us who've uttered, "There has got to be more to life than this," or you've been quietly questioning the life you're living. Or maybe a recent loss has accelerated the need for your life to change—a spouse choosing to leave, a friend ending a meaningful relationship, a job loss, a death of someone close to you, or any number of emotionally overwhelming events. If the loss has come as a direct consequence of your choices or actions, you may be experiencing increased confusion about wanting to make some much-needed changes, or the opposite—clarity—a deep-knowing that the time is now. You may find yourself reaching out in desperation as if you're losing something that's truly irreplaceable.

*You don't need to suffer to grow.*
*You don't need a bottom to change.*
*You don't have to be desperate to be different.*
*You can simply make a choice to evolve.*

Whether it's due to a quiet, inner questioning or a loud, external, traumatic experience—however you connect with a subtle desire or big push to initiate a change process in your life—you aren't alone. That shared, I've said for many years that you don't need to suffer to grow. You don't need a bottom to change. You don't have to be desperate to be different. You can simply make a choice to evolve.

Much suffering occurs as a result of unconsciously inflicting harm on ourselves and others before we choose to change. We lie or manipulate. We're rhythmically and unconsciously riddled with anxiety and fear. We react in ways that we seemingly can't hold back. Even if we're not addicted to any substance, we're similar to the addict who can't control their drinking or drugging, consistently seeking their next numbing agent or distraction. Oftentimes, we even create the distraction ourselves!

We often ignore the signs of disharmony in our lives. We neglect to realize that we have an issue until someone else helps us to see it, or until we have a physical or mental crisis. More specifically, we don't see where we could personally be playing a part in our own or others' troubles. On top of all of this, our society has made it easy to overlook our destructive behavioral patterns through the normalization of blame, distractions, desensitization, and apathy. There is much dis-ease, as well as societal, cultural, ancestral, and familial programming running each of us. This can take us away from leading a healthy, fulfilling, and joyful life. We could, in fact, name these states of compulsiveness, anxiety, and dis-ease as sicknesses.

*Our society has made it easy to overlook our destructive behavioral patterns, through the normalization of blame, distractions, desensitization, and apathy.*

My passion is to help where I once needed help. To support the sick in finding their innate wholeness. You may have heard the phrase, "Those who cannot do, teach," or "We teach best that which we most need to learn." For me, it's more accurate to say that I now teach best what I most need_ed_ to learn—before I sobered up, emotionally speaking. You'll understand what I mean by this in the coming chapters; but for right now, know that I understand how it feels to need help, to feel lost in knowing what to do, where to go, or whom to talk to. I remember looking for that perfect book that would help illuminate my path to emotional stability and functional relationships.

Thus, after years of self-work and guiding others to discover their path to Emotional Sobriety, I wrote the book that I most needed. This book is written primarily from an experiential perspective, meaning these are insights and perspectives gleaned through working with hundreds of people engaging in the process of attaining Emotional Sobriety, though I also weave both personal and scientific perspectives.

I'm now well-equipped to teach this, primarily because I was able to achieve massive personal growth, having begun with a rather large deficit. I initially blamed my continued emotional <u>in</u>sobriety on my inability to find the right teacher or book to "save" me. However, soon after my liberation, I realized that the delay in my process resided in my ignorance that I needed any help in the first place. This complacency had spawned an unconscious commitment within me to remain the same.

*The delay in my betterment did not reside in my inability to find the right teacher; it lived in the absence of knowing that I needed help in the first place.*

My invitation to you is to walk closely with me and complete the in-depth course of internal investigation outlined in this book. I've designed this, and the accompanying "The *You* You've Never Met Companion Journal," as a complete process to help you discover the *you* you've been being, which prepares you for the next levels of EMSO (Emotional Sobriety) Training. In the next trainings, you will be given the lifelong tools to demonstrate your Emotional Sobriety moment to moment—in your conversations, relationships, workplace, family life, and more. Though this book and companion journal offer the full preparatory curriculum, attending an EMSO Essentials Intensive will provide the additional support needed to begin this work. The more we see and sense one another—and choose to share the experience and our mutual desire to become emotionally sober, the greater success we all will have! This is also called "entrainment." Simply put, this means that if one person "gets it," the rest of the group will have a greater opportunity to understand quickly.

EMSO Training will allow you to clearly see how you've inadvertently adopted destructive personality traits, and the ways in which you continue to enact dysfunctional behaviors and negative patterns that may be hurting you and others. Or, if you're already aware of these, you can become free of these things that create pain for you and others. If your journey has already taken you to an in-depth exploration and removal of these, perhaps you picked up this book with more work to do.

Please allow yourself space to read each word of this text and let the concepts sink in. The contents herein invite you to a depth of seeking and self-searching that may feel overwhelming at times. The pace can be determined by how quickly you would like to complete your process. Some may feel the need to read it all in one go and complete the Take Actions in a short time span. They have a fire of desire to change as quickly as possible. This may not be the case for you, and that's okay. You may feel fatigue and need to rest between exercises. You may want to put it on your shelf for a couple of days at a time. Find the rhythm and pace that are right for you—for this is <u>your</u> life, <u>your</u> journey, and all of this is <u>your</u> choice.

*Moving at a more ardent pace produces the most promising results.*

That shared, I encourage you to read this in its entirety without distraction or skipping ahead. If you're someone who wishes to digest this as quickly as possible and make changes in an expedited fashion, this curriculum is designed to support you in moving quickly. I've noticed that when people stop partway through or move too slowly, they often become <u>more</u> aware of their problems. Then, without further training, may find themselves without the necessary tools to address those problems, thus experiencing a fall into greater deficit than where they began. They may become exhausted and unwilling to continue. Moving at a more ardent pace has proven to produce the most promising results.

Everyone who has ever taken on the task of a thorough internal investigation—and who has become emotionally sober—has met challenges along the way. If you aspire to become a more effective communicator, a better leader, more mentally clear, more emotionally balanced, or just simply wish to have a happier life with healthier relationships, this process will help you get there. If you want to walk the path toward lasting change, you must first recognize who you're being and where you're being held back. This is a path I've traveled, and I'll happily walk with you.

## Who's Doing this Work?

Every person on Earth can benefit from the utilization of EMSO Training. All people can benefit from waking up even more to who they <u>truly</u> are. This is a handbook for a new life—a real life—which assists you in experiencing more moment-to-moment clarity and levelheadedness in order to feel and emanate true peace.

I've coached and treated many people in my practice as a doctor, Strength & Rehabilitation Coach, Life Coach, and now as an Emotional Sobriety Educator. I've met and I've had the privilege of teaching and knowing numerous well-established, wonderful people from all walks of life including teachers, artists, doctors, inspirational speakers and thought-leaders, authors, professional athletes, parents, CEOs, and farmers. All are extraordinarily hard-working individuals, and some may even be considered very successful yet still had a difficult time managing their personal lives and personalities, both in their homes and professions.

In direct and open conversations, I've heard similarities in their struggles. Despite having a wide range of professions and unique backgrounds, all shared a common thread of suffering. Some felt alone and incomplete. Some couldn't "hold it together." Some felt broken in their bodies, riddled with autoimmune diseases, injuries, or chronic fatigue. Some were lying and hurting themselves or others. Some had carried childish tendencies into adulthood. Some had failed marriages, estranged children, or trouble finding love. Some were overweight, while others were starving themselves. Some were attention-seeking. Some were overwhelmed with anger and jealousy.

It became glaringly obvious that even with all of their successes, there was a large "gap in their game"—a missing piece of who they knew they could be. They expressed self-assessed defects in their character including dysfunctional behaviors, negative patterns, and destructive traits that created innumerable challenges that kept them from being able to be clear, levelheaded, and peaceful.

What I came to discover is that somewhere along the way, there was a misstep in their emotional development. They hadn't advanced to a level of emotional maturity that they imagined would come naturally with age. The gap in their <u>game</u> was created by a gap in their <u>growth</u>. They were missing the element of Emotional Sobriety.

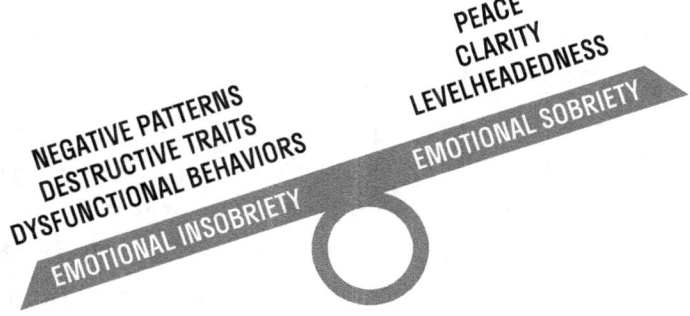

If you're reading this, perhaps you have this in common. Do you find yourself tipped more to the left side of this scale? Have you at some or many points in your life? Maybe you think of yourself as someone challenged in similar ways to these people? Take a moment and consider why you're here.

- Do you carry thoughts, feelings, or behaviors that create stress in your life or others' lives?
- Are there fears or pain that cause resistance and dis-ease in your life and relationships?
- Do you feel stuck or hopeless, or struggle with frustration or dissatisfaction that isn't easily overcome?
- Do you commonly wrestle with anxiety, depression, anger, self-pity, procrastination, or compulsiveness?
- Do you give yourself away or have discord in relationships?
- Are you more interested in keeping/sustaining your existing relationships (even if they're dysfunctional) than creating healthy ones?
- Do you use things outside of yourself to cope (social media, caffeine, drugs, alcohol, and more)?
- Do you find it difficult to stand up for yourself or have a voice?
- Do you often feel victimized or offended?
- Do you experience mood swings or sometimes get the sense that you are two different people?
- Do you need to be right in arguments?
- Do you feel a "gap in your game" even if you're successful in other areas of your life?
- Do you have a sense that you were meant for something greater, or to have greater capacities than you presently have?

If you answered "yes" to any of these questions, there are areas of your life that could be ready for an evolution. Most of us are unaware that we missed a step or more in our emotional development, and we aren't often offered a path other than the one we're already on. Until now. I'm not suggesting that these dysfunctional behaviors, negative patterns, or destructive traits are wrong or bad. Missing these steps is quite common, and you aren't to blame. No one is to blame, as we'll see in the forthcoming chapters. There will be no judgment of your current situation anywhere in this process—only _you_ having an observation of yourself and your life.

Take a few moments to allow yourself to become absolutely giddy about the concept of creating changes in your life! Open up to the potential for a huge upgrade in your capacity to handle things that may have previously felt impossible, now that you'll have a clear pathway; a community of support; and lifelong use of the training, tools, and resources available here.

*Open up to the potential for a huge upgrade in your capacity to handle things that may have previously felt impossible.*

This is a chance to have open, honest, and real relationships, not only with others, but with yourself. It's an opportunity to be balanced in situations that once caused you to spin, and to be a sounding board for others in need. EMSO Training allows you to be someone who can be relied upon in the most trying of times, and who rarely has to "protect" themselves thanks to your unassailable confidence. With Emotional Sobriety, you become the safest person in the room.

The current version of you may be keeping you imprisoned, but this doesn't have to continue. While it may seem as though <u>others</u> have been holding you back, in reality only <u>you</u> are responsible for your imprisonment. When I realized that it was only me who was ultimately responsible, I recognized that I was therefore my key to freedom. The one who's responsible is holding the key! The one who's responsible has the power to change the situation. I find incredible freedom in this.

This curriculum will show you where the key is buried inside of you— the key to unlock your cell door. Feeling truly free may be one of the peak experiences you can have in your lifetime. The intent of EMSO Training is for you to become free. I'll support you in learning how to run out of angst. I'll teach methods to remove resentment and anger. I'll encourage you to think only for yourself rather than thinking for others, and to become implicitly honest with yourself and others.

The curriculum gifted in these pages is a self-<u>work</u> book, rather than a self-<u>help</u> book, as it requires that you engage in a substantial amount of work to eliminate the harmful or destructive behaviors rooted in your habits. Yet through the work, you're naturally helped, or freed, from the prison.

You'll do this by observing your life and beginning to look at it from new angles. This can be quite challenging when you live the same way every day, using the same set of eyes. Through the "Coaching Moments," "Contemplations," "Intention-Setting Moments," "Do You Relate?" real-life stories, "Take Action" exercises, and ongoing "Practice Reps" herein, you'll come outside of yourself and look at your thoughts, feelings, and behaviors from above. If this sounds confusing, know that the curriculum clearly guides you to first explore, and then begin to stabilize, these new perspectives.

Like the people mentioned in this chapter who've risen out of despair and are now embracing their freedom, do you want to attain more clarity than you've ever had? Are you ready to discover and develop a newer version of yourself?

I lovingly encourage you to walk with me, inevitably becoming the *you* you've never met.

## 2

# The Me I'd Never Noticed

*Put your attention on what others are doing "wrong" and you're denied the opportunity to look at yourself and evolve.*

Humans are made of what we think (mental), how we feel (emotional), how we behave (physical), and the energy we emit (energetic). Whether we're alone or in a group, these are the four ways we demonstrate who we are. These are the things we embody and how others see us. Sometimes who we <u>think</u> we're being isn't who we're actually portraying.

In the past, there were times I believed I was cool and collected, and in reality, I was hysterical and dramatic—bearing resemblance to an unruly child. Or when I believed I'd been honest and of impeccable integrity, I later saw evidence of dishonesty and even manipulation. I behaved unconsciously in erratic, yet patterned, ways. I would lie about things due to my belief that the truth might be interpreted in a certain way by the other person. I jumped to conclusions and fought hard for my position. And through it all, I seemingly had no choice but to think, feel, and behave in these ways.

> *Sometimes who we <u>think</u> we're being isn't who we're actually portraying.*

Over time, my desperation to receive attention from others, and for them to declare that I was special and important, caused a huge amount of embarrassment and remorse in my life. My time and energy were consumed with distracting myself from feeling what was real in this ongoing effort to feel "good." I distracted myself and others as best I could to <u>avoid</u> being seen, while at the same time experiencing an overwhelming <u>desire</u> to be seen and understood. I was too disoriented to be really in whatever relationship that I was in, because to be in it would require being aware, secure, present, and available.

I made many attempts to survive in my day-to-day relationships. I was not actually the shiny version of myself that I believed I was. Although I would catch glimpses of the behaviors that were creating problems for me and others, I excused myself by exhibiting contrasting behaviors... being an overachiever, a hard-worker, and a "good" person. I didn't yet realize how deeply my problems ran. In the middle of an emotional outburst, I could sometimes see it, but even then assumed nothing was wrong with it and would usually defend myself right away. I could see only the blame flames before my own eyes.

A variety of activities helped keep me disconnected from reality. I kept myself continuously busy... frantically keeping all the dishes and laundry done, food prepared, and more, all under the guise that I was "taking care of things" and being helpful. In reality, I was keeping myself distracted from the present moment and from feeling what was real.

And it wasn't chores alone. I needed to be the object of everyone's affection. I smoked. I drank a little. I sought attention everywhere. I lied to get my way. At times I turned to excessive eating. When cell phones came out, I constantly used text messaging in order to be filled with the validation and distraction of receiving something back—another "hit." I watched T.V. excessively (dramas and rom-coms). I did pretty much anything short of hard drugs or excessive alcohol to achieve a change of state. I'd grown up watching soap operas, and I created my own soap opera to live inside of.

In romantic relationships, I was probably the least capable—jealous, insecure, and irritable. I was fearful and often distant. I lied to manage my dates' and partners' perceptions of me. I would think for them by translating what they said into what I thought they meant, or I'd simply decide what they were thinking in order to validate my fears. I didn't make any allowance for them to share their real feelings or critical thoughts, especially about me. I would focus on the "wrongdoings" of others and how they affected me, enabling me to never have to look at my own.

My life was a juggling act of energetic persuasion to maintain the moods and "safety" of the people around me, and my own internal state. The interesting thing is... I didn't do any of this intentionally. I didn't think, "I must keep busy or distract myself because I'm fearful of what I may experience if I stop." However, over time, I became quietly aware that my personal, familial, and romantic relationships were unhealthy and dysfunctional, but I didn't know why. I only knew that it wasn't my fault.

*I would focus on the "wrongdoings" of others and how they affected me, enabling me to never have to look at my own.*

It wasn't until I met my partner that I even realized I was stuck in this loop of dysfunction. His maturity in romantic relationships was like a language I'd never heard before, let alone spoken. He said things like, "We're partners, equals... I want to be able to talk through anything." This all seemed so out of the ordinary to me. Although his abilities and sensibilities were impressive and idealistic, I wasn't fluent in this language, nor was I prepared for the role of being his partner in this way. It was way out of my comfort zone at the time.

Before witnessing myself in this relationship, it hadn't yet been clear to me that I personally played a part in the unhealthy dynamics present in any of my past relationships. It was here that I first realized how I'd contributed to my past in destructive ways. Even when my intentions were to be "different this time," it seemed I had no control or choice in how I felt or behaved.

I was inspired by his awareness and connectability. The stark contrast between him and me was vivid, and I began imagining a continuance of pain in my future if I didn't change. It became obvious that I'd been ignoring hidden, emotionally reactive patterning and I'd not been aware of the driving force underneath it all. I wasn't awake.

I knew from an intellectual standpoint that no healthy relationship between two people can exist with even one unhealthy partner. Both people have to be healthy for the relationship to thrive. But I didn't experience this as anything other than a concept or ideal. I quickly realized that I didn't want to become a healthier person for this relationship alone. Rather, it was this relationship that made me aware that I had a problem, and began to see what my life would continue to look and feel like if I didn't make changes. My daughter was very young at the time and was also a great motivator. I knew she deserved the best mom I could give her, and we both deserved to live with more peace. I knew I had work to do.

Like most people, the concept of change was at first not only terrifying, but it seemed an insurmountable climb. I bounced between asking for assistance with my growth and demonstrating apathy or laziness that kept me believing that I was fine the way I was. At first, I wouldn't follow through with any real demonstration of new ways of being. Luckily, my partner was ever so understanding, even at my worst moments, saying, "I can see the true you in there." He gently let me know that even though I was struggling, he could still see my pure and whole heart as if it were as clear as day in front of his eyes. He understood that I was working on change and that it required me to go at my own pace. He believed wholeheartedly that I could change <u>anything</u> I set out to overcome.

With the huge project of healing myself, I realized I had to undertake the job of un-lying to myself. I didn't know any other way of being. I didn't know how to get to a place of honesty. Most important, even if I had a map, I still didn't believe that I could get there. I'd default to the norm of dysfunction and dishonesty, which would lead to emotional outbursts. I often felt there was no way to stop. The fact that I couldn't control myself, nor match my actions with my intentions, made me feel helpless, hopeless, and afraid.

Looking back from my new vantage point, I can honestly say that I was sick. While I characterize it as emotional sickness, I now know that we can't break ourselves up into little pieces. We are whole—one piece, one unit, one being. My sickness or "dis-ease" was all of me—my mental, emotional, physical, and energetic states. The biggest task I was truly undertaking at that time was to persuade myself from that "whole-istic" place to wake up and heal all the parts.

Since waking myself up and spending many years of my life and career doing this work to support others' wholism, I've become versed in the language of Emotional Sobriety—both in observing where it's lacking, and in aiding countless students in the detoxification and sustained change process required to attain it. The experience I've gleaned from coaching people toward Emotional Sobriety has also provided even more healing on my own journey, along with blessing me with the ability to continue to offer others the gift of transformation. I'm ready to support everyone and anyone who's ready!

*If I can do this, you can do this. For me, it wasn't only worth the time, energy, and temporary discomfort; it was the best decision I've ever made for my own life and the lives of those around me.*

Do you believe that there's something on the other side of where and who you currently are? Do you know how to get there when you haven't yet seen or even heard of it?

Together in these pages, and in the accompanying companion journal and online coursework, I share with you what I and many others have now done to "break the seal" toward unblocking the real you, or the *you* you've never met. You'll explore the complexity of emotional sickness which has many different expressions in each person. I know the common areas where you're likely getting stuck or where you may talk yourself into staying the same, and I'll assist you through all of the most difficult parts of this journey to the best of my ability. EMSO Training exposes you to the essential teachings of levelheadedness, clarity, and peace.

Perhaps, like many of the students who come to me, you haven't yet found the proper guidance to truly realize this place of wholeness that we talked about, or perhaps you haven't yet been pushed to a great enough degree.

One of the most sincere things I can convey to you is that if I can do this, you can do this. If hundreds of my students can do this, you can do this. For me, it wasn't only worth the time, energy, and temporary discomfort; it was the best decision I've ever made for my own life and the lives of the people close to me.

You may be where I once was. If so, EMSO Training is designed to support you in getting to a new place.

# Ignorant, Not Innocent

*We don't know what we don't know.
When we're not searching, we remain ignorant.*

As you can now see, the largest obstacles to beginning my transformation were: 1. I lacked a true belief that I had any part in my problems, and 2. I thought I was already okay in the first place. Because I thought I was already fine being who and how I'd been being, I didn't notice this other "me" that I could possibly become!

Due to the wide variety of emotional reactions I demonstrated, I realize that I, like many, was lost in self-absorption. I believed that I was the only person who had these issues, which became a viable excuse for me to keep them around. Though I experienced pangs of fear and anxiety, or sometimes felt waves of sadness, when I demonstrated these behaviors, I couldn't notice them as intuitions or invitations to change. In reality, these feelings were examples of self-protection or survival when I wasn't in any real danger at all. Though these emotional outbursts were creating pain for me and everyone around me, they were expressed as unconscious repeated responses. They had become more than habits. I was <u>addicted</u> to these ways of being.

> *In order to change who you are,
> you must first know who you're being.*

Yet with all of this seemingly obvious information stacking up to make the case that I needed to change, I still thought that it might be easier to simply stay the same and keep the behaviors, thoughts, and feelings that had kept me "safe." This is the vicious cycle that defined my journey and may define yours.

My biggest revelation occurred when I noticed who I'd <u>actually</u> been being compared to who I <u>believed</u> I was. When the distance between the two was revealed to me and another person close to me, and when the emotions that I couldn't feel previously were felt, there was no option but to change.

In order to change who you are, you must first know who you're being—realistically and factually. Without knowing who you're being, the path toward awakening, or even holistic self-improvement, can prove to be a long, and perhaps incompletable, journey. You can't edit what you can't see. Without seeing yourself clearly, you may stay locked in that vicious cycle.

Once you both know <u>and</u> feel who you've been being, and are open to others feeling you, you're ready to move forward in your life with greater self-awareness and self-responsibility. If you don't begin with these fundamentals, you may find yourself reading hundreds of books and parroting their inner wisdom without truly applying it to your life.

*You can't edit what you can't see.*

It's well known in human psychology, as well as learned through our lived experiences, that humans often continue to use survival tactics from childhood as a "go-to" in order to get what we think we need in our present, adult lives. If our sustained problems are proof that these tactics don't work, yet we still expect them to time and time again… well, that's like watching the same movie over and over and expecting a different ending, creating a spiral of insanity. I don't mean that we're clinically insane—rather, the kind of <u>insanity</u> that many of us experience—the feeling of being out of control or extremely unreasonable.[1]

On the flip side, sanity is therefore not merely the absence of mental illness. The way that I think of it is...

DEFINITION

**SANITY:** a comprehensive understanding of the self; the training and maintaining of the self, and the ability to have self-control, including control over our thoughts, emotions, and the way we respond to our inner and outer world.

Would you like to have a choice in how you behave, what you think, or even how you feel in any situation? Can you imagine being able to choose your responses, even in heated conversations? Let's explore a situation that may be familiar to you. Throughout the book you'll see "Do You Relate?" sections indicated with this symbol:

These are real-life scenarios shared by students, included for the purpose of helping you identify your own ways of being. The names have been changed for anonymity. You may also access these inspiring stories of transformation on the Levelheaded Talk Podcast.

DO YOU RELATE?

> Sharron arrives at the cafe where she meets with friends every other week for lunch. One friend starts complaining about how her spouse, yet again, did not clean up the kitchen and neglected to fill the gas tank. "Now I'm here and I don't have time to stop at the gas station. Can you believe it?!" There's a bombardment of complaints as Sharron and each friend jumps on board with additional stories of their spouses' latest mess-ups. The chatter of blame, name-calling, and irritability becomes overwhelming. When lunch is over, the whole table leaves feeling exhausted and frustrated, even though each of them arrived with a clear intention to simply have fun with friends.

If a friend of yours is hysterical, and you validate that frantic energy by becoming hysterical as well, you add to the distress. What if this were a real emergency situation? By matching the energy, you condone the behavior that caused the emergency. In the example shared here, the friends jumped into a problem, which added more problems, not only for Sharron, but for everyone in the group. When your response resembles the thoughts, feelings, or actions that created the upset or emergency, you're adding to the chaos. Now, your level of usefulness is no greater than the person in the emergency.

Do you see the impracticality of overreaction, emotional distress, and overall destructive behaviors in both an emergency situation and in your day-to-day life? Can emotional sickness—or insobriety—mimic insanity, or what are often labeled as mental disorders? Therefore, is it now possible to ascertain that true sanity is commensurate with Emotional Sobriety?

*When your response resembles the thoughts, feelings, or actions that created the upset or emergency, you're adding to the chaos.*

## So, Why Couldn't I Choose New Behavior?

Early on in my career as a coach and educator, I recognized that almost every one of my students had a beginning like mine, with similar dysfunctions, tendencies, and compulsions. Some may have even been offered psychiatric medication by their medical doctors. In my case, the pattern of lies, childish behaviors, and secrets made me sick in the first place, and my ignorance was what <u>kept</u> me sick. No medication was going to rid me of my secrets or take me out of my ignorance. What do I mean by ignorance?

DEFINITION

**IGNORANCE: unawareness; deliberately ignoring important information or facts about the self, including behaviors, beliefs, and treatment of the self and others.**

I know that if you're struggling with emotional insobriety, you may not even be aware of your condition—especially if someone hasn't yet reflected this back to you or if you haven't hit a bottom and had the realization yourself.

This lack of awareness is most often due to the two states I referred to at the beginning of this chapter:
- You don't see your part in your problems.
- You believe you're okay exactly as you are.

Two additional common mindsets that contribute to remaining ignorant of your emotional insobriety include:
- You're cradling a set of excuses that are allowable in our society.
- You tell yourself that you're unable to change due to your genetics.

Why was I unable to notice my sickness? I had elements of all four of these. My inability to perceive my sickness was well hidden behind my capacity to easily point blame at others. I could attribute any problems that arose in my life to everyone else. In part, it was also cloaked by my successes in other areas, including getting high marks in school and becoming a chiropractor at a relatively young age. Also, through my lens of interpretation, I was a good friend, sibling, girlfriend, and daughter! I was ignorant to the patterns of insobriety keeping me the same.

Let's explore these additional mindsets:

### Societal Normalization

My condition was invisible because it existed alongside others' similar issues. I didn't recognize my sickness because I was (and still am!) living in a time when emotional insobriety is a common and acceptable way of being in the world. I wasn't sharing much time with anyone I would have considered emotionally sober, or people who were "grounded" and coherent in their emotional expression, which didn't allow me to easily notice that there was any contrast. My feelings, thoughts, and behaviors were considered "normal."

Our society has normalized the deficiency of Emotional Sobriety such that it often flies under the radar. Being out of "emotional shape" is now acceptable, and maybe even glorified. Others' addictions and behaviors are serving as a distraction from our own, even containing entertainment value in popular movies, sitcoms, and now on social media. We have seemingly become desensitized to how widespread it actually is.

The commonplace nature of emotional insobriety often creates an easy excuse for us to remain irresponsible for our destructive emotions. However, merely because a behavior or emotion is common doesn't make it healthy or helpful.

### Genetics

I often hear statements such as: "I'm just this way," "It's in my genes," "I get this from my dad who was always criticizing everything and overreacting," "I know I'm just like my mother," "I have a hormonal imbalance," or "(insert genetic or personality excuse of choice here)!" It doesn't benefit anyone to focus on your supposed limitations as an excuse not to attempt change. To believe that how you currently are is the only way you'll ever be is simply untrue.

 DO YOU RELATE?

**In a moment of revelation, Jimmy shared: "When my wife asked me a question about my past, I became very anxious. I realize that I created a conflict to avoid the fact that I didn't know the answer, or I wished I had a different answer. I felt embarrassed and on edge regarding my secrets. I erupted with irrational frustration and guilt, and now have a screaming inner monologue which says, 'I don't know why she's wasting my time!'"**

This realization is conscious, but the emotions he described experiencing during the upset were unconscious, habitual survival responses to what might otherwise be a simple inquiry from someone who cares. In this particular case, he felt that his wife "asked too many questions." Instead of responding to the question, he stepped out of the present reality and quickly became confused and created a series of lies. During the interaction, he remained ignorant of his part in creating the emotional upset and can only blame her. Through EMSO Training, he's invited to slowly recount the experience and can then more clearly see that his emotional triggers are a response to shame and self-judgment of his own past actions.

With ignorance, we don't realize when we're lying, frantic, defensive, or needlessly afraid. We aren't present or vulnerable enough to see what's real.

In my case, as with many, I was unaware of my negative patterns, destructive personality traits, and dysfunctional behaviors. I couldn't name them as habits that needed to change because I was actually blind to the fact that I was even doing these things. I'm so grateful that someone could eventually get through to me and allow me to see myself.

*To believe that how you currently are is the only way you'll ever be is simply untrue.*

Many of my students develop the awareness that they need improvement because others have told them they do. Some even require convincing to meet with me for the first time; and even if they deeply look at the condition of their lives, they're still unable to see their own responsibility in having created it. There's a well of ignorance holding the troubling issues of their life.

Ignorance may seem like a strong way of describing this condition we find ourselves in, so let's explore what it really means. Ignorance commonly has three forms:[2]

- **Factual Ignorance** (lack of knowledge)—When information hasn't been offered to you nor has it been sought after.
- **Objectual Ignorance** (lack of familiarity)—Unacquaintance with an object; unfamiliarity with the problem, or not seeing the problem as a problem.
- **Technical Ignorance** (lack of understanding)—Absence of knowledge of how to do something; inexperience with the use of the tools that can correct the problem.

For the purposes of EMSO Training, I'm adding a fourth form of ignorance. While these forms of ignorance paint most of the picture, there are some of us who were, or are, adamantly opposed to even look to see if we have areas where we could be responsible for the condition of our lives. This is what I term:

- **Avoidant Ignorance** (lack of desire to know)—An intentional closing of the eyes.

Avoidant ignorance encompasses the first three and is responsible for so many people experiencing emotional insobriety and the problems derived from this. When I realized who I'd been being—with my own eyes—I woke up to the truth about me and the truth of what was around me. I could suddenly clearly see the absolute of what comprised me and my life. I remember it so vividly—the day I finally saw who I'd really been being for the very first time. When I <u>really</u> looked her in the eye, I decided to change. I decided to change, not because I hated her or because she was wrong, but because her behavior did not match my spirit—the me I believed I truly was deep down inside.

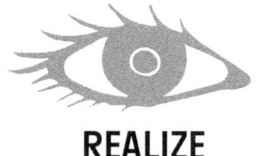
**REALIZE**

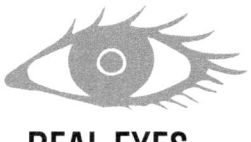
**REAL EYES**

Having a realization—or to realize—is to suddenly see what's actually occurring—to use "real eyes." This realization pushed me into an evolutionary process... and quickly! It's what encouraged me—or filled me with the courage—to embrace honesty, and it connected me with the energy to course correct and discover who I'd been being. It gave me the courage to actually attempt to overcome my patterns.

*When I <u>really</u> looked her in the eye, I decided to change.*

I was desperate for change. I used inspiration from all around me. I constructed a deliberate path to a new place. In other areas of my life, I'd been very focused and disciplined. Once I focused that discipline on finding the parts of me that weren't truly me and eradicating my emotional sickness, I was presented with the clear tools to change them. This has formed the EMSO Training that I now share with you.

If you feel nervous about this change, know that my life was filled with drama, chaos, resistance, and more when I began my journey. If you meet me today, you'll be introduced to the opposite. I was paradoxically later granted the nickname "Levelheaded Doc," as I now teach levelheadedness as a discipline. But it isn't only something we learn and practice, it's something we become.

# 4

# Common Misconceptions

*Knowing to pause before you react is Emotional Intelligence;
not needing to pause is Emotional Sobriety.*

Before we dive fully into the training process, there are a few misconceptions that we need to get clear on together. These are topics that are often thought to be the same, and I'll share what differentiates them. They include:

- Emotional Intelligence vs. Emotional Sobriety
- Being Clean vs. Being Sober
- Therapy vs. EMSO Training

## Emotional Intelligence vs. Emotional Sobriety

In addition to having an intelligence quotient, or IQ, research indicates that humans also have an emotional intelligence quotient, sometimes referred to as our EQ, or simply EI.[3] Let's see how this plays into our lives.

Emotional Intelligence is most commonly defined as "the ability to understand the way people feel and react and to use this skill to make good judgments and to avoid or solve problems."[4] It's the act of being intelligent about them and instilling the necessary attention skills to ensure that you know <u>what</u> you're feeling and <u>when</u>. In addition, it also spans using this awareness to know when you should act a certain way to relieve stress (e.g., exercise) before your emotions get the best of you and you end up in emotional overwhelm.

I therefore most simply define it as:

DEFINITION

**EMOTIONAL INTELLIGENCE:** awareness of your emotions.

Though this intelligence is incredibly important, it isn't a complete solution. It doesn't solve the issue that your emotions are capable of "getting the best of you" in the first place.

Awareness of your current emotions and patterns offers no real lasting salvation. Dispersing your energy into something external by expressing that emotion is a temporary bandage. That emotion will come again. As will its power over you. Although a necessary practice and skill, an <u>awareness</u> of emotions isn't enough to experience lasting freedom.

For example, simply being aware that I'm overweight won't provide me with a real solution for changing my weight. A real solution here requires desire, intention, and action. In this case, it requires generating a desire to shift my weight, choosing to recreate my mindset around food, and then consistently choosing to eat and exercise differently. I'd need to actually become someone different. The person I am now is overweight. The person I'll become won't be. So, the same way I'd need to become someone different to overcome my weight issues, I'd need to make the same level of change to my issues with emotional overwhelm.

So then, what is Emotional Sobriety? I'm often asked this question because this term hasn't had as much attention in the recent years. Let's break it down. There's a broad foundation to the definition of sobriety. Most people think of sobriety only as a state of recovery after a drug or alcohol addiction. Someone who's sober could be identified as: "One who doesn't do drugs or drink alcohol." An example may be the friend at the barbeque who used to have nine beers before driving home, but who's now drinking iced tea instead and is therefore considered the "sober driver."

The dictionary <u>first</u> defines sober as: "sparing in the use of food and drink; not addicted to intoxicating drink; not drunk."[5] You've probably heard a person claim, "I've been clean and sober for 10 years!" Since this isn't a book specifically about drug or alcohol addiction, why are we talking about sobriety? Let's look at some of the subsequent definitions to get a more complete picture.

Another definition of sober is: "marked by earnestly thoughtful character or demeanor, unhurried, calm; marked by temperance, moderation, or seriousness; showing no excessive or extreme emotion, or prejudice."[6]

Some synonyms of sobriety include:

- Clear-headed
- Sensible
- Dignified
- Steady
- Down-to-earth
- Commonsensical
- Self-controlled
- Factual
- Realistic
- Objective
- Low-key
- Matter-of-fact
- No-nonsense
- Rational
- Logical
- Straightforward
- Well-considered

*Emotional Sobriety is just that—a levelheaded, balanced, and reality-based state of being.*

Notice that none of these synonyms mention an abstinence of drugs or alcohol, rather they're states of being, or character traits. I'm not suggesting there is a "normal" or "right" way to be and behave. Though some of these synonyms seem colorless and bland, I want to impart that "sober" is not synonymous with being callous or boring. You'll still feel your emotions. You may experience intense passion or have hilariously goofy moments. I assure you that all of your most adored traits can remain part of your expression. The primary difference is that once you achieve Emotional Sobriety, you'll be selecting, feeling, and expressing yourself <u>consciously</u> and <u>realistically</u>.

These traits describe someone of reasonable and rational emotional character, or as we explored in the last section, someone who's "sane." Emotional

Sobriety is just that—a levelheaded, balanced, and reality-based state of being. It's the best foundation upon which to build a joyful and abundant life—a sustainable and unshakable place for growth in all areas of your life.

In my career, I've met with many people who were chemically addicted to drugs, alcohol, or prescription medication. Given the fact that they'd already taken the step to come to my office, most of them were already aware of their problem, yet every person continued to actively demonstrate their addictions. With alcoholics, for example, nearly every person I met was extremely intelligent and could comfortably share their knowledge and understanding of their addictive patterns. But that didn't keep them from drinking, nor did it disable their ability to get drunk once enough of the compound was in their bodies.

*You can be aware of your emotions and your predisposition to having them, and still become inebriated under their influence.*

The same goes with the emotionally unsober. We may become aware of all of our patterns of behavior in relation to a certain emotion, and even know when we're experiencing this emotion. But once the emotion presents itself, we still become engulfed by it and lose control regarding the behavior that follows. When we rely upon awareness alone and don't follow up with conscious action, we ignore the fact that this emotion is capable of "taking us out" and is still allowed to make an appearance. Again, awareness of our emotions is the first step in us overcoming them, but it's not the entire solution.

You can be quite intelligent in regard to the effects that drinking alcohol has on you and still become inebriated under its influence. In the same way, you can be aware of your emotions and your predisposition to having them, and still become inebriated under their influence.

Emotional Sobriety is therefore a combination of Emotional Intelligence and training yourself to not simply outsmart your emotions, but to overcome them. Emotional Sobriety gives us such levelheadedness that almost no situation can create destructive emotional responses because it's no longer our habit to have them. Emotional Sobriety is not a temporary tool to manage our emotional overwhelm. Emotional Sobriety is a <u>solution</u>—a state of being—which requires becoming someone new.

### DEFINITION

**EMOTIONAL SOBRIETY:** to be rid of the filters, beliefs, and subsequent emotions that cause our belligerence; to remove the offensive chemistry that promotes our triggered behaviors; to be able to experience all of our life and relationships with levelheadedness, clarity, and peace.

Emotional Intelligence, combined with dedicated work, elicits the mental and energetic change leading to Emotional Sobriety. Going through such a mental and energetic change rewrites your subconscious programming and removes the habit of destructive emotional responses. Being emotionally intelligent may be similar to being the bright-eyed student taking a new course, whereas being emotionally sober is to become the professor of that course.

## Being Clean vs. Being Sober

Now that we better understand the distinction between Emotional Intelligence and Emotional Sobriety, it's essential to distinguish the difference between being clean vs. being sober.

As we just established, many people hear the word "sobriety" and think that it's only about recovering from drug and alcohol dependence. I propose that people who were once drinking and/or using drugs in an unhealthy amount, and have now stopped have become "clean," but not necessarily "sober." Getting clean is something to celebrate, yet it isn't the finish line.

Someone who refrains from drinking, drugs, sugar, and the like, is abstaining. This abstinence is what creates a clean state. But what about the thing that made them drink, drug, or binge to this level in the first place? What about the thing that made them reach for the substance?

In the EMSO community, we understand that sobriety isn't the absence of drugs and alcohol. Sobriety is having internal clarity, levelheadedness, and peace. This is what keeps us from needing to reach for something such as beer or pills as a "Band-Aid."

It is to annihilate the component of ourselves that makes us behave in ways that we don't consciously choose. The behaviors can be anything from drinking all day to just getting in a fight with our partner.

I believe, in fact, that emotional insobriety is the common contributor to most alcohol, drug, and other addictions. I also believe that all addictive behavior is the <u>symptom</u>, not the problem, and nearly all addiction comes from the same biochemical sickness, only with different symptoms.

With this idea in mind, drug, alcohol, gambling, relationship, and other addictions are not really the primary problem. Therefore, removing them cannot be the sole solution. Our distractors are most often in place due to our emotional (biochemical) addiction, which we'll explore in great detail in this book. We're addicted to the substances as a secondary dependence—a dependence that we've created in order to feel something different than what we're addicted to feeling. Therefore, from now on I'll refer to these as secondary addictions.

*I also believe all addictive behavior is the <u>symptom</u>, not the problem, and nearly all addiction comes from the same biochemical sickness, only with different symptoms.*

Perhaps we aren't addicted to the distractions we think we are! In other words, we use these "aids" to release us from the bondage of our pain and discontent. They're only a symptom of our primary emotional, biochemical addiction. These distractors are something we've trained our bodies to crave to no longer feel what we don't want to feel. Is our problem really drugs, food, social media, alcohol or compulsive promiscuity, or are these only secondary distractors? What if they're not the distractions you cannot live <u>without</u>, but the emotions you feel inside you that you cannot live <u>with</u>?

If we felt competent, content, free, and joyful, would these addictions even begin in the first place? I propose that there would be no desire for a change of state, and even if there were, it wouldn't be due to a thought that something is lacking or that we're in too much pain.

In my experience working with exogenous addicts, this has been the case. Self-admittingly, they didn't begin using drugs or alcohol while in a state of levelheadedness, clarity, and peace. Thus, if the emotional challenges came first, after they overcame their addiction to an external substance, they remained in continued deficit due to their remaining emotional insobriety, and they simply found themselves reaching for something else to take that chemical's place—another secondary distractor. Or, they'll return to their original distractor that delivered them away from their disturbing emotions.

This continued emotional deficit is how a "recovered" alcoholic or a drug addict can still end up relapsing. It was quickly made apparent that no matter the addictive substance or compulsive habitual behavior, the cause of the sickness was the same: their addiction to discontentment, confusion, resentment, low self-esteem, fear, shame, and more.

It's imperative that those who are here to attain Emotional Sobriety really understand the difference between getting clean and true sobriety… that the common definition of sobriety be removed from our culture, and that we understand that sobriety is a very concept from than getting clean. Otherwise, there will continue to be a belief that abstinence and a program are the pinnacle of recovery, and without the removal of this belief, we have a false sense of security and are more likely to relapse.

Someone whom I dearly love—who was quite active in a twelve-step recovery program—died from alcohol addiction. This was a massive catalyst for me to develop this curriculum. I knew that we could take someone from addiction recovery all the way to true, lasting sobriety. We lose people in recovery when they don't know how to handle the pain in their life, and they go backwards to reach for the thing that they believe will annihilate their suffering. It "worked" in the past, and the body and brain remembers that. I know that we're called to do better for each other. This is when I asked for not only the answer for myself, but in finding that answer, I knew I had found his as well. I asked myself, "If he had EMSO would he still be alive today?" The answer came back to me as a resounding yes! I firmly believe that with true Emotional Sobriety, this person would not only be alive today, but he would be teaching this with me as well.

Getting or being <u>clean</u> is abstinence, with a commitment to no longer reach for that unhealthy compound or activity. Using willpower (or a higher power) to do so, the addict may remain in suffering. Getting or being <u>sober</u> is the transformation of someone whose maturity allows them to navigate situations and relationships that were once impossible, with ease and understanding.

### Therapy vs. EMSO Training

The third misconception I often hear is, "I see a therapist, so why would I need EMSO Training?" A therapeutic relationship often supports changing a person's emotional state in the moment they're in session, and even grant them with some tools to self-soothe, reframe, or medicate, which can change their emotional state in some capacity when not in session. EMSO is a once-in-a-lifetime opportunity to explore every facet of your past and present, and uncover the beliefs that are keeping you addicted to your emotions.

*In EMSO Training, you train to become the person you were made to be, not the person or child that trauma made.*

EMSO Training isn't therapy, nor is it counseling. I don't have any negative thoughts around anyone who goes to therapy, as I believe first and foremost that it's important to have someone to talk to. However, like getting clean, I don't believe that therapy is a long-term solution to our overall emotional pain.

In a therapeutic setting, we tend to contemplate the trauma, the circumstances, the current and past situations, and our struggles in them. We're either medicating ourselves or talking about our trauma over and over, sometimes about the trauma specifically, and other times about the circumstance in our adult life that resembles a childhood trauma. By doing that, we're merely marinating and becoming more of a product of that trauma. I've become curious if therapy offers a long-term solution.

In EMSO Training, you train to become someone different. It provides massive shifts in your emotional state offering lifelong results that you often don't gain solely from therapy, meditation practice, or medication. You train to become the person whom you were made to be, not the person or child that trauma made.

# 5

# Emotional Belligerence

*The loss of self-control while under the influence of emotion is Emotional Belligerence.*

It's important to note that while most of us are emotionally unsober on some level, there are also cases that I've witnessed within my career and in my personal history that I refer to as Emotional Belligerence. We become emotionally belligerent when we're quickly flooded with emotions and have an over-the-top reaction to an event or comment. We're not stumbling on our <u>feet</u> as if we're drunk on alcohol; we're stumbling in <u>life</u>, and we seemingly have no power of choice, making "mistake" after "mistake." If you've ever experienced being inebriated, either on medication, drugs, alcohol, or another substance, you may relate to the sense of being inside a fog of unreality, of feeling as though you're here but not really connected to the present. You've become massively intoxicated. The same is true when we're <u>emotionally</u> belligerent.

*We're not stumbling on our <u>feet</u> as if we're drunk on alcohol; we're stumbling in <u>life</u>.*

As we'll learn in great depth in the next part of the book, this flood of "emotions" is actually a flood of chemicals in the body, and we're literally now under the influence as a "blind drunk." We cannot reason, listen, or think straight. If you've had the feeling of not being able to hold yourself back when you're angry or been too threatened to make a new decision to behave a certain way within that moment, then you've been emotionally belligerent. You've become sick with behavioral compulsions, which are dictated by your wild emotions.

Have you experienced times in your life that were sideswiped by emotion and were unable to control your behavior? Or even your thought process?

So have I.

When we've reached the stage of Emotional Belligerence, we no longer have the power of choice. This requires extra work to unravel, and don't worry, you'll learn how!

DEFINITION

**EMOTIONAL BELLIGERENCE:** to become overrun with harsh biochemicals, emotionally "drunk," losing the power of choice regarding behavior, along with the inability to be corrected until the chemistry changes on its own.

## Signs of Emotional Belligerence

While a majority of the subsequent chapters deal with emotional insobriety and the components of what I've termed an Intoxicated Identity, it's important to acknowledge the more extreme cases of emotional insobriety that take this form of Emotional Belligerence. We're at our peak of seeking to control our environment whilst being completely out of control ourselves. The common symptoms include:

- Being excessively flustered
- Speaking in circles
- Acting hysterical; being unable to maintain control or volume of voice
- Being overly dramatic
- Exaggerating; greatly overstating something to make the point carry more weight
- Compulsively lying
- Demonstrating outward rage

- Consistently thinking for others, thinking about what others are going to say next, or wondering what they're thinking
- Repeatedly choosing predictably unhealthy relationships
- Excessively using substances to change your emotional state
- Expressing feelings of intense shame or shaming others
- Slandering or attacking others
- Violently defending oneself

Ironically, Emotional Belligerence may often feel more like a lack of emotional stamina rather than an excess of emotions. This may be fatigue due to an overproduction of the chemical (e.g., adrenaline, cortisol, norepinephrine, and more). In various situations, you may come up against more than simply a "loss of words" or balance; you may become a volcano of anger and say things that you wouldn't intend to say if you were capable of more clarity. Or you may speak repetitively in circles until you feel satisfied that these emotions are appeased, getting what they want from you, and everyone around you. You've essentially become a slave to these emotions when they're in charge and you feel helpless.

# 6

# EMSO Training

*Any change you desire can be achieved through training.*

Welcome to this in-depth process that came out of the many years of personal and professional experience living and guiding others toward Emotional Sobriety. It has become my life's mission to support as many people as possible in EMSO Training. It's reaching people across the globe and is now provided in three phases:

- **EMSO Essentials** (provided in this book and the companion journal, as well as in an online course curriculum)
- **EMSO Practicum** (second-tier training to practice EMSO)
- **EMSO AP** (third-tier training on advanced practices)

While my intention was to provide the comprehensive training inside "The *You* You've Never Met" and the companion journal so that as many people as possible could easily receive it, I also realized that there needed to be opportunities to go deeper and receive additional support. Thus, I've added new support tools in this revised edition, a new chapter on "secondary addiction," as well as additional opportunities to train alongside and with the support of others. Please join the EMSO Community at **liftedacademy.com** and on social media **@levelheadeddoc** to stay abreast of additional offerings. Consider joining an upcoming online training as you're reading along in the book. We can also pair you up with an "EMSO CO"— a co-pilot, colleague, companion, confidante, comrade—who's at a similar stage in his/her EMSO Training. This isn't a sponsor/sponsee relationship; rather, a peer-to-peer one. Some who may have a rather large deficit or are going through a particularly challenging time as they're reading this curriculum have opted to engage one-on-one with an EMSO Coach to complete their EMSO Essentials. Whatever format is best for you, give yourself the time and space to devote to it.

*One at a time doesn't take much time,
when we're each responsible for our own lives.*

After attaining Emotional Sobriety in my life, I was blessed with the desire and opportunity to work with others like me. Over many years of guiding women and men through this essential process, I've assisted them as they engaged the training and undertook the challenge of becoming someone new. With each success story, I was astonished as I witnessed the power of metamorphosis and humbled by the pull of addiction in those who weren't yet ready to overcome it.

A coach or a very experienced mentor is necessary in the process of changing ourselves, as is a supportive community. This is particularly true in the beginning of this process when we're becoming aware of our deficits and addictions. We'll bump up against our belligerence and want to indulge in old thought patterns, behaviors, and of course, emotional expressions. This is why I'm here with you now. Our accompanying trainings will allow you to walk side-by-side with others going through this process so that together, we can go deep and truly change our long-standing emotional insobriety.

In short, EMSO Training is a detoxification process of the chemistry that you're used to making. Having gone through the process of changing my biochemistry and becoming emotionally sober, and having sat with many others who have as well, I know the common patterns that your mind and body uses to block your success.

I'll share what you might butt up against during the process of change... where your chemistry will try and pull you back into the old ways. I'll sense where the gaps are in your sobriety, integrity, and overall maturity (i.e., thinking, feeling, or behaving, based on your childhood program). I'll notice when you're lying to yourself. Unlike some who may let you alter the path to change, negate the value of your past as it is, or not invite you to take responsibility, I'm going to push you further than you may have been pushed before, as pushing past your current state is the only way to truly overcome your problems.

Together, we'll begin our transition to a healthier humanity by recognizing the presence of our patterns and the prevalence of emotional insobriety. We do this first as individuals, and if we take it upon ourselves to do our own deep and lasting healing, we can then help others around us. Similar to having our own oxygen mask in place before we can help the person next to us on the airplane, let's bring awareness to our own behaviors, thoughts, and feelings, and begin to change the ones that are harmful. Once we've achieved our own wellness, we can naturally create a constructive ripple of awareness and transformation all around us. One at a time doesn't take much time when we're each responsible for our own lives.

EMSO Training promises the opportunity for you to have far fewer negative emotional responses, and in turn allows you to be present without external influences altering your mood, behavior, or ability to clearly communicate. You may end the experience of drowning to the point of despair, or participating in irreversibly harmful conversations or actions, including the pulls of all of the other aforementioned addictions.

*When you become emotionally sober your emotions will not, and in fact cannot, control your life anymore.*

For me, this metamorphosis was life-revolutionizing, and it has the potential to revolutionize your life as well. Doing this training was not only the greatest gift I gave to myself, but also to my daughter and everyone around me. Truly healing yourself is the greatest gift you can give to everyone in your life… to your parents, your children or future children, your partner or future partner, your friends and acquaintances, your co-workers… literally everyone who can see you, talk to you, and feel you will be affected by your sobriety.

Each aspect of EMSO Training will create a unique opportunity for you to truly see the current version of you and make a conscious choice if that is who you wish to be going forward.

When you become emotionally sober, your emotions will not, and in fact cannot, control your life anymore. You'll be the keeper of your own mind and body.

I invite you to seek further clarity alongside the community of others who are already embracing their own massive transformations. Join me in remodeling the emotional stature of humanity by starting with yourself!

EMSO Training follows what I call The 4A Formula:

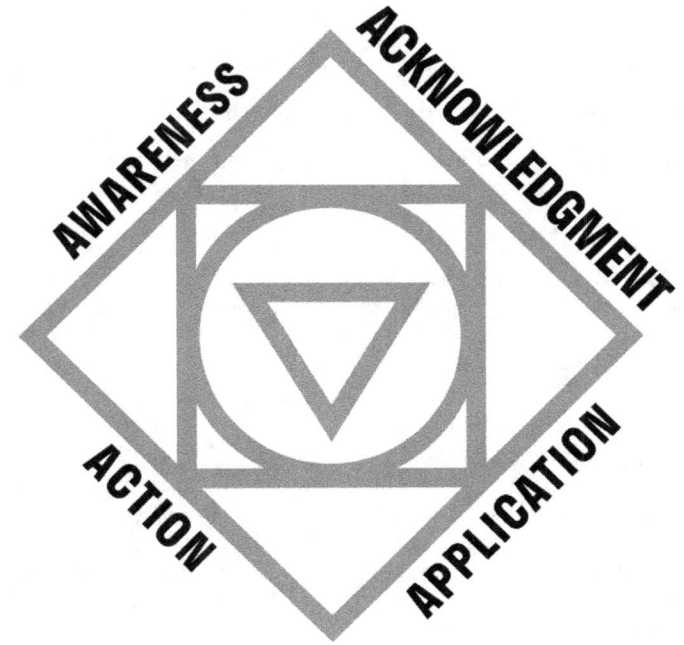

The first-tier EMSO Essentials Training, as outlined in this book and the companion journal, is an inward journey and is structured as follows:

- **EMSO Foundations**—grows your awareness of the *you* you've been being and exposes your Anatomy of Emotional Insobriety.
- **EMSO Investigations**—gives you an opportunity to deeply acknowledge and accept the *you* you'd never noticed and its impacts on all the parts of your life.
- **EMSO Repairs**—continues the acknowledgment part of the formula by inviting you to heal with humility using The 4Rs, which shape the *you* you're revealing.

The second two components of The 4A Formula—the practical and outward action and application of your Emotional Sobriety—is briefly introduced in this book, and then shared in great detail during the follow-up training called the EMSO Practicum.

**Introducing Pause Points:**

In addition to the "Do You Relate?" stories I've already introduced, the following "pause points" invite you to stop and contemplate something, read aloud, or perhaps pull out the companion journal to complete an exercise.

DO YOU RELATE?

Again, these are the real-life stories from students of Emotional Sobriety. Pause as you're reading, and feel into the person who's sharing and ask yourself, "Do I relate to this? Is this how I would react or respond in a similar situation?"

COACHING MOMENT

While I can't sit with you one-on-one as you read the pages of the book (though I have with some students!), these moments offer you the opportunity to feel my presence as your coach on this journey. They're the "I've been there/done that too" moments to remind you that you're not alone, and we're all the same.

### INTENTION-SETTING MOMENT

These are great moments to slow down, connect to your future self, and be still before a big push forward. I recommend speaking these out loud if you're able, and if not, simply read aloud in your head.

### CONTEMPLATION

Throughout the book there are moments to pause and contemplate a set of questions. This doesn't require writing anything down. In fact, it's important that you <u>don't</u> write your responses to these. Rather, sit quietly and simply read and contemplate internally. Then, feel what you feel and think what you think. There's no need to share them with anyone.

### TAKE ACTION

These are the exercises. Each time you see this Take Action symbol, get out your pen or pencil and find a quiet place to write. You're welcome to write directly in the book as I've provided some space for each one here. However, this work is designed to be accomplished along with the "The *You* You've Never Met Companion Journal." I highly recommend obtaining your personal copy to organize your process. Each Take Action is in the journal with plenty of space. Most students find that working with both is more effective for attaining Emotional Sobriety.

Also, you're prompted throughout the book to visit your member page for complementary, downloadable PDFs and audio recordings of several of the contemplations to support your journey: **liftedacademy.com/tyynm**.

Let's complete your first Take Action by recognizing that who you've <u>been</u> may not be who you truly <u>are</u>, as evidenced by your suffering in life. None of us were born to suffer or to create suffering for others. EMSO Training is here to unblock or unveil who you really are. The first exercise is an opportunity to begin this process by seeing which emotionally sober trait or traits you wish to attain. Whatever traits you wish to have are the real you underneath the "rubble." For the purposes of this book and forthcoming exercises, I've developed a series of graphics to depict the most common forms of each component. These distillations came from working with hundreds of students over more than a decade, and observing what they uncovered inside themselves, as well as my own journey to Emotional Sobriety. Each graphic also appears in the companion journal.

Throughout the EMSO Training curriculum, you'll be invited to look at various aspects of "The Real You." Remember, this is the *you* you've never met... the one that is already within you, waiting to be revealed. This book contains the first three access points to this *you*. Let's begin!

 TAKE ACTION

**THE REAL ME, PART 1:**
**COMMON TRAITS OF AN EMOTIONALLY SOBER PERSON**
As a contrast to where you may be beginning, look at the graphic below. It contains what I commonly see in people who've become emotionally sober. Ask yourself: "Which of these qualities do I wish to attain?" (Yes, it can be all of them!) Circle as many as you wish, and write about why you circled them:

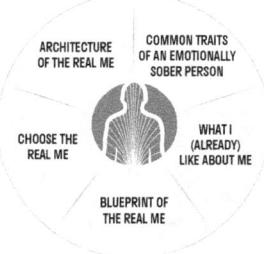

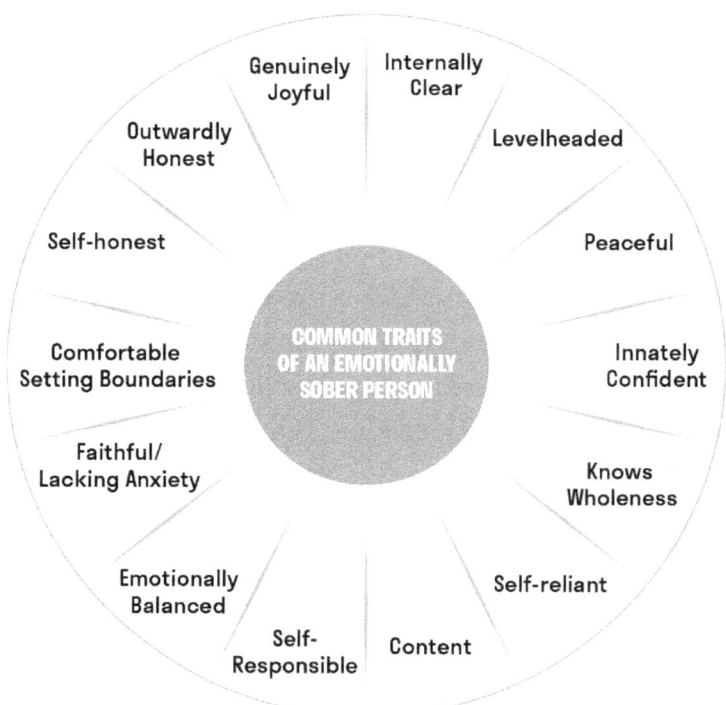

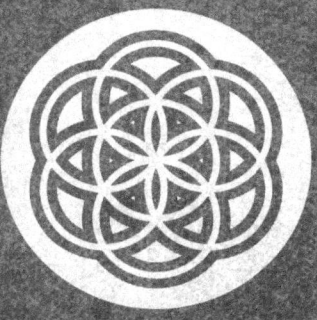

# EMSO FOUNDATIONS
### THE *YOU* YOU'VE BEEN BEING

# 7

# Early-Age Trauma

*You aren't breakable.*

In order to deeply engage the process of attaining Emotional Sobriety, we'll first develop your Emotional Intelligence and help you become aware of how you became emotionally <u>un</u>sober. How did you become the *you* you've been being? How did most of us develop these destructive patterns, dysfunctional behaviors, and negative traits?

Because emotional insobriety is now such a common way of being—and as I shared, so widely accepted in our culture—I've uncovered the common cycle that I believe creates this condition. When you put together the six concepts in this section, you discover what I call your Anatomy of Emotional Insobriety.

To unravel the cycle, we begin where our insobriety seemed to begin... with trauma. Here's how I define it:

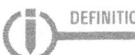 DEFINITION

**EARLY-AGE TRAUMA:**
<u>any</u> event that creates a hard change in your emotional status... a stark contrast to the feelings you had before the event; a moment that changes or influences what you believe to be true about yourself and the world around you in a negative way.

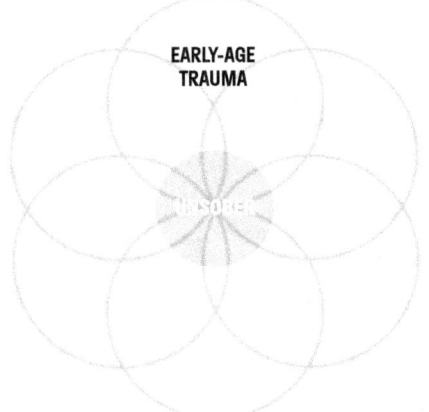

EARLY-AGE TRAUMA

Early-Age Trauma is often such a shocking and crashing experience that it creates a crack, separating you from your perceived sense of security. Due to the rapid and sudden injury, I believe trauma to be a fracture. I don't think of trauma as an unhealable, final break. We don't break from trauma, yet the remaining fear, anger, sadness, and more may lead us toward the <u>belief</u> that we have. In fact, we're often so fractured by our earliest trauma(s) that we seem forever changed by them, or we block them out and have no real memory of them. What we don't forget is our <u>response</u> to the traumas... who we become because of them.

In his book, "Healing Trauma," Peter A. Levine, a renowned psychologist and leader in the field of stress and trauma defines it as "the often debilitating symptoms that many people suffer from in the aftermath of perceived life-threatening or overwhelming experiences."[7] The U.S. Department of Health and Human Services names them "ACEs"—Adverse Childhood Experiences.[8] In my experience, whether major or minor, we <u>all</u> have experienced some form of Early-Age Trauma. Depending on your age and emotional maturity at the time, traumatic experiences can significantly block your emotional, intellectual, and spiritual growth. We'll find out how they severely affect your physical biochemistry as well.

For our purposes, we'll explore the experiences that occurred before the age of 20—and often very early on in life (ages 0 to 7)—before we had the capacity to fully think and speak for ourselves. I characterize trauma in four distinct ways:

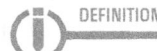
### DEFINITIONS

**OBSERVED TRAUMA:** witnessing an impactful or dissonant event.—e.g., listening to your parents fight as a chlid and feeling unsafe or insecure.

**PERCEIVED TRAUMA:** judging the intention of someone else's action.—e.g., witnessing your father leave your mother and believing it's because of you/your unlovability.

**INFLICED TRAUMA:** trauma inflicted upon you by someone or something.—e.g., rape, physical abuse, mental or emotional abuse, etc.

**DELIVERED TRAUMA:** trauma that you as a child inflict upon someone or something.—e.g., bullying another kid at school, being verbally abusive to a sibling, etc.

No matter what the trauma, whether absorbed by us or delivered by us, it births the development of beliefs about ourselves, which begins the crack in the foundation of our self-esteem. In EMSO Training, it's essential to become aware of the effects of your Early-Age Traumas of all types, in order to be able to fully emerge from their hold on you and understand where you've carried their effects over to your current life.

*No matter what the trauma, whether absorbed by us or delivered by us, it births the development of beliefs about ourselves, which begins the crack in the foundation of our self-esteem.*

For example, you may be easily offended, triggered to feel sadness or shame, or have unexplainable tendencies that others don't. You may have deep patterns of Emotional Belligerence. Whatever the severity of your patterns, these are all things that you can remedy with the right knowledge and by connecting the <u>how</u> and the <u>why</u> behind them.

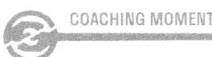
**COACHING MOMENT**

> It doesn't matter how old you are. You're allowed to look at this, even if it happened 40, 50, or 60+ years ago. You may have an early childhood experience that you've been camouflaging, or you recall the event itself but can't connect it to the true effects it's had on your life. This is often demonstrated with repeated self-talk such as, "Yes, that happened, but it's not a big deal."

I've sat with 50-year-old men who thought they were completely free of all of their blocks and had looked at all of their difficulties. Maybe they still had some things they were "hung up on," but had no idea what was still lingering within them and keeping them from advancing to the level where they wished to be. They were stuck and couldn't learn the masterful teachings they desired to learn and live a resistance-free life. Once they clearly saw the trauma that they'd endured and/or delivered, and felt safe enough to "look there" more deeply, they realized why they tended to be a certain way in their lives today. Once they connected the two, they were able to begin the process of all-encompassing growth.

Let's focus on the most common traumas I find with my students—all of which can be one-time events or chronically endured throughout our early years.

**COACHING MOMENT**

> It's important to note that the contemplations in this chapter may elicit strong emotions—emotions you may not have been able to express or process in a smaller, younger body. For now, simply hold the perspective that although you've experienced this in your past, it won't need to define your future. Let me take you through these safely and slowly to help you collect the truth about your trauma. When I did a similar exercise, I imagined I was undertaking it with a trusted friend or confidante right there with me. If that's an idea that appeals to you, utilize this method to ease this process as much as possible. If you need assistance, sit with an EMSO Coach, your EMSO CO if you have one, a therapist, or trusted friend.

**CONTEMPLATION**

**PEEK INTO MY PAST**
Glance through the Common Early-Age Traumas in the graphic on the following page. Do you notice any that jump out as a description of your personal experiences? Are there others not listed here that you've experienced? Remember, you don't need to write anything down at this point, as you're merely contemplating this.

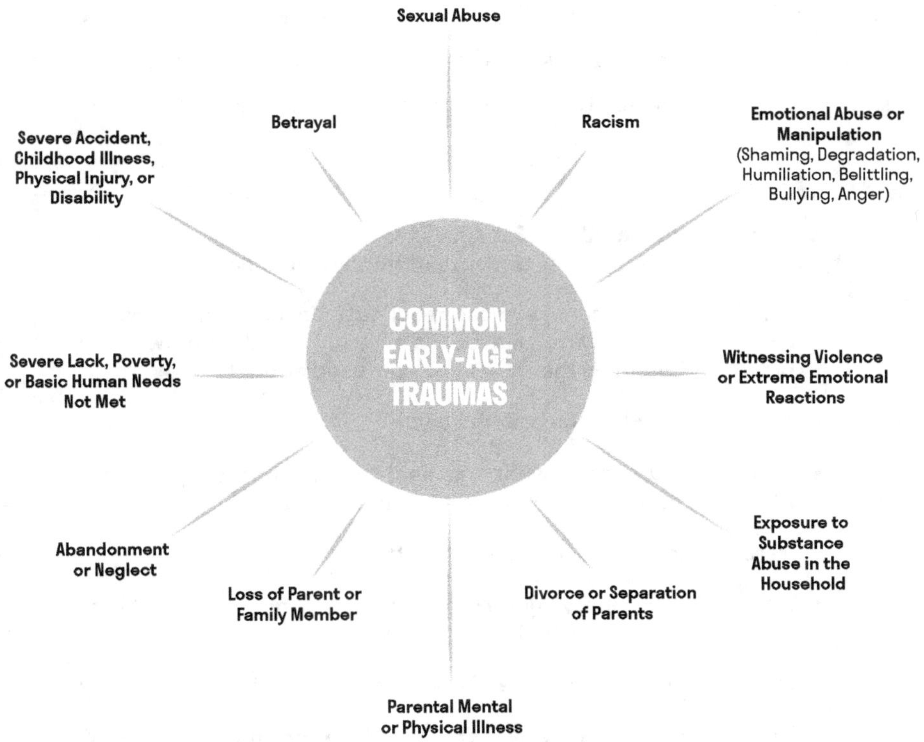

**COMMON EARLY-AGE TRAUMAS**

- Sexual Abuse
- Betrayal
- Racism
- Emotional Abuse or Manipulation (Shaming, Degradation, Humiliation, Belittling, Bullying, Anger)
- Severe Accident, Childhood Illness, Physical Injury, or Disability
- Severe Lack, Poverty, or Basic Human Needs Not Met
- Witnessing Violence or Extreme Emotional Reactions
- Abandonment or Neglect
- Loss of Parent or Family Member
- Divorce or Separation of Parents
- Exposure to Substance Abuse in the Household
- Parental Mental or Physical Illness

(Add any you experience by drawing more lines out on the graphic above.)

Most traumas are presented at such a young age that we naturally forget them, block them out to ease confusion, or are even prompted to bury them by someone who either inflicted or witnessed the trauma.

Most often, your life between ages three to five contains the first recollectable trauma. A trauma that you experience during this time will most likely be a simple memory—a quick flash or a sudden "knowing" about what occurred.

We recall the feeling more than the details. It's not particularly <u>healthy</u> to keep your childhood traumas buried into adulthood, but it's <u>common</u>. Give yourself the time to really recollect the moments that you thought you never wanted to feel or think about again. Once you look at them, you may see that they've always been so close to the surface, or what I often describe as "the things right behind your eyes." These traumatic events are the moments after which you pulled back or away from life in some way, and developed compensating behaviors to not have to experience that trauma <u>ever</u> <u>again</u>. Or you developed strategies to brace yourself or be ready were it to happen again.

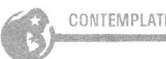 CONTEMPLATION

**RECALLING MY MOST NOTABLE EARLY-AGE TRAUMA**
Again, without writing these down, contemplate quietly:

- What's the first trauma you can recollect? Maybe it's a glimpse of memory or a "knowing." Maybe it's an event you thought was "no big deal," but know that it left you confused at the time.
- What happened to you or around you?
- What did you sense—what was said to you/what did you hear? What did you see? Where there any smells around you?
- Were you standing, lying down, or sitting?
- What did the energy feel like? (Is someone hiding something? Are they nervous? Mean?)
- What was the feeling you felt? Confused? Terrified? Embarrassed?
- Did the trauma escalate over time? Did it happen more than once? Did it become more confusing?
- Did anyone protect you?
- Did you tell anyone? How did they react? Did they get angry? Shame you? Did you feel misunderstood?
- What primary feeling did you feel after this that has carried over to today?

It's also okay if you don't recall most of these things, as you're just beginning. You'll have a chance to explore deeper later on in the process. For now, it's simply important to become aware that you (like all of us) have experienced Early-Age Traumas that set some patterns in motion. Let's gain an understanding of the consequences of these experiences in the subsequent four chapters.

# 8

# Trauma-Influenced Self-Beliefs

*What you feel in each situation is derived from
what you believe to be true about yourself.*

When we're faced with a trauma at a young age, we adapt differently than we would if a trauma is experienced as an adult when we have a fully developed and capable body. As a result of Early-Age Trauma, we're left with only our child-self's thought process and inability to understand what happened to or around us. Using this child's interpretation, we decide that what happened is about us and because of us.

We believe our interpretation of what that event(s) meant about us, thus adopting a traumatized "identity"—a sustained belief that we're now unworthy of love, unimportant, unheard, last on the list, disgusting, powerless, that we don't belong, or that we're an embarrassment. We subconsciously need to agree with these beliefs about ourselves in order to be ready for the next "attack" on us. We're rarely able to have an original thought or belief about ourselves and our world. We think that we need to lie to please others, that it isn't safe to stand up for ourselves or have a voice. Sometimes, we become overly aggressive or mean-spirited. With unresolved trauma, or insobriety, we experience difficulty creating our own version of ourselves, as we have little access to what's real for us.

Once we believe our self-beliefs are exposed, we develop patterns of behavior and emotions to protect ourselves. These behaviors and emotions will continue to keep us in "victim mentality" well into adulthood. We fall into a cycle and think it's a normal lifestyle, but it's a trap—all stemming from the beliefs formed after our trauma.

To continue exploring your Anatomy of Emotional Insobriety and build your understanding of who you've been being, you first need to explore what your specific beliefs are. These are what I've termed Trauma-Influenced Self-Beliefs.

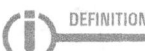

DEFINITION

**TRAUMA-INFLUENCED SELF-BELIEF:** a belief adopted about ourselves that becomes part of our identity as a remnant snapshot of our Early-Age Trauma; with unresolved trauma, the self-belief becomes the internalized "story" of who we are and what we expect the outside world believes about us as well.

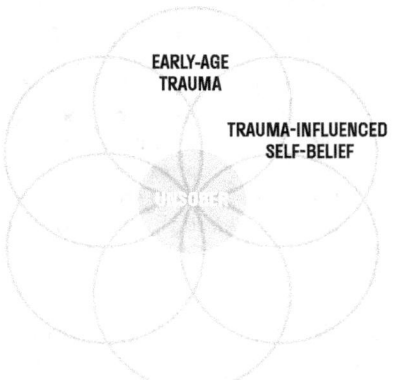

You looked at your trauma so as to have the opportunity to recognize the beliefs that were created due to the trauma—and held onto as truth about yourself. This is essential, because these beliefs are the root cause for your emotional insobriety. If these beliefs aren't really true, then we're believing a lie about ourselves. The byproduct of our Early-Age Trauma has left us with an interpretation from the imagination of a child, or perhaps the result of the brainwashing inflicted by an abusive person in our early lives.

Regardless of how we rooted these beliefs deep within our psyche, we all have them. Believing something about ourselves that's not necessarily true is the universal reaction to trauma. Many of my students have completely contrasting childhoods and still came into adulthood with the same Trauma-Influenced Self-Beliefs. When we have these beliefs and react accordingly, we're protecting ourselves by creating another persona. When we do this, we begin to veer off track of becoming our real self—the one we were born to be.

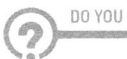
DO YOU RELATE?

When Gino met with his EMSO CO, Terry, they noticed that even though they'd each experienced very different childhoods, they were incredibly similar in which beliefs they took away from them.

Gino had an "overprotective" and controlling mother, who would remind him daily of his incapacity to do things for himself. As he grew into a young man, his mother continued this theme and whenever Gino wanted to increase his confidence, his mother would say that if he tried, he would get hurt, fail, or embarrass himself.

Terry, on the other hand, had a father who would put her in positions that forced her to perform on-the-spot, expecting perfection. If she didn't win the awards or get the "good" grades, she was reprimanded. Both have come away with the Trauma-Influenced Self-Belief: "I'm inadequate," and translated the theme of their existence to be "I will never be enough. I can't do anything right."

Now we understand the second component of your emotional insobriety, so let's apply it directly to your personal experience. Again, through many years of supporting people through to their Emotional Sobriety, I've uncovered these as the most common Trauma-Influenced Self-Beliefs.

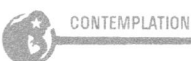
CONTEMPLATION

**WHAT ARE MY TRAUMA-INFLUENCED SELF-BELIEFS?**
Without writing anything down, review the most common Trauma-Influenced Self-Beliefs on the following page, and ask yourself:

- When under the influence of my biochemistry after an Early-Age Trauma, what did I interpret the event to mean about me?

- Which belief(s) did I create about myself due to this trauma(s)?

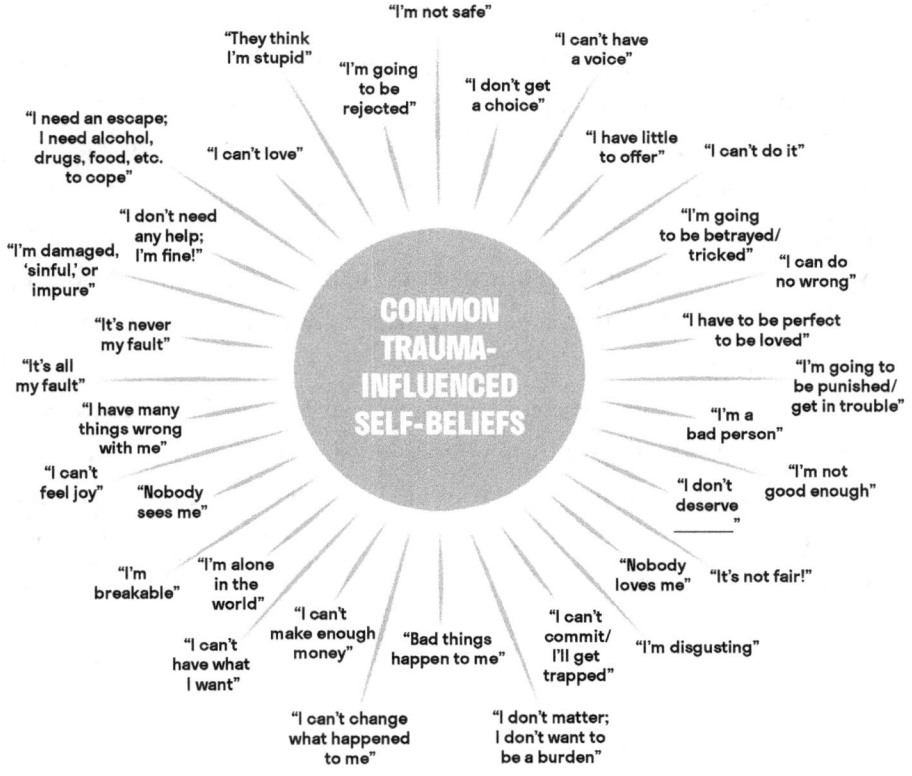

(Add any you experience by drawing more lines out on the graphic above.)

In the next chapter, you'll learn about the component that intensely and chronically triggers these beliefs, and allows for the release of emotions, or biochemistry, that intoxicates you. These beliefs have been toxic to your identity and to your life, and when you unbelieve the lies you've sustained about yourself, you'll remove the central component that sustains your emotional insobriety. Once this belief is unbelieved, you'll be free from the emotional addiction that comes from it.

Your Trauma-Influenced Self-Beliefs are the pinnacle of learning about your Anatomy of Emotional Insobriety. Your self-beliefs are the root of your cyclical life problems, yet the least known or understood without training.

We're going to change that! You're going to become aware of your self-beliefs that sustain your insobriety and be able to see not only where they interfere with your peace, but also overcome them completely, leading you to sobriety.

If you can <u>really</u> see the truth about yourself, you'll recognize how your interpretation of something that happened to you wasn't really about you. When you can understand that while the event may have had an impact on you, your insobriety permanently shifts to sobriety. With this incredible life change, you'll find the person you were made to be, rather than what trauma made you to be.

Trust me, these self-beliefs are toxic to your identity, both because they keep you from living an authentic life, and because of what happens when they're repeatedly validated. They're of the utmost importance to know about within the framework of your Anatomy of Emotional Insobriety, as they'll become the center point from which you'll train.

# 9

# Trauma Filters

*Filters are the thieves of your reality.*

The purpose of a filter is to change a product from what it really is to something different. Filters change what's really there. Filters alter light. When utilized, filters are how you receive and interpret the world around you. With photo filters, we alter light to make something appear different from what we're actually looking at in the moment. With their use, we change the original—or real—experience into something else. When we utilize filters, we create a different perception of what's <u>actually</u> occurring.

*Trauma Filters collect everything about your current experience as if it were the same as the trauma you initially experienced.*

Trauma Filters, the next primary component of emotional insobriety, are formed unconsciously after your Early-Age Trauma to attempt to repeatedly "prove" your Trauma-Influenced Self-Beliefs both to you and to the rest of the world. Thus, you'll notice that they're often identical in theme to the beliefs themselves. In other words, you continue to believe these things about yourself until they become the primary lens through which you view yourself and the world. Trauma Filters collect everything about your current experience as if it were the same as the trauma you initially experienced.

Everything tends to be filtered through the lens of your biggest trauma. Through it, you'll see the past reappear in the present. In fact, you'll unknowingly look for it too.

DEFINITION

**TRAUMA FILTER:**
an unconscious barrier put in place after an Early-Age Trauma to validate our Trauma-Influenced Self-Beliefs by collecting events that are familiar to our past and adapting the picture of everything, allowing for repetition of our memorized feelings of trauma.

EARLY-AGE TRAUMA

TRAUMA-INFLUENCED SELF-BELIEF

TRAUMA FILTER

If your primary Trauma Filter is, for example, unworthiness, you'll go around unconsciously collecting the "proof" that you're unworthy from your surroundings. What you see, what people say and do, and even what you imagine they're thinking, are interpreted to help corroborate your self-belief, thus solidifying the filter. For example, if you're looking at life through the filter of danger, then everything you perceive becomes more "evidence" of the world being an unsafe place, specifically for you.

DO YOU RELATE?

Bobby shared with me: "She took another call when we were discussing something important to me. It's obvious she doesn't think I matter!"
Trauma Filter: <u>Unimportance</u>

Your Trauma Filters not only bring your emotions and reactions to the front line, they manipulate everything you do, think, and witness. Depending on the nature of your trauma, you may even experience your entire environment through the dimmed window of your particular filter. As we'll explore in great detail in the next chapter, this filter allows for the repeated production of the same biochemistry of your past trauma. It's therefore part of maintaining your emotional addiction. This filter disconnects you from your real light and ability to see with clarity. It becomes a self-protecting lens, and doesn't allow light to be shed on the reality that's actually happening around us.

CONTEMPLATION

**DO I HAVE THIS FILTER?**
Review each of the following Trauma Filters and repeat to yourself with each one: "Do I have the filter of _____?" Are there others not depicted here that you may have?

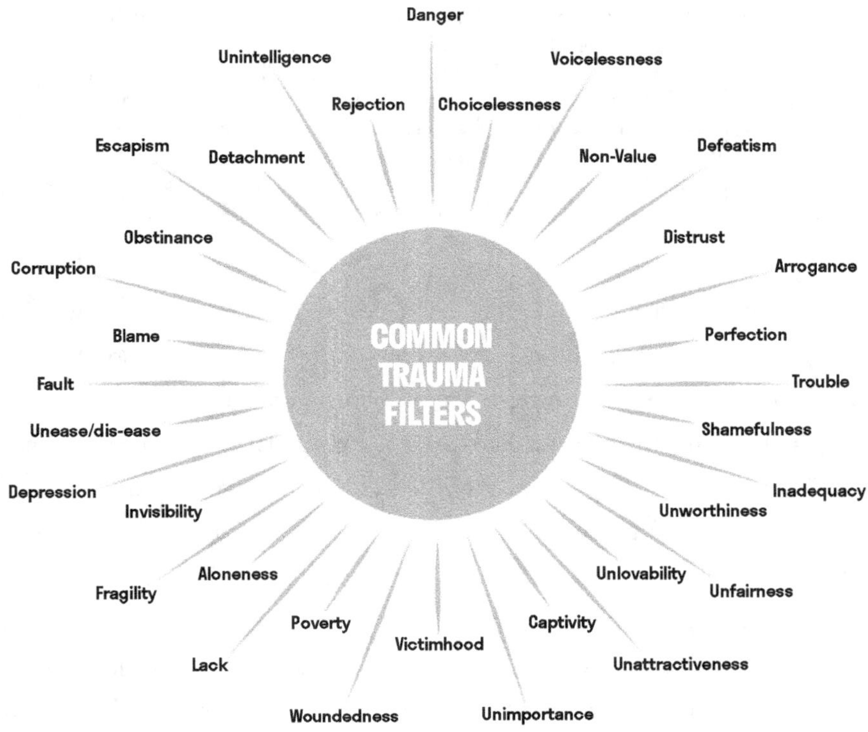

**COMMON TRAUMA FILTERS**

- Danger
- Unintelligence
- Voicelessness
- Rejection
- Choicelessness
- Escapism
- Detachment
- Non-Value
- Defeatism
- Corruption
- Obstinance
- Distrust
- Arrogance
- Blame
- Perfection
- Fault
- Trouble
- Unease/dis-ease
- Shamefulness
- Depression
- Inadequacy
- Invisibility
- Unworthiness
- Fragility
- Aloneness
- Unlovability
- Unfairness
- Poverty
- Captivity
- Lack
- Unattractiveness
- Woundedness
- Victimhood
- Unimportance

(Add any you experience by drawing more lines out on the graphic above.)

You'll place your filter over any given situation, conversation, text message, email, letter, and even non-verbal communication such as body language, facial expressions, or actions. In each instance, you'll make it match the theme of the filter, thus "validating" your self-belief. Again, everything gets filtered through what you <u>believe</u> to be true—what you've been telling yourself (or being told by others) about you that may not <u>actually</u> be true.

DO YOU RELATE?

> Through a series of coaching sessions, Cindy discovers that her Early-Age Trauma was sexual abuse. During the abuse, she developed resonating chemicals in her body that possibly became associated with the emotions of shame, embarrassment, and fear. She quickly formed self-beliefs including: "I'm worthless," "I'm only of value if I have sex," and "Sex isn't safe." This type of abuse created the Trauma Filters of unworthiness and distrust, which she's lived with since that initial trauma. These beliefs about herself will resonate and have become evident in all of her relationships and situations due to these filters being in place. Thus, she doesn't only feel the possibility of being harmed in some way again by future sexual partners, but also by her friends, co-workers, family, teammates, and more. It has become her primary lens.

We not only create filters from our <u>own</u> traumatic experiences, we also collect them from the past trauma of those who influence us the most. This is one way we carry on tendencies from our families and ancestors. Because we are wired as humans with a desire to survive longer and more reasonably within our "tribe," or our "growing-up family," we'll unconsciously add the primary filters that our family members use in order to continue the success of our species and our particular lineage.

Thus, if we make our filters from our own traumas while growing up <u>and</u> we adopt the most severe filters from the people around us (put in place by <u>their</u> traumas and/or learned filters), could it even be that our predisposition to dis-eases like depression and anxiety aren't really genetic... but contagious? Is our being around others affected by these filters enough to capture us within the same net?

When we come from a traumatized place of lack or insecurity, we're exposed by our weakest link in the chain of our human existence—our insobriety. Remember, our filters are responsible for maintaining our self-beliefs. They serve as the "security guards" that protect our image of ourselves and our biochemical makeup so that our body and brain think we're safe. They show us only what our trauma made us believe about ourselves, not what we truly believe deep down.

We may even become desperate for those around us to disprove our beliefs of unlovability or unworthiness by begging for love or affection. Yet we'll inevitably use these same people to prove that we're indeed unlovable, unworthy, or unimportant. Our Trauma Filters communicate both verbally and non-verbally, ensuring that we're proving our self-beliefs in all interactions—with friends and even people we meet one time!

COACHING MOMENT

> You've taken an initial peek into your Early-Age Traumas, Trauma-Influenced Self-Beliefs, and Trauma Filters. At this stage, you may feel overly tasked, or you may be feeling open and curious to explore further. Either way, I offer you my sincere congratulations and encouragement to keep moving! It's important for you to know that you're not broken or damaged. You're not bad for having these beliefs or filters. You're now being offered an opportunity to become aware, finally begin to gain capacity to work more easily with them, and eventually rid them from your life completely.

Next, let's gain a deep comprehension of what our Trauma Filters influence: Strong emotional reactions that inspire certain behaviors that demonstrate a version of ourselves that we don't wish to be. This keeps us locked within a loop of false beliefs and filters, over and over again, thereby solidifying our emotional insobriety.

# 10

# Biochemical Addiction to PANE

*There are chemical addicts, and there are biochemical addicts.
And we might not be so different.*

Your Trauma Filters will make your body create the chemicals it's addicted to making, to allow you to feel the feelings you're addicted to feeling. Now, let's gain a deeper understanding of our feelings, our chemistry, and the nature of the one addiction I believe we all have. I call it our Biochemical Addiction to PANE—our Predominant Accompanying Negative Emotion.

We use the acronym "PANE" to consolidate a big concept into one memorable word. Also, this gives our brain relief from the word "pain," which is something we naturally want to look away from. In EMSO Training, we must look in order to uncover our biochemical addiction. We're giving "pain" a new identity—a more objective space to begin to remove its power or hold over us.

*Your filter will make your body create the chemicals it's addicted to making, to allow you to feel the feelings you're addicted to feeling.*

As we explored, most of us consider an addict as someone who's addicted to drugs or alcohol, whom medical professionals diagnose as "chemical addicts." Though I've coached many people who've struggled with drug addiction or alcoholism, I don't have firsthand experience with either. I do, however, understand how those who are addicted got there. As I've shared, I used many external substances (T.V., texting, chores, staying busy, some alcohol, and more) in response to the perception that something was lacking in my life. Like a drug addict, this belief of lack created an emotion that then caused me to seek a distracting behavior. The distraction wasn't the sickness; it was a symptom of the sickness—in this case, a symptom of lack or incompleteness.

Science has shown us that the emotions we feel are in fact, chemistry—our biochemistry. A basic example is that in many cases, fear is a chemical like adrenaline. The adrenaline rush is the physical feeling that comes after our fearful thought or threatening experience. Fear is therefore the emotional response.[9] Emotions are <u>endogenous</u> biochemicals. They're made within (en) the body. On the other hand, drugs, pharmaceuticals, alcohol, food, and more are <u>exogenous</u> chemicals that are made outside (ex) of the body. Internally or externally made, they're both chemicals. I believe people become addicted to both types, and for predominantly the same reason.

*The distraction wasn't the sickness; it was a <u>symptom</u> of the sickness.*

For many years, I'd suggest that compulsive liars, gamblers, people with OCD, infidelity patterns, or extreme hysterical jealousy were behavioral addicts, without chemical dependence. I'd often label them as "non-chemical addicts" as they weren't addicted to drugs or alcohol, yet were still suffering with compulsive addictions. The concept of emotional addiction was revealed to me via the findings of the latest neuroscience and biological research. It described perfectly what I'd been seeing over many years in behavioral addiction, but proved to me that my previous theory was incorrect. Behavioral addicts are chemical addicts too, whether or not they're addicted to drugs or alcohol, or even use them! Given the prevalence of Early-Age Trauma and the universal pattern that follows these experiences (the onset of self-beliefs and filters), it's clear that most, if not all of us, are chemical addicts—biochemical addicts.

### Here's How it Works

When we have an experience, especially a traumatic one, the body creates a designated chemical, which we identify as an emotion or a feeling. This chemical is in place to help us remember the experience. For a majority of our memories, we may only recall a small portion of the details, and in fact we may not be able to recall much of it accurately. However, the feeling quickly becomes the most dominant part of the memory. When we relive that memory or choose a specific thinking pattern in relation to this experience, we make this same chemical again and again. Eventually, our bodies will even make the chemical in response to simply thinking the thought, without requiring a new experience to trigger it.

Again, this biochemical will be felt in us as an emotion. The same rule applies if we think a negative or stressful thought about a future event, or something occurring in the present. For example, if we choose a fearful thought, stress chemicals will be released into our body for survival. Alternately, with enough time making these emotions, the chemicals will be made in the body even when we don't think a fearful thought. We'll begin habitually making the chemical without a thought or experience to trigger it, yet we still express the intense symptoms of the associated emotion. Our brain has automatically matched this chemical with a thought of fear felt in the past.

*This biochemical will be felt in us as an emotion.*

In other words, after the first chemical release in response to a fear thought or feeling, it doesn't matter if you have the thought or feeling again; the intensity of the emotions will be experienced simply in response to the free-flowing biochemical now in your bloodstream. Of course, this doesn't apply only to fear. It could be anger, anxiety, self-pity, judgment, or any thought that's synonymous with the biochemical that was previously created. The thought can cause the chemical, or the chemical can cause the thought!

As I learned from one of my favorite teachers, neuroscience researcher and acclaimed author, Dr. Joe Dispenza, we naturally become reliant on stress chemicals to remain in homeostasis, or stability. Determined by which emotion we experience most, the body becomes skilled at making the chemical on its own, and more important, becomes reliant on it being there for its seeming survival.[10] After time, not only has the associated emotion become normalized as part of our personality, but our body becomes predisposed to making and depending on this biochemical.

Are we at the whim of our body's chemical cravings?

Yes!

Our body is now under the impression that it cannot live without obtaining access to this chemical. We're now chemically addicted via emotional chemistry. We may therefore now name it what it is—not <u>behavioral</u> addiction, as many in this field have in the past, rather <u>biochemical</u> addiction. Here's a simple definition:

DEFINITION

**BIOCHEMICAL ADDICTION TO PANE:** addiction to chemicals created within our body that can intoxicate our thinking and behaviors, which our body becomes chronically addicted to making.

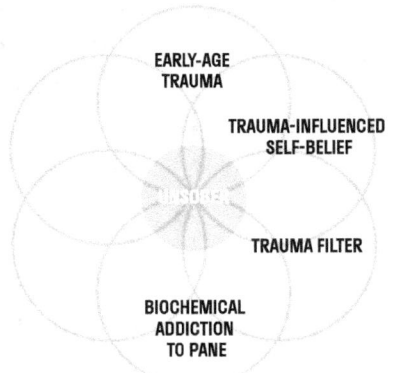

Now that you've begun investigating your Trauma-Influenced Self-Beliefs and Trauma Filters, you can see that the validation of these beliefs causes an eruption of chemistry in the body. Our PANE is a product of our trauma and the beliefs we're left with. Your Trauma Filters will allow your body to create the chemicals it's addicted to making, to allow you to feel the feelings you're addicted to feeling.

I've created the following graphic to depict what I've noticed as the six most common PANEs in my students. The outer ring represents how we'll often access each of these emotions. We'll use this throughout EMSO Training, so no need to study this quite yet!

CONTEMPLATION

**WHAT PANE AM I ADDICTED TO?**
Review the six common PANEs (Predominant Accompanying Negative Emotions), and their associated forms. Identify the emotions you feel in response to this prompt: "When I notice my self-belief (e.g., 'I'm unworthy. I'm unlovable, etc.'), I commonly feel this emotion."

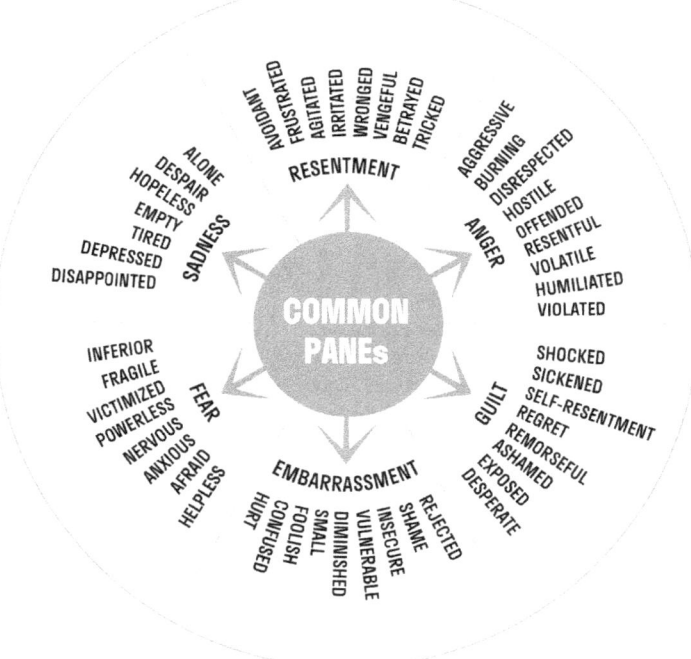

If our biochemical addiction is the recurring habit of feeling fear, anger, resentment, and other challenging emotions, has our dependence on this chemistry forced us to remain subject to the <u>feeling</u> of trauma forever? Is it possible that we develop an addiction to feeling the specific emotions that substantiate our subconscious beliefs—that we're inadequate, unworthy, unseen, uninteresting, unsafe, and more?

You may be asking: "But why would I be addicted to feeling 'bad'? If bodies naturally want to find balance, why would it stay addicted to a negative emotion? I don't want to feel pain! At least drinking or 'happy' drugs give me a 'good' feeling, so it makes sense I'd want more of them. I don't want more negative emotions at all!"

I understand the absurdity of how this sounds. It seems that we become addicted to drugs, alcohol, sex, food, and other compulsive behaviors because they give us the "hit" of happy hormones such as serotonin, dopamine, or oxytocin and help us feel "good." Like the hormones created during drug or alcohol use, we become reliant on the chemical reactions taking place in our bodies due to emotions as well. If our bodies naturally make these "emotion" chemicals after traumatic events and are left with mechanisms that perpetuate and sustain the release of these chemicals, they then "think" that they must keep making them for our survival. Even though we don't feel <u>good</u>, we feel <u>normal</u>. We feel like we've always felt, and that's what our brains and bodies desire more than anything—normalcy. As we all know, the good feelings from the other addictions wear off, and eventually we're merely seeking to feel "normal" from their use as well.

*In my experience, with few exceptions, <u>all</u> addictions begin within the body, before any exogenous substance or experience is even sought after or introduced.*

When we feel emotions that are compulsive, unconscious, and repetitive, such as an insistent overproduction of adrenaline, this is biochemical addiction. These are manifestations of our emotional insobriety.

There are exogenous <u>chemical</u> addiction and endogenous <u>biochemical</u> addiction, and they're not so different. In my experience, with few exceptions, <u>all</u>

addictions begin within the emotional body, before any exogenous substance or experience is even sought after or introduced.

This is also a common opinion shared by EMSO students who are in drug or alcohol recovery. They state that they began to use drugs or alcohol (exogenous chemicals) to make them feel different emotions (endogenous chemicals). They're using exogenous (external) chemistry to change their endogenous (internal) chemistry.

Additional examples of external chemicals include cigarette smoking, compulsive or binge eating, pharmaceutical drugs, excessive coffee drinking, and more. Our emotions are influenced because these external chemicals change our internal chemical makeup. That "different" feeling being sought after by the aforementioned addicts is tied to a desire to be removed from their current internal environment. They begin to believe in and physically depend on this state change. In the same way, we begin to believe in and depend on the state change that comes from believing our Trauma-Influenced Self-Beliefs, which perpetuates our biochemical addiction to PANE.

Remember the basic cycle? We first experience trauma as young children and our bodies create a chemical. That chemical's primary purpose is to store the memory of that event. This doesn't have to be a monumental event. It doesn't matter how seemingly "small" it is (a trauma is a trauma). What matters is that each time we have a stressful experience or think a stressful thought, our bodies create the corresponding chemical to match the event or thought. Eventually we don't even require a thought or event, as the body simply thinks it needs that chemical to remain stable. We make this chemical indefinitely unless we consciously overcome it. This phenomenon of biochemical addiction leads to actions of protection and reaction—behaviors that are often destructive.

Are we also then stuck in a cycle of repeating the same thoughts and behaviors in order to keep the body's chemical state at status quo? Are we simply surviving in the state we're used to? Do we keep creating the same chemical (e.g., adrenaline) to sustain the same addictive emotion (e.g., fear)? Are we filtering a thought of potential threat and making a matching chemical (e.g., fear, anxiety), or are we making a chemical (e.g., adrenaline) and matching it with a worst-case-scenario thought?

Here are several glimpses of what this may look like:

DO YOU RELATE?

Little Johnny witnesses his parents fighting. Stress chemicals are made. Judy is physically abused or abandoned. Again, stress chemicals are made. These events are equally translated by the body as trauma.

The next time something remotely similar occurs, or when Johnny or Judy has a memory of the stressful event later in life, they will have the same biochemical response to the fear, which is the body's way of preparing them to handle the potential trauma. They generate the same physical chemistry alerting them to the event's threat: "This could be happening again! You're in danger! Run and hide, or fight!" Eventually, they're experiencing chronic (continual) stress due to unresolved trauma.

The following example outlines what I call "Feeling Flow 1" and "Feeling Flow 2." This framework is explored in much greater depth in subsequent parts of the curriculum, but it's essential to have a basic understanding that while sometimes our addiction flows top-to-bottom beginning with a thought (as we've explored in great detail), at other times it begins in the body.

DO YOU RELATE?

**FEELING FLOW 1:**
**THOUGHT-TO-FEELING PHENOMENON OF BIOCHEMICAL ADDICTION:**
Let's say Sarah is having dinner with her romantic partner. After dinner, she's in the kitchen doing the dishes and looks over to see him on his cell phone with an unfamiliar look on his face. Due to a previous trauma that had left her with a deep-seated insecurity, she's impulsively thrust into the idea that there's a threat on the other side of the phone. She assigns a meaning to the look on her partner's face ("He must be having feelings for someone else") and quickly decides how she thinks it's going to affect her ("My partner is going to leave me!"). Bam! The fear chemical releases, which may lead to her throwing a fit, manipulating, yelling, or excessively crying. She has a fearful thought that releases the fear-based chemistry her body is so eagerly willing to make, thanks to her past traumatic experience.

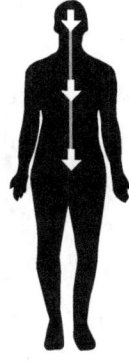

**FEELING FLOW 2:**
**FEELING-TO-THOUGHT PHENOMENON OF BIOCHEMICAL ADDICTION:** Alternatively, while washing the dishes, Sarah suddenly feels a surge of a stress chemical within her body, which she translates or labels as "fear" (or intuition). Now her brain matches it with a corresponding thought ("My partner is going to leave me!"). She then follows this feeling/chemical by looking over and interpreting a certain look of "passion for another" on the face of her partner, which may lead to the same behaviors (throwing a fit, yelling, or hysterically crying). She's made the chemical of fear due to her bodily addiction to making it, and her brain then matches it with a fearful thought.

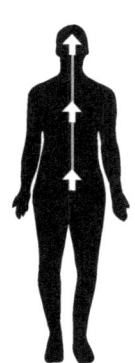

Both of these scenarios originate from low self-esteem, insecurity, jealousy, attention-seeking, and compulsive neediness, most likely generated from a previous trauma, and not necessarily with this particular partner or even in a prior romantic setting. Maybe she'd experienced abandonment or rejection early in life.

Remember, trauma creates the initial crack in the foundation of your self-esteem. Thus, you're now more susceptible to feeling unsafe, even with the people whom you choose to be with because you think they help you feel safe. You're going to have that same feeling you had when you first experienced the trauma, despite the current circumstances being different.

*Avoiding triggering situations isn't a long-term solution.*

With Emotional <u>Intelligence</u>, you may be able to see that this was an overreaction, but the subconscious memory of the emotional trauma causes the chemical response, even in a completely different setting, and you lose conscious control. This is because with unresolved trauma and the addiction to the biochemistry created after the event, you aren't yet emotionally sober.

I'm often asked if certain situations should be avoided to deter our biochemical reactions. I respond with a question: "If I'm an alcoholic, do I need to stay far away from any place I might encounter a drink <u>forever</u>? If I'm a person who's constantly jealous, would I need to <u>never</u> see my partner talk to another person?" In the initial stages of an intentional change process, we may want to consciously avoid the situations we don't yet have a handle on, especially if we're hurting ourselves or others—but avoiding triggering situations isn't a long-term solution.

Using avoidance as a solution is attempting to change the <u>situation</u> in order to not have the feeling, as opposed to changing <u>who we're in relationship to our feelings</u> and <u>why we have them in the first place</u>. When you become a different person with Emotional Sobriety, no situation could make you behave or feel like the previous version of you did. For example, seeing your partner talking to another person wouldn't engulf you with fear, not even for a moment. With EMSO Training, you'll become a different person in relationship to your previous issues.

If a former alcoholic is now truly sober, both clean of alcohol and emotionally speaking, they'll be able to walk into a bar, smell the booze, and not even consider or be tempted to drink it, as the previous version of them would have. It's no longer in their makeup. The chemical addiction and behavioral habit of drinking haven't left <u>them</u>; rather, <u>they</u> have become a person who no longer has those addictions.

The same goes for the emotionally unsober. When you overcome your past pain and change who you are regarding that pain, nothing outside of you can make you behave or feel in the ways you once did. When becoming emotionally sober, your addiction doesn't leave you. You leave the addiction.

*When becoming emotionally sober, your addiction doesn't leave you. You leave the addiction.*

As with avoidance, we need to look at other ways of coping or distracting. We may add medicines or drugs to "cope" with our underlying emotional chaos. Some of these added chemicals can make us behave even more erratically. Others may make us seem more emotionally stable, but are we just experiencing forced numbness?

All exogenous chemicals—birth control pills, hormone replacement therapy, performance enhancers, street drugs, alcohol, prescription painkillers, and even in some cases psych medications—are there to alter our emotional state, instead of us changing our state of being. Added chemistry won't take away our trauma. With these substances—which are meant to help us—are we creating an <u>exogenous</u> chemical addiction to "cope" with our <u>endogenous</u> chemical addiction? We often don't have a solid enough emotional platform to be taking these substances and we're rarely capable of doing them responsibly when we haven't yet uncovered our pain and changed who we are in relationship to that pain.

A real solution is created by changing who you are, not by avoiding the problem. If you're seeking an escape from feeling your PANE by means of a chemical or compulsive behavior, then when you're no longer seeking an escape, you won't have a reliance on that chemical or behavior.

### COACHING MOMENT

Now that you know that your emotional insobriety is actually an endogenous biochemical addiction, you may be concerned that you can't overcome it. Changing your mindset usually seems easier than changing your physical biochemistry.

However, it's through the actions and practices you engage in EMSO Training that you actually <u>do</u> create new neural pathways, new fiber tracts in your brain, and a new "garden of emotions" in your gut microbiome, such that the old ways of being no longer have a hold on you. The old chemicals stop being produced. You aren't the person you used to be, nor the one who identifies with them. You're free.

The first step at this stage is to become aware that: 1. You have a need to overcome your biochemical addition, and 2. You have the support and knowledge to get there. Can you feel this possibility?

You <u>can</u> reprogram your brain and biochemistry. Where you've been the least capable in your life you can become the most capable.

When it comes to biochemical addiction, you can overcome any of it. It's not situational. When you're truly different and have attained mastery in Emotional Sobriety, no outside situation can make you go back to who you once were. You can change. Knowing and believing you can change—and then doing the work to actually change the biochemical response in the body—genuinely liberates you from the addiction.

*You can reprogram your brain and biochemistry, and where you have been the least capable in your life you can become the most capable.*

Look at it this way: Our addictions are habits, and habits are skills. Give anything both repetition and time, and you make a habit! Anything that you repeat and attain mastery over becomes a skill. The same way you've practiced addiction, you can practice sobriety. I've found that most people enjoy doing what they're good at. When they're skilled at something, they tend to want to continue doing it, even if the skill is a destructive habit. They have a track they're on, and they run efficiently on that track. The same is true for emotional responses and behaviors. It's natural to also want to keep your learned skills honed in these departments—especially if you believe at some level that they're keeping you safe.

In short, if you're going to overcome your biochemical addiction, the first step is to generate awareness around it by investigating why you have it, and then by making real, lasting changes. Once your addictive skills are witnessed and their causations are chipped away, you create space for new skills. Thankfully, you can relieve the body of biochemical addiction through the active practice of Emotional Sobriety, which, once attained, allows you to incorporate even more advanced teachings.

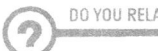

DO YOU RELATE?

Anna shares her transformational story: "When I was a little girl, I had low self-esteem, and often thought I was being ignored and unloved. As soon as I was alone, I would eat—specifically, sugary treats. I learned that this worked well to alter my feelings of loneliness, anxiety, and sadness. It felt like I was receiving something when I ate. It seemed to make me feel better. I became used to it, and I realized that I didn't cry as much, or feel as nervous about anything when I knew there were treats nearby. I could even hide them!

It created a familiarity, and what felt like stability. It's something I chose so frequently that after the first couple of times using it, I didn't even need to think in order to choose it again (it had become a skill). This skill followed me into adulthood, and as an adult, even when I found myself alone (not necessarily lonely), I would automatically think it was time to go find a sugary treat.

I realize now that the problem wasn't the sugar in the treats. My behavioral and chemical addiction was based on the choice to numb my emotions. I had made this pattern, route, or pathway in my brain to crave sugar to "feel better." It wasn't there from birth. It wasn't my genetic predisposition or something I learned from one of my parents.

For a period of time my body had become reliant on this chemical that created the sensation of numbness around my emotions, because it had been fed it over and over, and repeatedly expected it.

Now, I think differently, feel differently, and simply give my body something different than sugary treats, and keep repeating this new process. Today, my body expects something different than sugar because I <u>became</u> someone different. I don't feel loneliness, anxiety, or sadness in the first place, so I no longer crave sugar. My (exogenous) addiction to sugar was remedied by overcoming my (endogenous), biochemical addiction to PANE.

How did I do this? Training and receiving coaching to stabilize my personality changes were utilized to attain Emotional Sobriety, leading to the relief of my behavioral or exogenous addictions. For a simple example, when I first engaged in my change process, every time I was alone, instead of eating sugar I sat in a chair and meditated, or I put on headphones and danced around for a few moments. Over time, I retrained my brain and body to respond differently to being alone, and no longer associated it with sadness, anxiety, or loneliness, and therefore removed the urge to eat sugar. Instead, I even began interpreting being alone as an opportunity to have fun or take care of myself! I have developed new skills and am on the pathway to mastering my Emotional Sobriety."

In the coming chapters you'll find exercises and practices that can take you to the next level of your personal growth or evolution. If you've been challenged to retain elements of your personal growth, can't seem to find the right teacher(s) or support, or have reached a barrier to your next expansion, this is the next chapter of your life. When you've completed this process, you'll meet a new *you*—the *you* that's been buried under the rubble of beliefs and behaviors that weren't yours to begin with—the *you* that had (naturally) become addicted to certain biochemicals. Then, the exponential growth begins... and expands in greater ways than you could have ever imagined.

There are so many people who struggle with emotional insobriety all while being successful in so many other areas of their lives. As I've shared, I was one of them. Can you now see that this is the most common form of addiction on the planet?

I want to warn you that initially your body isn't likely to enjoy the changes you're about to undergo. Your body's chemistry has been working to maintain these skills for a very long time and believes it's doing exactly what you've asked it to do. Your body has been the loyal friend you've trained it to be. It doesn't know how you're mentally and emotionally tormented day to day, as it doesn't have the ability to recognize that you may no longer need the chemicals it made in response to your past trauma. It's simply doing what it thinks you need it to do, based on various input (or lack thereof), or what you surround yourself with. Remember that your repeated thoughts, behaviors, and feelings continue to engage the old chemical pathways, and you've likely been thinking, behaving, and feeling similarly for a very long time. If you're asking your body to change suddenly, it may think you've "lost your mind." Let's just say you and your body may have some disagreements as you begin your journey to Emotional Sobriety. Stick with it, and the physical freedom, too, will come.

# 11

# Emotionally-Triggered Behaviors

*Who we became because of trauma isn't our fault,
but definitely our responsibility.*

You're now in closer contact with who you've been being through contemplating your initial traumas and the subsequent beliefs and filters that you unconsciously developed in order to stay "safe." Next, we find out how these created the compulsive, repeated behaviors you find yourself enacting now. These are the most obvious symptom of our emotional insobriety, as they can even be witnessed by others. We call them Emotionally-Triggered Behaviors, or ETBs.

**DEFINITION**

**EMOTIONALLY-TRIGGERED BEHAVIORS:**

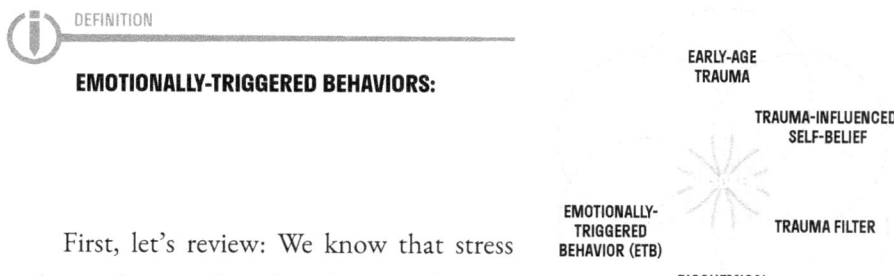

First, let's review: We know that stress chemicals are released within our bodies, 1. at the onset of a trauma, 2. habitually as a result of a present threat, and 3. continuously, even without any real cause. When we feel the flood of the chemical in our body, we experience and label it as one or several emotions. Now we're experiencing chemically-induced symptoms, which, as they persist, support us in locking in certain beliefs about ourselves and lenses through which we view the whole world around us (not only the potential threats).

Now, what happens after the intoxication of the emotion is felt? These symptoms are followed up with behaviors, which, like our beliefs and filters, are also in place to "protect" us when in danger. Though these behaviors are learned and become mastered skills over time, they eventually become so habituated that they are acted out compulsively in the moment the chemical is released.

We respond to the burning acidity of anger, pangs of fear, or the suffocation of shame. Because the emotion triggers the behavior, it can appear that we don't have a choice other than to react.

*It's a re-action—a re-creation of a past action, a habit, or a survival mechanism—designed to bring us what we perceive as an optimal outcome.*

We interpret an incoming message or action through one of our Trauma Filters, which can create a triggered reaction, and then often discord in our relationships because we're under-resourced when we're responding. Our brain has interpreted something or someone as a predator, so the incoming message or action is already skewed. This "predator" could even be a well-meaning spouse or friend. Now, jostled by a hostile emotion, we may feel threatened, angry, or hurt. We feel the need to protect ourselves and we retaliate with a negative or harmful behavior—a reaction. It's actually a <u>re</u>-action—a re-creation of a past action, a habit, or a survival mechanism—designed to bring us what we perceive as an optimal outcome. However, the outcome is often <u>de</u>structive rather than <u>con</u>structive.

And the tricky thing is that this perceived predator isn't even necessarily reminding us of the specific emotions associated with our original trauma. By this point, we don't need a reminder because we're always ready to battle it. We immediately create a rebuttal for our safety. We may instantaneously lie, defend, or argue. We may become a flame of jealousy or suspicion. We compulsively re-act based on what our filter has us see, or what someone else has taught us to feel.

You can think of some of these ETBs as a skunk's spray—a chaos-inducing mechanism emitting a scattering of disharmony around us, leaving a "stench" and creating a fence line for our safety. For the emotionally unsober, we produce an energy field of incoherence and destruction because our ETBs are created during times when we've closed our hearts and gone into defense mode —"protecting" ourselves from feeling what's actually there (fear, embarrassment, etc.).

On top of this, these behaviors often sway our communication in order to alter our surroundings to further enhance the "protection" we think we need. Even in something as small as an argument over the dishes, these behaviors can create such a strong confusion in the room that everyone can feel the remnants of the blast.

DO YOU RELATE?

> After Marley's outburst, her husband, flush-faced, walked away. You could cut the tension in the room with a knife.

This book focuses on the seven most common ETBs: defensiveness, childishness, jealousy, self-centeredness, judgmentalism, dishonesty, and secondary addiction. You'll learn about these in greater detail in the subsequent chapters as you begin to explore your life in relationship to each of them.

These behaviors arise from such strong compulsions and knee-jerk responses that you usually feel you can't control them. There may <u>not</u> be a control button on your ETBs! Do you feel like you have a choice in how you behave when you feel emotionally triggered?

Behaviors that are created by your reactions, as opposed to your choices, make you a puppet in your own life. However, it's important to note that not <u>all</u> behaviors are reactive. You can, and will, learn how to respond rather than react to situations, even triggering ones!

Here's the distinction I make:

**DEFINITIONS**

**RESPOND:** behave by choice or intentionally.

**REACT:** behave compulsively, seemingly without choice; a pre-programmed act or behavior.

**DO YOU RELATE?**

Jean shares: "At the age of six, I overheard my mother in hysterics, screaming and throwing a tantrum after my father came home and mentioned his new female sales partner was attractive. I recall my mother sobbing and questioning my father like he was on trial... accusing him of betraying her, hurting the kids, and even questioning if he had been unfaithful. She was out of breath, and I could feel her negatively charged energy seeping through under the door. My father yelled back at her and told her she was crazy, and that all he said was that someone was attractive. It wasn't a big deal to him, but to her it was as if her actual life was being threatened. Once I became an adult, although the memory of the event was not clear, that feeling of threat did not leave me. Now, every time I perceive that my husband is even possibly looking at another woman, I freak out."

Jean's story doesn't seem overly traumatic, yet a powerful set of beliefs were established—"He might betray me," "I'm of less value to him if he's mentioning someone else's attractiveness," "I'm not good enough"—which set her up for viewing the world through the filters of distrust and danger. Her mother's behavioral reaction to the threat of betrayal had become a learned behavior to support Jean's "survival." She may continue to have strong hysterical and emotional reactions, based on her mother's experience, around the issue of her own partner being attracted to another person. These filters also likely extend into her professional and other familial and friend relationships. To Jean, her husband will likely be unfaithful, regardless of his level of displayed trustworthiness. Or if he <u>does</u> think another woman is attractive, it definitely means that he's no longer attracted to her. This creates discord in Jean's relationship because she, too, screams and throws tantrums when she feels his attention is elsewhere or if he's being dishonest. Even if her husband <u>is</u> honest and committed to her, she's filtering through that lens of distrust—feeling her biochemical emotion of fear—and thus reacts accordingly. Even though she may lose her relationship if she doesn't stop, when she feels threatened, she'll continue to emotionally react in the same way that she witnessed her mother that first day. This takes away her opportunity to have a real connection and relationship with her husband and disallows him the same. He and Jean will have a difficult time merging and experiencing true intimacy when there's a fence line of her pain in the way.

Because we subconsciously believe that ETBs protect us, we protect them. In fact, we feel entitled to have them and we react in the ways we do because we feel we've been the victim of our past traumas or hardships. They become so habitual that even when we find ourselves in a safe place, we'll be internally persuaded to filter it as dangerous or create our own chaos in order to match these trauma-filtered expectations.

Although your ETBs aren't chosen consciously, and they may even be epigenetically inherited or learned from those around you, it's still your responsibility to change them. Through your EMSO Training, you'll engage a broad and deep search for the behaviors that aren't of your choosing, and you'll have the opportunity to choose to change them. You can then observe your ETBs at their onset and your new intentions can inspire different, chosen behaviors.

*Although your ETBs aren't chosen consciously, and they may even be epigenetically inherited or learned from those around you, it's still your responsibility to change them.*

Let's share our first intention-setting moment. Read this aloud or in your mind:

INTENTION-SETTING MOMENT

**"I desire peace in my life. I choose to be rid of the filters that create triggering emotions within me. I now choose to be responsible for my behavior. And to be responsible for my behavior, I must first be responsible for what I'm feeling."**

However, awareness alone of your ETBs won't give you Emotional Sobriety. You don't get the results without doing the work. Did you hear me? Do the work and you'll reap the rewards!

While overcoming my own ETBs, I often feared that the finish line was too far away, and at times thought that I could never get there. I was overridden with the exhaustion created from battling my Emotional Belligerence, beginning to observe my Trauma Filters, and feeling ashamed and disheartened each time I would revert back to displaying an ETB. I was exhausted at the thought of doing more training. The idea that one day I could change a triggered behavior and not see the other person as a threat or predator seemed impossible. The possibility of feeling so whole in who I was that the chemical wouldn't even release in me to create the reaction seemed fantastical. It wasn't until completing the entirety of this deep self-investigation and training that I was not only able to attain what I had long hoped for myself, but to far surpass it. Now, I'm peaceful, levelheaded, and clear, and you can be too.

I learned that our interpretation of what we're capable of is extremely muted compared to what we're actually capable of doing. The muting device that makes you believe you can't go any further is an ETB itself! If they're doing their job to keep you the same, these habitual behaviors will seem to come out of the dark even louder than before. This is the phenomena of biochemical addiction—chronic biochemically-induced emotions, Trauma-Influenced Self-Beliefs, Trauma Filters, and ETBs... try to get rid of them and they'll make you see all the reasons why they think you shouldn't.

Thus, while now is a great time to invoke perseverance and commitment, it's also a time for incredible patience and gentleness. Invite in support so that you have a softer-than-usual place to land when these chemicals flare up. This isnt a time to start a new project other than this one. Trust that you will soon be equipped to notice your emotions as they're arising, observe your behavior in the moment, and consciously choose something different.

*ETBs... try to get rid of them and they'll make you see all the reasons why they think you shouldn't.*

Here's a glimpse of what you may experience in EMSO Training. The following table allows us to see the difference between a reactive ETB and a consciously chosen response to any given trigger or situation:

| I REACT THIS WAY: | I RESPOND THIS WAY: |
| --- | --- |
| Re-playing/acting out previously learned behavior after a triggering event | Displaying real, honest, and thoughtful behavior after a triggering event |
| Compulsive/Not chosen | Deliberate/Chosen |
| No identity/Role-playing | Chosen identity |
| Fear-based | Reality-based |
| Dishonest | Honest |
| Exclusive | Inclusive |
| Unempowered | Powerful/Empowered |
| Destructive | Productive/Cooperative |
| Repulsive/Negative | Attractive/Positive |

Remember, each and every one of your ETBs (and the biochemistry that initiates them) has an opportunity to be both captured and eliminated from your personality when you mobilize this training. First, you'll develop the capacity to become aware of your thoughts, feelings, and behaviors, taking note of your actions and the emotions that come before them. You'll begin to access your true feelings during conversations, when recalling memories, and when making decisions, and you'll start having a subtle but important internal dialogue that includes inquiries such as, "How am I <u>really</u> feeling right now? Are there any self-beliefs that are triggering familiar emotions within me? Are my behaviors a result of this?"

The following contemplation gives you a glimpse into your capacity to demonstrate responsibility and command over your ETBs, so that you and others may one day no longer suffer from having them in your life. This requires making EMSO Training a priority in your life. It means being humble when you're tempted to fight, and open when you're tempted to hide. It takes commitment to becoming more and more aware, and I believe that's exactly what you're here to do.

*ETBs deny you the very thing you're attempting to achieve by using them.*

CONTEMPLATION

**OBSERVE AN ETB**
First, identify someone in your life with whom you're presently having a challenging time connecting. Read through the following and take these questions with you into the next setting that includes them—perhaps tomorrow at work when you're around a challenging co-worker, or the next time you visit an argumentative or triggering family member. Go into the interaction without trying to force anything to happen. Simply take a mental note of the following:

- What were you thinking? What did you notice in the interaction? (Thoughts)

- How did you feel? And how did you perceive the other person felt? (Emotions)

- What did you do? (ETBs—see the graphic on the next page*.)

*The ETBs graphic represents the seven most common. I find that, while there are many other ways of describing various behaviors, they may all be narrowed down to these. Thus, there is not an invitation to write-in additional at this point.

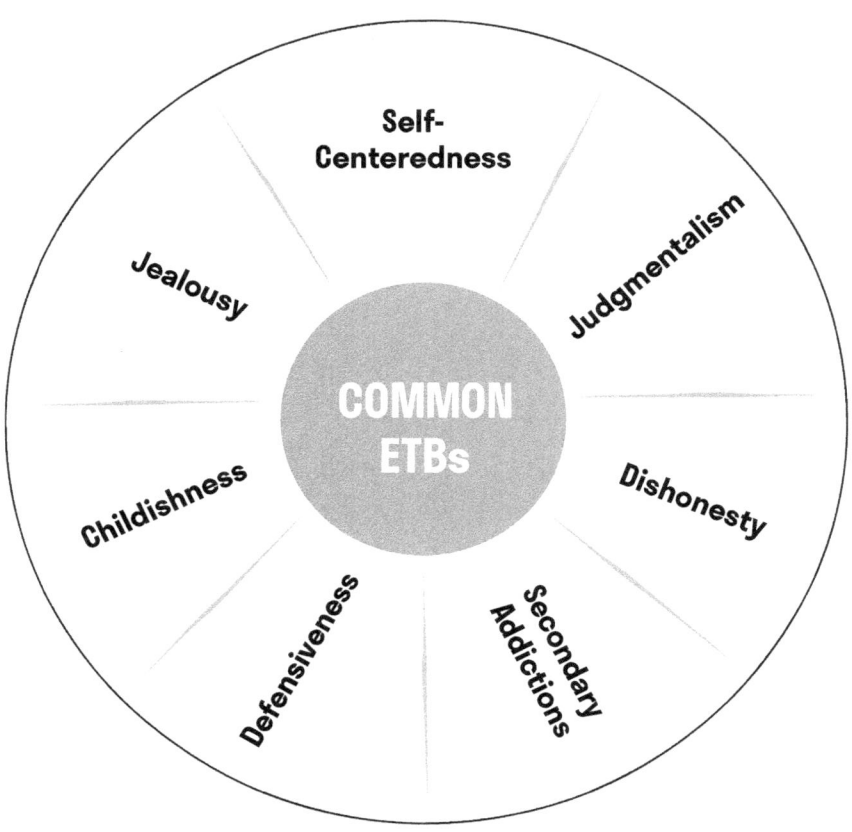

You now know that having ETBs is a normal response to your unresolved traumas. You may be beginning to realize that they're no longer acceptable or desired. ETBs destroy your ability to build trust in relationships. They cause separation and pain. ETBs deny you the very thing you're attempting to achieve by using them. They deny you the peace, comfort, and safety you're seeking. Identifying and then eliminating your Trauma Filters, which cause ETBs, will actually be what save and protect your peace. These actions will allow for the possibility for real connection through personal security.

**12**

# Intoxicated Identity

*When something controls how you feel, it controls you.
Choose who you are.*

I introduced you to the concept of ETBs (Emotionally-Triggered Behaviors), which are demonstrated after the stress chemicals of PANEs (Predominant Accompanying Negative Emotions) are released into our bodies. We know that these biochemicals, in addition to our Trauma-Influenced Self-Beliefs (which are validated by Trauma Filters) are created as a survival mechanism after Early-Age Trauma. Because this has been occurring unconsciously for most of our lives, it has in essence formed our entire personality. We learned to be emotionally unsober in order to survive what happened to and around us in early age, and it has stayed with us as a continued survival mechanism. So, if we didn't purposefully create these reactions, are they a part of our real identity? Is it possible that we're intoxicated by emotions and lessons that shaped our identity to one of basic survival? Does this mean we may lack our own chosen identities?

 DEFINITION

**CHOSEN IDENTITY:** how we present ourselves to the world based on who we've chosen to be—our values, beliefs, thoughts, feelings, behaviors, personality traits, how we speak, our level of energy, and our capacity to transform our energy depending on the situation.

All of this (and more) makes up our identity, yet we rarely choose our way of being consciously. As I've shared, when you were young, you patterned after what you witnessed around you. This was necessary for your survival as it made you cooperative in your community and understood in communication within your tribe. It's important to ask some deeper questions at this juncture; however:

- What is your personality founded upon?
- Are you being yourself, or are you being who you were taught and incentivized to become?
- Are you living as the real you when you're unconsciously behaving, feeling, and thinking based on your Early-Age Trauma?
- Are you living from your real identity when you're enraged with resentment and anger, throwing tantrums, and judging others or yourself?

Despite it being one of the most sacred opportunities we have as a human, the majority of people around you don't have personal or carefully chosen identities. Instead, they're mirroring or re-enacting their past and their family's past. They think what they were told to think. They believe what they were told to believe. They're feeling the same emotions that they most experienced in their family circles, via the predominant biochemical patterning.

For example, maybe you lived within an angry family, a depressed family, or an anxious family, and now, despite not having an angry, depressed, or anxious partner or children of your own, you find yourself naturally in these states. In addition to the influence of your early traumas, add in the ingredient of the familial mirroring that naturally occurs, and you easily form additional Trauma Filters and ETBs. Now you have a reactive, traumatized personality. This recipe creates what I term an Intoxicated Identity.

 **COACHING MOMENT**

**Intoxicating chemistry has sustained your Intoxicated Identity. I urge you to take a moment and recognize that who you became because of trauma was a child's way of surviving. Now that you're more grown up, you can begin to develop new ways of living and go far beyond mere surviving. You're not alone in this! We're all the same, having all had Early-Age Trauma in one form or another, leading all of us to an Intoxicated Identity.**

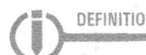
**DEFINITION**

**INTOXICATED IDENTITY:**
becoming someone we didn't choose as a result of our Early-Age Traumas and the <u>reactions</u> and confusion from these experiences; to lack a chosen identity due to emotional insobriety; to take on a role in life rather than living as our chosen self.

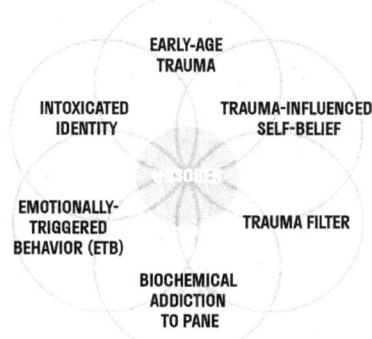

When the foundation of your identity is based on fitting in with a social crowd or ensuring that others like you, you'll end up mimicking others. Furthermore, because this is your community and everyone around you is essentially seeking to feel connected and understood, you unconsciously inflict pressure on yourself to be dishonest, childish, or defensive in order to fit in. Each of you has adopted a role or way of being in the group and you each reinforce this role by needing the same things over and over from one another.

This may sound like a drama that you're perpetuating, but the reality is that you simply may not yet know how to be the truest version of yourself. Thus, you're continuously guessing what you believe others want you or need you to be. This is a natural part of the cycle, and it's my mission to assist in the unraveling of the Intoxicated Identity.

**DO YOU RELATE?**

**Jessa mimicked her older sister for her entire life. She unconsciously patterned after her as she saw it as an opportunity to get closer to and be accepted by her. The way she narrowed it down was that she did it to be loved by her. Jessa said she also felt she would get more power from mimicking the person that she observed "always got what she wanted" from their parents and other authorities.**

**So, she spoke like her, dressed like her, and believed what she believed. She even acted the same way as her sister in friendships and romantic relationships. She became dishonest to keep up her role and was constantly under her own pressure to be something that she wasn't.**

> Can you see how this would lead to her stumbling within a cycle of dissatisfaction in her life and relationships? She wasn't getting what she wanted out of her life because she was living her sister's life. At age 26, she was really feeling the destructive nature of not having developed her own identity, so she made the decision to start cleaning up her life. She urgently cleared away a lifetime of debris. She exposed her now raw identity with possibility. She hand-selected all of the traits that she most wanted for herself. She practiced diligently and applied everything to her life as she became a new person. Once deciding to change, however, her sister became severely depressed and felt dejected.
>
> When Jessa decided to make an identity for herself, it translated to her sister as rejection. The mimicking made Jessa's sister feel important and empowered, along with attaining perceived control over Jessa, and giving her a sense that she could protect Jessa this way. Jessa's changing created change in the relationship, and now Jessa's sister felt self-conscious when Jessa erased the false bond of mimicking.
>
> Once discussed, Jessa's older sister realized that she'd <u>also</u> been mimicking—their mother! They both spoke to their mother about this, whom they discovered was also unhappy and dissatisfied with her life—the mother noticing how she had mimicked <u>her</u> own mother in many ways and made decisions based on what her mother would have wanted or expected of her. I wouldn't be surprised if there were generation after generation of this same story within this family.
>
> Soon, these three women were all working on rebuilding themselves. They were each able to develop a truer identity and continue to work together on their reality-based relationships. It's still a challenge for them not to fall into old patterns, and sometimes they're emotionally triggered by each other, but now they can laugh about it.

When mimicking someone else's identity to gain power, the power won't be your own. True power cannot be mimicked—it's personal. You'll therefore be continually dissatisfied with your life if you're mimicking someone else's or being what someone else decided you should be. With this dissatisfaction, you may try harder the next time, leading to an ongoing cycle of discontent.

In addition to families, this also occurs within friendships and romantic relationships. Think of relationships that are primarily motivated by the desire to be a part of something rather than a sense of curiosity or energetic connection—the ones where there is a desperation to feel accepted or fit in.

I call these Forced Relationships. These are not relationships based on authentic connection. In these relationships, there will be a buried resentment due to the fact that your friends or partners aren't feeling satisfied. This dissatisfaction is born out of the fact that you're stifled by your intoxicated disposition of lacking identity. You may each unknowingly blame the other for your discontent, yet continue to be unable to identify many of the real dynamics at play.

An example of an Intoxicated Identity forming would be when a child asks an authority figure a simple question, and they (the parent, guardian, teacher, etc.) react with hostility. This creates startling confusion for the child. The child is witnessing the authority figure react negatively to something that the child wanted to talk about or have clarified. Since the child is going to be on the receiving end of the authority figure's ETB, this consequently teaches the child to go mute, to never speak about this topic or anything close to it, ever again. It causes the child to avoid saying, asking, or telling anything that may become a highly uncomfortable confrontation for them in the future—ultimately creating aversion and fear for the child to speak his/her truth or inquire for truth from the adult, thereby deepening his/her overall confusion. This confusion and inability to speak contributes to the intoxication of the child's identity from there on out. Also, based on what we've discussed above, this child will more than likely grow up and be identical in behavior with his/her own children, while still struggling within him/herself to search for truth.

If we reenact what we saw from the past, does it mean that <u>all</u> of the personality disorders and negative conditions in our lives are the responsibility of our family members, caregivers, and other teachers or mentors? Can you simply blame others who came before you for all of your problems?

No.

*They're not to blame. No one is to blame. Not even you.*

Whomever you mirrored—the people you learned from while growing up (family members and non)—were mirroring someone from <u>their</u> childhood. The people they were mirroring were mirroring from theirs, and they from theirs, and so on down the line. It's been a continuous cycle. They're not to blame. No one is to blame. Not even you.

You can now be responsible for it all, and when you're responsible, your Intoxicated Identity can come to an end. If you aren't choosing how you <u>feel</u>, you aren't in control of you. If you aren't choosing who you're <u>being</u>, you aren't choosing your life.

If you're someone who claims to be aware of the limitless nature of consciousness and how this transcends personality, I want you to know that it's not my objective to limit your expansion of consciousness by asking you to be myopically attached to the idea of your identity. However, unless you're going to be living in isolation, you'll have human interactions and thereby the potential for insobriety patterns to show up. Thus, knowing you can have an identity that's chosen—and choosing it—is the next bridge to Emotional Sobriety.

You can now see others as an example of what you may want as a part of your identity, rather than how you must act in order to fit in. You can surround yourself with people you feel are powerful in strength, honesty, and vitality. Then you'll still be able to create your own identity and be aided in the transformation through conscious energetic entrainment and inspiration, versus unconscious mimicry.

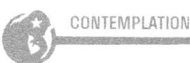 CONTEMPLATION

**IDENTITY MOCKUP**
Ask yourself the following questions and contemplate your responses:

- What does the new version of me think, feel, and do?
- What are my values and qualities?
- What are my greatest virtues?
- How do I walk, dress, and speak? (You can even think about what you wish to smell like!)

- How do I feel in their romantic partnership (if I choose to be in one)?
- How do I talk to children?
- What foods do I choose to eat and why?
- How might other people describe this new version of me?
- How does this new version of me behave...
  - in an emergency situation?
  - when given feedback?
  - when given a gift?
  - when I meet someone for the first time?

Do you believe you may have an Intoxicated Identity? Are you looking forward to creating and choosing a real and chosen identity for yourself? I understand that the opportunity to choose a new identity can be at once both incredibly empowering and intimidating. We'll do this together once you get further along in this process and reach a place where you can easily build your new identity. With the tools provided, you'll decide who you want to be and embody it in every aspect of your life.

## No Identity. No Integrity.

Committing to your own identity begins to build your integrity. An integrity-based identity is expressed when you're being the same person in every situation, with every single person. You're always you. To be anything else would be to lack integrity. Saying different things to different audiences would be to lack integrity. In this case, you're being more than one person and acting out a part or role. You're an actor. Your emotions have become intoxicating and have coerced you out of choosing to be yourself. Your belligerence, nervousness, or patterns have convinced you that you need to be someone else.

Once you have your chosen identity and are easily sticking to your values and your highest choices, only then are you able to maintain your integrity in any situation and in every relationship. Relationships based on insecurity (i.e., Forced Relationships) demonstrate your dysfunctional, impostered, or intoxicated identification. This would look like choosing to have a relationship because you don't want to be alone. Or clinging to a friend with whom you can't be honest because you think you don't have any other options. Especially if you're mimicking someone else, this can lead only to a destructive outcome.

Almost every single person I've worked with has initially proclaimed that they already have their own identity. They say that they're always the same person around everyone. They even brag to the point of being "brutally honest" or "not afraid to speak up in any situation." We're going to take a sincere look at this and see what I'm talking about. Because during their EMSO Training, each of these same people was shocked to see that they were indeed playing a role and being different people in various situations.

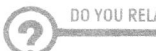
DO YOU RELATE?

Neal is having tea with his cousin. She shares with him that she doesn't enjoy having his children over to play with her kids anymore because they use profanity around her kids and that's not acceptable. Neal doesn't share any feelings or reveal how upset he is and plays it off as if it's no big deal to him.

Later at home, Neal tells his husband what a terrible person his cousin is, and with the attitude of "good riddance," shares that he doesn't care anyway. Inside, he's actually hurt and would like to keep the relationship going but feels too embarrassed to continue and definitely can't speak confidently or directly with his cousin about the issue.

You don't need to cause a scene or "set someone else in their place," but if something that triggers you is worth complaining about to someone else, it's worth discussing directly with the person as well.

*If you leave a situation feeling smaller than when you went into it, then your Intoxicated Identity was in the driver's seat.*

Now let's explore from a different perspective. Imagine you and your best friend are out to lunch together. You're sharing opinions and perspectives, and you outwardly agree with everything they say, when in actuality, you don't share the same opinions. In this case, you're sacrificing your real identity to fit in or be liked or accepted by them. In a more historical or time-concentrated relationship, such as with a partner or relative, you may do it to "keep the peace," yet how peaceful did you actually feel while doing that?

If you leave any situation feeling smaller than when you went into it, then your Intoxicated Identity was in the driver's seat. In moments where you <u>outwardly</u> agree with what you don't actually agree with on the <u>inside</u>, you're not giving the other party, nor yourself, the courtesy of your integrity. You're hiding your real self and managing others' perceptions of you. You're creating a false image of who you actually are and what you actually believe. If you're doing this in any area of your life, then you're lacking integrity, due to the absence of having a chosen identity and the courage to demonstrate it in any circumstance. If you don't come to the table as your real self, you're misleading others, and this is destructive for your relationship.

Most of us lie more than we think we do. When you begin to pay attention to your dishonesty throughout the day, you'll notice this is true. If you find yourself needing to constantly shift and sway to meet the requirements of the status quo in your relationships (business, romantic, and familial), then you may be lying many times per day to yourself, and/or to others. Without a solid identity, lies <u>have</u> to happen, especially white lies and half-truths. A half-truth is actually a whole lie.

You may find that in many areas of your life where you lack integrity, it may be evidence that you lack an integrity-based identity. With no identity, you have no integrity. They're interconnected.

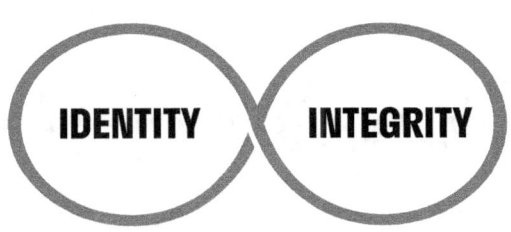

Prior to going through the process of choosing a personal identity, you're managing everything and nothing is real. For instance, if your thoughts include, "What will they think if I say this? Wear this?," then you're preoccupied with how you'll <u>appear</u>, not with who you actually <u>are</u>, and there's no longer room for reality.

I recall saying and doing things that weren't true. I remember feeling emotionally overwhelmed in the moment because I didn't know how to stop once the flywheel was set in motion. I became so out of touch with reality that I would say things without realizing what I was saying. There were times that I would say something and not remember what I'd just said. There was little balance nor reality—only confusion. I didn't know it at the time, but I didn't have my own chosen identity!

I didn't know who I was, and therefore couldn't embrace who I <u>really</u> was in every moment, every circumstance. I wasn't respecting myself because I didn't know how to respect myself, or even know that this was important. I was giving up who I wanted to be to satisfy or appease others, and to play a role that fit into their picture of who I was. I now know that not only was lying disrespectful and inconsiderate to others, it was a slap in the face to myself as well. When we attempt to appease others, we're literally guessing what would appease them. We're guessing what we should lie about to make something appear different than it really is, instead of just letting it be what it really is. We're twice removed from reality, meaning we're already living with an inauthentic identity, and on top of it, thinking for others, from an unclear, dishonest place.

Can you now see that having integrity isn't only being honest with others? It's our wholeness, confidence, and committment to being honest with ourselves. Integrity can be defined simply as:

DEFINITION

**INTEGRITY:** the state of knowing you're whole, entire, and complete, regardless of the circumstance.

When we're lacking integrity, there's something in the way—a Trauma Filter derived from an initial crack in the foundation of our self-esteem. When we're constantly filtering, we're under the illusion that we're broken and no longer whole. However, integrity isn't only something we receive from committing to our chosen identity; it's also knowing we're already whole, and then living from that place forever.

Do you recall my utter disbelief that I could become someone different—someone clearly sober-minded and confident? I had no idea how to create a new identity! At that point, these words came to me: "It's absolutely freeing to know that I can create a new me, a truer self, and that the real me is simply waiting to be uncovered from my emotional insobriety. The terrifying part is only that I've never done it before. Now, I make the decisions. Now I get to live." Let's try the following on for size. Either read the statement above, or create your own using this framework:

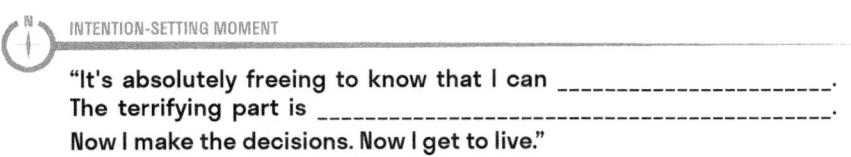

INTENTION-SETTING MOMENT

"It's absolutely freeing to know that I can _____.
The terrifying part is _____.
Now I make the decisions. Now I get to live."

This was a turning point for me. I jumped into that new territory, and I invite you to do the same. By committing to creating the *you* you've never met, you'll become an individual with your own identity, and you'll never have to lie again for any reason—not even those little white lies that seem harmless! You won't have to lie to get what you want, or to fit in. You'll already have everything you need, and maintaining the status quo will no longer be your aim.

Looking at my past feels like I was living in a movie. When your "movie" ends, you won't have to play any roles anymore. You'll easily say to yourself and others, "My movie has ended. I can be honest at all times, even if it's hard and vulnerable. I tell the truth where I've once lied, and I now deal with the consequences. As I don't sit in my past, I can be me in the now."

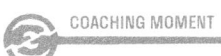 **COACHING MOMENT**

I won't assume what you're feeling at this point, but in case you're struggling, know that most of us who sought out this remodeling at times felt exacerbated, furious, fearful, confused, and lonely. Yet at the same time there's a first glimpse of the person we hadn't noticed before. I know you can expand even more than you already have. Hang in here with me. Envision the others who are completing this same process. They're enduring what you're enduring on the journey of self-discovery. With this discovery, you'll be given the tools for self-recreation.

You'll build a version of you that will allow you to be *you* around everyone. You'll maintain your highest principles, speak your word, and maintain your word. You'll sincerely be one person in every setting—ever growing, but consistently one whole person. Being yourself means selecting and working diligently on creating your identity, then maintaining this identity with integrity.

You can't have integrity without an identity.

# 13

# Case Studies: Trauma Filters & ETBs

You've probably heard the saying, "You're only as strong as your weakest link." Your filters are your inner weakest links, and as I've shared, everything is filtered through your biggest trauma. The messages you received because of these filters will inevitably precede an Emotionally-Triggered Behavior (ETB). This is why it's important to investigate, discover, and then remove our filters.

Perhaps you want more connected and joyful relationships, greater physical and mental health, and more time to enjoy your life. Trauma Filters contribute to your lack of trust in others. Another person cannot say, do, or think anything about you that you'll fully believe, or even receive as constructive feedback, if it contradicts your filter. When, for example, you're in the ETB of self-centeredness, every action or inaction is "about" you and specifically driven through the filter, causing your reaction. This often makes it difficult to advance in your profession, attain whole health, and simply live in peace, clarity, and levelheadedness.

Let's go back to our example in Chapter 9 of the trauma of sexual abuse, during which Cindy developed resonating beliefs of "I'm worthless," "I'm only of value if I have sex," and "Sex isn't safe," and the Trauma Filters of unworthiness and distrust. Her remnant emotions of shame and fear, as well as these beliefs about herself, have likely made their way into all of her subsequent relationships and experiences on some level. They've become the filter through which she views her reality. They've now become her weakest link. What she sees and hears as she goes throughout her days, all line up with these filters, further validating her self-beliefs. In most cases, this is the beginning and continuation of internal tension, when she's arguing for the situation to match what she really believes about herself, regardless of what the truth is. Her behaviors, or ETBs, likely include the need to control situations in order to prevent the potential of being abused again, as well as jealousy of others who seem to have the "ideal relationship."

Let's look at three additional scenarios of the way Trauma Filters create ETBs, and how we worked with them in sessions with students:

### Case Study #1: Romantic Relationship

Jeremy: "I'm often afraid that my partner will cheat on me or leave me for someone else."

With Trauma Filters in place, Jeremy becomes a "detective" of his partner's actions, words, and intentions, finding it nearly impossible not to filter every situation to match what he believes about himself and his world, regardless of what the truth is. He compulsively sorts through her purse when she's not around, looking for evidence of betrayal. He observes the way she talks to other men and how she behaves around them. He gets angry when he thinks there's something hidden behind her intentions.

Everything Jeremy's partner says or does—and all that Jeremy sees—is filtered through this lens. It keeps him "safe," so he's not saddled with a potential surprise. He's protecting himself from being re-traumatized (can you guess his Early-Age Trauma?). In addition, his filters look for ways to validate him for believing what he thinks will happen. It "proves" that the worst-case scenario that he believes to be a certainty is right around the corner. It gives him permission to continue using his energy to hold onto fear and that it's worthy of being used... that the weight of his neediness is worth carrying. To reiterate that he's unsafe in his relationships and that his heart is going to be broken.

**Early-Age Trauma:** Betrayal
**Self-Beliefs:** "I'm unsafe, I'm going to be tricked."
**Trauma Filters:** Danger, distrust, rejection
**ETBs:** Childishness, jealousy, judgmentalism

### Case Study #2: Close Friendship

Becky: "I know that my friends are talking about me behind my back, and this makes me anxious."

Because Becky sees the world through her particular lenses (again, can you guess her Early-Age Trauma?), she becomes sure that her friends are all going to end the relationship or go on their own paths without her. So she chooses to retreat and stop calling anyone, getting more into reading books and watching movies at home alone every night, along with a bag (or two) of chips.

She's now ready for everyone in her life to therefore leave her behind. Everything they say or do, and all that she witnesses happening around her, has to be filtered through this lens of insecurity, unworthiness, and certain rejection. Because she then reacts by pulling out of the relationships, it further "proves" that she's right... that she actually is unworthy of love and friendship, and that she has nothing to offer.

**Trauma:** Abandonment
**Self-Beliefs:** "I don't matter." "No one cares."
**Trauma Filters:** Inadequacy, unworthiness, rejection
**ETBs:** Defensiveness, self-centeredness, secondary addiction (to sugar)

As you can see, the common Trauma Filters often overlap, resulting in a very cloudy lens. If it sounds difficult to look further, remember that these filters have created reactions within you that may have harmed you or others, engorging you with chemicals of emotions such as guilt, fear, or embarrassment. Let's first discover what your individual filters are, thus beginning the essential process of changing your lens, and thereby your biochemistry.

Let's explore one more common scenario to support you, further learning the language of Emotional Sobriety.

### Case Study #3: Codependent Relationship

Anita: "My father was an alcoholic and couldn't care for himself or manage his depression. I took on the role of being the savior of the family… because I'm the strong one."

Anita believes she failed her father because he ended up dying of alcoholism. An unfillable hole was created within her that says, "I'm useless unless I can save others." She adapted to the environment she grew up within, and she took on the role of the one who's in charge—the one who must fix others' problems. She's managed to maintain this role throughout her life and into adulthood. She easily attracts people who need her to "save" them or care for them, and Anita compulsively gives herself away in these relationships to prove her value and usefulness. Contrary to this, she also easily finds all the reasons why she's not useful, which then perpetuates the cycle of her addiction.

**Traumas:** Exposure to substance abuse in the household, Parental illness
**Self-belief:** "I have to save everyone or I'm a burden."
**Trauma Filters:** Inadequacy, non-value
**ETBs:** Defensiveness, secondary addiction

In these three scenarios, we see several of the common Trauma Filters in action, shining a light on the beliefs we have about ourselves and how these have created the reactive ETBs that we can't seem to control.

Later in Part 4, we'll engage a deep self-investigation that exposes those hidden defective links in your chain of wholeness. You'll witness them with intense readiness to remove them, and in that same breath you will remove them. Envision your chain as remodeled into a whole and complete chain of solid integrity. Remember, you're not broken. You're not "bad" or "wrong" for having these experiences or these resonating symptoms. You're simply now being offered an opportunity to deal with them in a new way—to free yourself from their attempt to keep you the same.

# 14

# Find My ETBs

*The things you use to survive are keeping you from living.*

Of all the components of emotional insobriety, the most obvious symptoms are your Emotionally-Triggered Behaviors (ETBs). In this chapter and subsequent chapters, we'll explore each of the most common ETBs in greater depth and identify which ones have unconsciously become part of your identity. If you have a copy of the companion journal, get it out now, along with your pen or pencil, and let's find out who you've been being.

 **COACHING MOMENT**

**This may prove to be a challenge. How humble and observant can you be for yourself as you begin to gain awareness of your ETBs? You likely didn't intend to behave in these ways, but how much honesty can you bring to this exploration, knowing that in order to change them, you must first become aware of them? Let's see what you're actually demonstrating in order to find out where you are. When you become challenged by any of this process, choose to be honest with yourself and hold yourself responsible instead of looking for external excuses.**

Any change you desire can be achieved through training. First, you have to know where you stand. We're looking for proof of ETBs, chronic negative biochemical addiction, and evidence of compulsive habits. Emotional Sobriety isn't easy to objectively measure, as it's a subjective topic. Thus, I designed the following exercise to reveal as accurately as possible where you are in your Emotional Sobriety.

No one else is going to do this for you, and no one else <u>can</u> do this for you. You're the only one who has access to the truth about what's really going on inside of you. You're the only one who can dig through the deepest and darkest corners of you. If you can lie to others, you'll have unhealthy relationships, but if you can lie to <u>yourself</u>, you're in real trouble. Get honest with yourself now, and this will become much simpler.

You'll see the lie-truth meter below dotted throughout the book. I call it a Self-Honesty Checkpoint. It's a chance to stop and evaluate inwardly: "How honest am I being with myself in my life right now?" Is your inner critic blocking you from looking deeper? Are you afraid someone may find out what you're about to discover about yourself? Each time this symbol appears, put an "X" on the line somewhere between "lie" and "truth" to indicate your self-assessment:

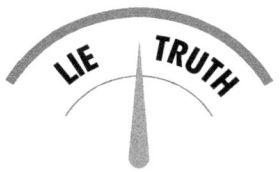

Be kind to yourself as you engage further in EMSO Training. I'm here to remind you that this isn't about you <u>judging</u> yourself. It's about you <u>observing</u> yourself. Look at the examples I draw out and see if any of them sound familiar or resonate with you, either in your past or present. Feel for any rising fear, sadness, anger, embarrassment, or other emotions while engaging in your next Take Action exercise. Allow yourself to see and acknowledge truthfully if these resemble pieces of your personality.

Also, remember that this is <u>your</u> life and no one else's. So please don't get distracted by placing others' names next to these ETBs. You may catch yourself saying things such as, "Oh, my ex did this all the time!" This isn't about your ex, your family members, your partner, your co-workers, or your friends. This part is about you and only you.

The following exercise outlines the ETBs that correspond directly to your personality—the behaviors that stem from your emotional addictions, which may cause you to act out and harm others. As you may recall, an ETB may be more related to a personality defect, or a secondary addiction, such as drinking alcohol or scrolling on social media when you feel the negative emotions we're speaking of. Let's look specifically at which ETBs you enact, which are caused (without your choice) while under the influence of your emotions.

We begin with defensiveness because it's usually the strongest force at play. Without awareness that you're exhibiting defensiveness, it can easily serve as a roadblock for you in continuing this process. When you feel defensiveness during this and the subsequent exercises, become aware of it as something that may be blocking you. By increasing your awareness of it, you may find the ability to work through it. If you cannot overcome defensiveness, you'll struggle moving forward with your exploration of the other ETBs. So be brave and honest, and attempt to release defensiveness as you complete this exercise!

Take a deep breath...

COACHING MOMENT

Don't beat yourself up. Each of these are very common forms of emotional insobriety that you can delete from your personality!

TAKE ACTION

**FIND MY ETBs**
Are any of the common ETBs part of your current identity? Fill in the square next to each statement that applies to you.

*REMINDER: All of the Take Action exercises offered in this book also appear in your "The *You* You've Never Met Companion Journal," with extra space for writing. Most students prefer to go through this book with the journal alongside it.

1. **Defensiveness: When threatened, I tend to...**
   - ☐ have a bodily reaction (tighten physically, get a lump in my throat, have stomach tension).
   - ☐ mentally spin (feel fear or worry, need to justify, talk repetitively or compulsively, question or think obsessively).

- ☐ yell or lash out at the messenger.
- ☐ cry uncontrollably and/or feel like crying.

If you have one or all of these, you have tendencies toward defensiveness. This ETB is a symptom of emotional insobriety.

2. **<u>Childishness</u>: I notice that I sometimes…**
   - ☐ argue to get my way.
   - ☐ shame others.
   - ☐ slam doors.
   - ☐ hit, slap, punch, scratch, and/or bite.
   - ☐ give people the "silent treatment."
   - ☐ have a compulsion to control who gets the "last word" in an argument.
   - ☐ lie to not get in trouble or to get my way.
   - ☐ throw tantrums (even in public places, making a scene).
   - ☐ say "It's not fair!" or "It's all your fault!"
   - ☐ keep harmful secrets (mine or another's).
   - ☐ am unable to speak (voiceless).
   - ☐ complain or whine.
   - ☐ excessively cry or display overly dramatic behavior.

If you have one or all of these, you have tendencies toward childishness. This ETB is a symptom of emotional insobriety.

3. **<u>Jealousy</u>: I often…**
   - ☐ roll my eyes and "huff" when I notice any attention going away from me.
   - ☐ cause a scene.
   - ☐ pick a fight or criticize.
   - ☐ yell or become aggressive.
   - ☐ shame or play emotional games.
   - ☐ threaten ending the relationship.
   - ☐ destructively compare myself to others.
   - ☐ feel pain when someone else does well or has what I want.

If you have one or all of these you may have tendencies toward jealousy. This ETB is a symptom of emotional insobriety.

### 4. Self-Centeredness: I find that I sometimes…
- ☐ think for others (assume I know what someone else is thinking, feeling, saying, or doing).
- ☐ overtly direct others to play the roles I want them to in my life.
- ☐ passively direct others to get what I want from them.
- ☐ have expectations of others (demanded or unspoken).
- ☐ interrupt or talk over other people (in argument or in general conversation).
- ☐ gossip or slander (as participant or initiator).
- ☐ use "emotional leverage" (attempt to impact others' emotional states to get my way).
- ☐ get easily offended and/or embarrassed.
- ☐ project what I'm "guilty" of onto someone else.
- ☐ am in self-pity/victimization.

If you have one or all of these, you may have tendencies toward self-centeredness. This ETB is a symptom of emotional insobriety.

### 5. Judgmentalism: I notice that I tend to be…
- ☐ critical of others.
- ☐ critical of myself.
- ☐ avoidant of others who have a different point of view.
- ☐ argumentative when another isn't living or thinking as I would.
- ☐ racist, sexist, ageist, etc.
- ☐ judgmental of others for being "guilty of that" as I was reading the above statements.

If you have one or all of these, you have tendencies toward judgmentalism. This ETB is a symptom of emotional insobriety.

## 6. Dishonesty: I notice that I...
- ☐ lie to myself.
- ☐ lie to others (about anything).
- ☐ manipulate others by lying to or about them.
- ☐ am "sneaky."
- ☐ omit select information.

If you have one or all of these, you have tendencies toward dishonesty. This ETB is a symptom of emotional insobriety.

## 7. Secondary Addiction: I tend to frequently...

**use exogenous (external) chemicals, including...**
- ☐ drugs (marijuana, cocaine, heroin, pills, etc.).
- ☐ alcohol.
- ☐ nicotine.
- ☐ food.

**use distractions, including...**
- ☐ phone scrolling, texting, social media.
- ☐ T.V. and streaming (aka "binge" watching).
- ☐ gaming.
- ☐ dating sites.
- ☐ chronically entering into new relationships.
- ☐ mental fantasies (revenge, romantic, sexual, etc.).
- ☐ work/hobbies.
- ☐ trading one addiction for another.

**behave compulsively, through...**
- ☐ self-injury (cutting, anorexia, bulimia, extreme exercise or diet, etc.).
- ☐ vanity (obsession with appearance; taking daily "selfies," posing/posting for attention, excessive plastic surgery, consumed with looking in mirror, judging body or looks).
- ☐ an inability to be in silence (repetitive chatter, laughing as a defense mechanism, changing topics to deflect, "scatter bomb").

- ☐ isolation/hiding/rebelling.
- ☐ hoarding.
- ☐ spending (shopping, gambling, gift-giving).
- ☐ OCD/repetitive thoughts or actions (body tics or twitches, coughing or sneezing fits, excessive cleaning or hand-washing, turning lights on and off, numerical obsession, etc.).
- ☐ violence (bar fights, street violence, violence for entertainment, gaming).
- ☐ voyeurism/stalking.
- ☐ sex (excessive pornography, affairs, etc.).
- ☐ being restless (not sitting in the same place for long; continuously wanting to move geographically).

If you have one or all of these, you have tendencies toward secondary addiction. This ETB is a symptom of emotional insobriety.

In this curriculum, I use these seven common ETBs, as they are the most common root symptoms of emotional insobriety. Most behaviors fall under one of these categories. As you do the real work through this curriculum, any unwanted behaviors that reside in you may naturally fall away.

Do you now have a sense that you have yet to attain or master Emotional Sobriety? Are you wondering what to do now that you've grown your awareness? The answer is that you go deeper, you listen, you hold onto this awareness and see where it takes you—where it takes us—together. To do that, you'll need to know what you're <u>actually</u> feeling, explore each of the ETBs in greater detail to know what you're <u>actually</u> doing, and uncover <u>why</u> you feel and behave the way you do.

# 15

# What Am I <u>Actually</u> Doing? Feeling? And Why?

*Ask yourself again and again.
Then ask again.*

Let's take your awareness one step deeper. Your Emotionally-Triggered Behaviors (ETBs) are reactions derived from your emotions. It's easier to know why and when you're experiencing ETBs by accessing what you're actually feeling and why.

Since we're biochemical addicts and this is still relatively new information, how can we know which emotions we're experiencing since we've been having them since childhood? How can we know that what we're feeling is "abnormal" if it's been our norm?

It may seem warm and cozy to stay in what you've known, yet imagine that the *you* you've never met is excitedly inviting you with arms reaching out to follow them into the future. They've already figured it out and they know it's safe there. Let me help you discover how to feel what's real for you.

## What Am I <u>Actually</u> Doing?

The easiest way to access what you're actually <u>feeling</u>, is to first develop the capacity to identify what you're actually <u>doing</u> (ETBs), and unwind the pattern from there. You've now been introduced to some behavioral patterns that you may not have previously noticed in as much detail. These behaviors may have seemed like they were a part of your personality, as they've shaped a part of your current identity. It may feel like "you," but what if you knew that these behaviors were really only a byproduct of your biochemical addiction and mental patterns that you've held since childhood, and that they could be changed?

The next way you'll begin to understand your most common symptoms of emotional insobriety is through continued awareness of your ETBs.

TAKE ACTION

**BEHAVIORAL AWARENESS**
Now that you've made an initial assessment of your possible ETBs, let's practice identifying which specific behaviors you displayed during three recent triggering experiences.

## SITUATION 1:
The last time I felt threatened or overwhelmed, this happened:

I reacted by (ETB)

## SITUATION 2:
The last time I felt threatened or overwhelmed, this happened:

I reacted by (ETB)

## SITUATION 3:
The last time I felt threatened or overwhelmed, this happened:

I reacted by (ETB)

Think about how many times you've tried to solve a problem with an ETB. Now think about how many times an additional problem arose because of that ETB. When you behave without clarity there seems to be no solution, only repetition of the same problem. This is because the same way of thinking tried to <u>solve</u> the problem that <u>caused</u> the problem. The dysfunctional behavior that's supposed to help you survive in this experience of possible loss will actually cause the loss. By practicing knowing what you're really feeling, doing, and thinking, and discovering new emotional states, behaviors, and beliefs, you'll regain trust in yourself, which will begin to repair the crack in your self-esteem.

 COACHING MOMENT

**Choose to search for your innermost honesty and gain your own trust through action by caring for yourself before asking someone else to care for you.**

## What Am I <u>Actually</u> Feeling?

Now we need to address what triggers the behavior... your Predominant Accompanying Negative Emotions (PANEs). As you learned in Biochemical Addiction to PANE, your emotions are really chemicals, and with EMSO Training you'll gain access to your real feelings. If you sustain a lack of emotional awareness, you'll often be disconnected from the behaviors that follow them. These emotions/biochemicals turn you into what trauma made, not who you were made to be. Who you were made to be is unblocked, authentic, and clear.

This is a dominant disconnect in an emotionally unsober person. If you don't understand your own true emotions, then how can you expect someone else to understand your feelings and know how to respond accordingly? If you misunderstand your <u>own</u> feelings and then share them outwardly, it often leads to confusion and a reaction you don't expect from others—both for the person hearing it and yourself, as you'll sense the behavior or response you're receiving from the other person doesn't match what you're feeling. This is due to lack of communicating what you're <u>actually</u> feeling.

What if your anger is really just embarrassment? What if your depression is really just fatigue and a sense of hopelessness around feeling this painful chemistry for so much of your lifetime?

*It feels like "you," but what if you knew that it was really only a map of your biochemistry and mental patterns that you've learned since childhood, and that it could be changed?*

Not truly knowing what we feel can create misunderstandings in communication and dishonest relationships. It also keeps us from knowing where we are in our development and what we actually want in our lives.

Because we've become so dissociated from our true emotions, many therapists and coaches use a "wheel of emotions" to simply support the identification of which emotions are <u>actually</u> being experienced. In Chapter 10, I introduced you to the six most common emotions—PANE: Predominant Accompanying Negative Emotions. Gaining the capacity to be aware that you're experiencing a feeling, and then to name your accurate emotion is an example of building Emotional Intelligence, which is an important first step. What we'll learn later in EMSO Training is how to <u>choose</u> the emotion you wish to feel inwardly and share outwardly.

Notice the word "feel." An emotion, or feeling, is a physical, chemical, and sensory message. How does a thought affect the way your body feels? Which emotion does this bodily sensation elicit? That's the first feeling flow I want you to start observing as you complete the next exercise.

TAKE ACTION

**EMOTIONAL AWARENESS**
Use the three situations from page 113 for this exercise. Let's find the real, underlying emotion that you may have been feeling at the time of these events. For example, was your anger or sadness really embarrassment or fear?

How did this experience really make you feel? How do you feel now when you think of it?

Continuously ask yourself: Is it possible that this isn't the real feeling? Can I look deeper?

Reference the common PANE graphic on page 70 to support you in identifying the specific emotion.

## SITUATION 1:

During this situation, I used this behavior (ETB): _____

because I was experiencing the emotion (PANE) of: _____

_____.

## SITUATION 2:

During this situation, I used this behavior (ETB): _____

because I was experiencing the emotion (PANE) of: _____

_____.

## SITUATION 3:

During this situation, I used this behavior (ETB): _____

because I was experiencing the emotion (PANE) of: _____

_____.

DO YOU RELATE?

Ruth shares that when she sees her partner talking to someone she believes he thinks is attractive, her body feels tingly, tense, and numb. Also, her heart feels tight and her throat starts to close up. She begins to feel her hands sweat, and her vision becomes different. Some of the time her ears begin to ring. She feels this way because she's experiencing the emotion of fear.

She's experiencing fear because of her Trauma Filters of unimportance, rejection, and inadequacy, which correspond to the Trauma-Influenced Self-Beliefs of "I'm not enough," "I'm going to be left out," and "I'm not important to him."

These filters and beliefs stem from an Early-Age Trauma of abandonment (Perceived Trauma where she felt abandoned when she was often left home alone at younger than 5 years old while her [single] mom went to work).

She now knows that she felt this way when he said this because of her Trauma Filters of rejection, unimportance, and inadequacy. She translated his actions to mean something that seemed true for her —"I'm unworthy, I'm not important, and I'm going to be left alone."

Ruth acknowledges that she saw the event through her Trauma Filters. When she reviews her partner's actions again <u>without</u> these filters, she now sees that he was merely talking to another person. Ruth realizes that she's a grownup now and can take care of herself, and she knows she's important to him because he said she was, and he shows it daily. She knows that she's safe in the present moment.

COACHING MOMENT

Remember that <u>all</u> of your learned reactions, including your moments of intense Emotional Belligerence, are survival reactions. This means that if you're behaving erratically, you're attempting to survive something. Biologically, your body cannot easily tell the difference between a life-threatening predator and a simple perceived threat like the one depicted in Ruth's story. You must choose to learn to discern the difference between a real life-threatening situation and a learned, pseudo-threatening situation. Your emotional insobriety seems normal and necessary, until you learn to choose.

CONTEMPLATION

**MY PRIMARY EMOTIONAL ADDICTION**
Ask yourself: What is the negative feeling that I suffer with most of the time? Is it similar to the emotion that I felt when I experienced my Early-Age Trauma(s)?

Take another look at the common PANE graphic on page 70 to discover the closest match to what you're feeling throughout most of your daily life. What emotion are you <u>most</u> addicted to?

### Why Am I Feeling & Doing This?

Now that we've explored what you're really doing and feeling, let's begin to uncover why you do these things and why you feel these feelings. You may first be asking, "Why me?!" Remember, you're not alone.

If the chemical released in your body is interpreted as your emotions, then you know that the chemical is merely affirming some dysfunction within you. Without the dysfunction, there will be no stress chemical made. We know that the dysfunctions come from Early-Age Trauma, when you began to develop false beliefs about yourself and the world around you. By reviewing the filters that were built from these experiences, you'll find a part of the code for getting all the way clear of it.

For example, you've learned that if you can find out what's really behind what appears as anger in your body, you'll discover that it's triggered by a filter such as unimportance. This came from a trauma that was inflicted upon you, that you observed and perceived as trauma, or that you inflicted upon someone else.

Again, we've also memorized feelings from our family members. Although we don't blame our families for imprinting their emotional patterns and behaviors onto us, we must understand where our dysfunction came from.

If you can't recall choosing a specific response to an emotion that arises within you, then it was most likely observed, downloaded, and learned from somewhere—either during a traumatic experience, from your family, or through a cultural influence such as T.V., movies, or social media. Behavioral learning is our subconscious mind applying all the information from our surroundings so we'll best survive in our tribe. Even your parents learned this way. But how?

From ages 0 to 7 we're in a hypnotic brainwave pattern that allows for easy learning of language, behavior, reaction, and survival.[11] How does Mom react to this? How does Dad manage this? What do we eat? What level of volume do we use when speaking? How do we manage energy? Who's the leader of the family? By watching our parents, siblings, and other community members, we can learn what they know and predictably live at least as long as they have due to downloading their same behaviors. We unconsciously say to ourselves, "If it's worked for them this long, it will work for me too."

I want you to remember that since your parents and community were also programmed from a young age, unless they've done the hard work to improve their Emotional Sobriety, it's likely that the patterns that were downloaded into you are the same behaviors that were handed down to them. This isn't usually a chosen learning. Your subconscious mind takes it upon itself to be your "note-taker" as you grow in your older childhood years. Once you're out of this brain-wave pattern, there's more to be learned, yet most of your ETBs have already been carefully and safely stored for when you need them again, thereby making it seem nearly impossible to reprogram these patterned reactions.

When you're in a state of survival or threat, these emotions, reactions, and behaviors will come right out to the forefront, revealing to the world what you were taught as a small child. It's quite spectacular that your subconscious mind has this capacity! Yet you can also make quite a spectacle when you behave like an angry three-year-old when you don't get your way. They're the things you seemingly have no control over that cause harm to yourself and others, and they're doing you no good in your life now that you're an adult.

Through many years of supporting students to identify and then eradicate their ETBs, I've observed not only their commonality of identification, but also their similar origins—similar "whys" and "whens" that these ETBs most often present themselves. In other words, while you may think your life experiences are utterly unique to you, we can often trace them to similar Early-Age Traumas, which then creates a somewhat predictable pathway to developing a nearly identical set of Trauma-Influenced Self-Beliefs and Trauma Filters. Wouldn't it make sense, then, that we could find similar pathways to freedom as well?

Let's take the next step with the same scenarios you've been working on in the previous two Take Actions and uncover the real "why" for your emotional insobriety in these moments. It comes back to the belief you hold about yourself, derived from Early-Age Trauma. In later stages of EMSO Training, you'll learn that changing the Trauma-Influenced Self-Belief, therefore, is the crux of your training.

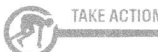
**TAKE ACTION**

**BELIEF AWARENESS**

Let's find out why this situation triggered you by looking for the Trauma-Influenced Self-Belief that it "validated."

ETBs are brought on by PANE, and you feel this PANE because you interpret a situation to mean something about you. This is a Trauma-Influenced Self-Belief.

By answering this same question again and again, your true self-belief may be revealed.

Using the same scenarios from your Behavioral and Emotional Awareness exercises, continue by increasing your Belief Awareness.

## SITUATION 1:

What did I interpret the situation to mean about me?

And if this were true, what would that mean about me?

And if that were true, what would <u>that</u> mean about me?

## SITUATION 2:

What did I interpret the situation to mean about me?

And if this were true, what would that mean about me?

And if that were true, what would <u>that</u> mean about me?

## SITUATION 3:

What did I interpret the situation to mean about me?

And if this were true, what would that mean about me?

And if that were true, what would <u>that</u> mean about me?

There's more to the "why" than meets the eye. This is a sneakier, more subversive reason for your behavior that will help increase your self-honesty when practiced with diligence. This practice allows for you to access even more of who you've been being from many different points of view. I call it checking motive.

When you behave with ETBs due to your PANE via validated Trauma-Influenced Self-Beliefs, you may feel like two people: 1. the one who's good-hearted and well-intentioned, and 2. the one who's thinking and behaving in ways the former "never would." The latter is your Intoxicated Identity.

TAKE ACTION

**MOTIVE AWARENESS**
Become a detective and trace the very thoughts you were thinking (your internal conversation with yourself) around the time of the behavior. In each of the scenarios, what was the real motive behind your behavior? What were you hoping to accomplish?

**EXAMPLES:**

- "I told him I was going to the movies because I knew he wouldn't attempt to call me during those hours, and I could be with the other guy."
- "I said I needed to go buy toilet paper but (underneath) I knew I was really going to buy beer."
- "I mentioned that I was single so that they would overhear and know I was available."

## SITUATION 1:

I know I behaved by being _____.
I did so specifically by _____.
This seemingly solved my problem by _____.
When I really think about what I was hoping to accomplish by doing this, I know my real motive was to _____
_____.

**SITUATION 2:**
I know I behaved by being _____.
I did so specifically by _____.
This seemingly solved my problem by _____.
When I really think about what I was hoping to accomplish by doing this, I know my real motive was to _____
_____.

**SITUATION 3:**
I know I behaved by being _____.
I did so specifically by _____.
This seemingly solved my problem by _____.
When I really think about what I was hoping to accomplish by doing this, I know my real motive was to _____
_____.

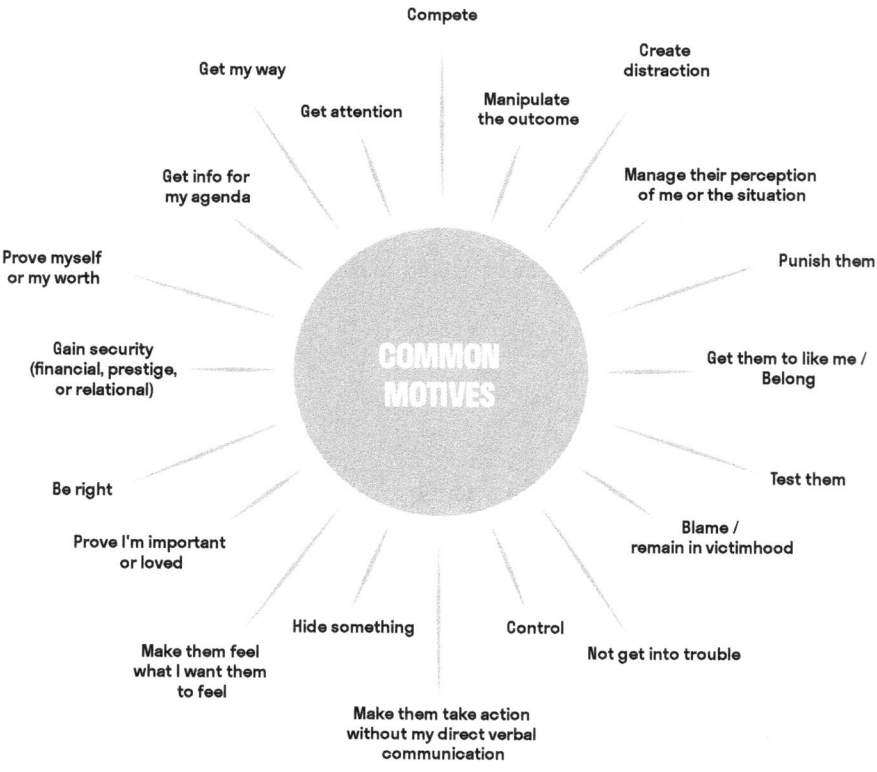

(Add any you experience by drawing more lines out on the graphic above.)

The behaviors, emotions, beliefs, and motives you identified with in the above Take Actions likely permeate much of your life and relationships. Self-criticism, dishonesty with yourself, and self-judgment may stop you from continuing this process more than anything else. You might be thinking, "I can't believe I do that!" or "I now realize just how belligerent I've been with my friends and family. How can they even love me anymore?" or "It's too late for me... I can't possibly pick up all the pieces of my past. It's just too much." If you're anything like me, overcoming your aversion to honestly look at yourself requires repetition and consistently increasing your courage.

Thus, it's time for another Self-Honesty Checkpoint. Am I being honest with myself as I reflect on the work I've completed in this chapter?

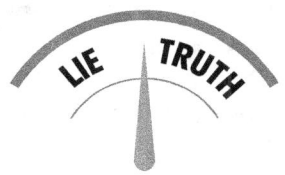

Let's dig deeper for the reasons we behave in the ways that we do. These are the reasons that are within our own mind at the time of the behavior. The following in-depth Take Action is going to alert you to the possibility of your having an ETB that you may not have recognized in the last exercise. It also serves as a reference point to further uncover what has created the *you* you've been being. (Remember, this is also in the companion journal.)

 TAKE ACTION

**REASONS FOR MY ETBs**

After finding which ETBs you demonstrate, look to see the reasons <u>why</u> you specifically may be behaving in these ways. As you read each of the statements on the following pages, mark the squares next to those that sound the most like you when you demonstrate that ETB.

**Fill in all that apply:**

1. **Defensiveness:**

   **When I have a bodily reaction (tighten physically, get a lump in my throat, have stomach tension), it's because...**

   - ☐ I'm guarding by building "a fence"—others can't enter and I can't get out.
   - ☐ I feel the need to block my truth from being spoken.
   - ☐ I feel fear of speaking up.
   - ☐ I think that "I can't speak my truth because I don't know the truth," or because "I won't look perfect by being forthcoming."

   **When I mentally spin (feel fear or worry, need to justify, talk repetitively or compulsively, question or think obsessively), it's because...**

   - ☐ I feel fear of being rejected, not being loved, or "not being picked for the team."
   - ☐ I'm emotionally dependent on the criticizer to like/love me.
   - ☐ I assume that if I'm not seen as perfect, I'm not lovable.
   - ☐ I'm worried about others.
   - ☐ I assume that the worst-case possibilities are an absolute reality.

   **When I yell or lash out at the messenger, it's because...**

   - ☐ I have an "I don't like you if you don't like me" attitude.
   - ☐ I'm angry at myself for not being perfect or for getting caught.
   - ☐ I'm angry with others for not protecting my illusion of perfection.
   - ☐ I feel frustrated not knowing how to communicate, or I'm too tired to fix it.
   - ☐ I need to reject them before they reject me.

**When I cry uncontrollably and/or feel like crying, it's because...**

- ☐ I'm being rejected and I'm alone, tired, and exhausted due to not being able to achieve perfection.
- ☐ I feel hopeless and/or helpless.
- ☐ I'm attempting to get what I want; get attention.
- ☐ I'm attempting to create sympathy from another instead of receiving their punishment.
- ☐ I'm scared of not being seen as perfect or not being loved.

If you're lashing out and hurting someone else for trying to tell you something about you, or out of fear that what they say or do means they don't like you, that's defensiveness. Are you ready to clear defensiveness? It takes practice, but trust me, you can eliminate this nasty little habit from your life forever!

## 2. <u>Childishness</u>:

**When arguing to get my way, it's because...**

- ☐ I'm committed to a certain emotional state and opinion, and I'm determined to change the other person's stance.
- ☐ I'm holding a motive to win or be right.
- ☐ I'm attempting to control someone else and get what I want.
- ☐ I'm outraged when there's contrast in what I want or believe should be.

**When I'm shaming others, it's because...**

- ☐ I've brought my experience of shame as a child into adulthood.
- ☐ I want them to feel the same way I think that they made me feel.
- ☐ I feel shame myself but can't name it as such, so I shame others to match my unspoken shame.
- ☐ I have the perception of being on "higher ground"/being more powerful than others.

### When I slam doors, it's because...

- ☐ I'm "shutting the other out."
- ☐ I want to manipulate others emotionally.
- ☐ I have feelings—without voicing directly—"I'm angry and feel hopeless in this argument. I may not want to be alone, but I can't be with you."
- ☐ I'm noisily letting others know that they're wrong, in trouble, or being punished.

### When I hit, slap, punch, scratch, or bite, it's because...

- ☐ I'm attempting to "tear someone out of their own skin" so they'll see my side.
- ☐ I'm unable to communicate.
- ☐ I want to feel "power over" another person.
- ☐ I don't know what else to do with my frustration.

### When I'm giving someone the "silent treatment," I'm really thinking...

- ☐ "If I ignore you, you may see what you're missing."
- ☐ "You may worry about me instead of being angry with me."
- ☐ "Perhaps my withholding of love will make my point and create desperation in you."
- ☐ "If I'm quiet, you'll think of how you've wronged me, and I'll think of how you wronged me too."
- ☐ "My feelings are more important than yours."
- ☐ "I'll build a stronger argument in my head to 'win' the next time we talk."
- ☐ "I need no self-examination nor do I seek responsibility for the conflict."

### I have a compulsion to control who gets the "last word" in an argument because...

- ☐ I believe that if the other party has nothing further to say, that means I win the argument ("the defense rests" attitude).
- ☐ I don't seek resolution or connection through conversation.

### I lie to not get in trouble or to get my way because...

- ☐ if I tell another this untruth about me, they'll see me the way I desire them to see me, and I'll have perceived control over the situation.
- ☐ I don't want to be punished for what I think I did wrong, or what I believe others will think is wrong.
- ☐ I don't want what's here (reality) to be true.
- ☐ I want to get out of something or to become more likable.
- ☐ I want to blame others for my own discrepancies.
- ☐ I feel threatened and afraid of loss, so I have no choice other than to manipulate others to get the outcome that I want.

### When I throw tantrums (even in public places, making a scene) it's because...

- ☐ I'm "screaming for attention."
- ☐ I want to divert attention away from the truth.
- ☐ I'll do anything to keep the status quo.
- ☐ I can't have a mature conversation.
- ☐ I don't know how else to be seen or heard.

### I say, "It's not fair!" or "It's all your fault!" because...

- ☐ I'm struggling to maintain control.
- ☐ I believe I should get my way, or I deserve to get my way.
- ☐ I'm assuming my needs should come first, but I don't voice my precise needs.
- ☐ I'm neglecting to remove myself from chronically imbalanced situations.
- ☐ I have expectations of others.

### I keep harmful secrets (mine or another's) because...

- ☐ I'm avoiding "getting in trouble" or protecting someone else from getting in trouble (usually someone with power over me).
- ☐ I can't freely share my harmful or embarrassing experiences with others.
- ☐ I'm protecting myself or others or protecting an image of a desired reality.

### I'm unable to speak (voiceless) because...

- ☐ I'm afraid of what might happen if I speak and can't protect myself.
- ☐ I don't believe in myself.
- ☐ I don't know how to use an honest voice in certain situations.
- ☐ I think "I don't have the right to have a voice."
- ☐ I'm unable to communicate well.

### I complain or whine because...

- ☐ I'm attempting to make others feel small.
- ☐ I'm relaying information of discomfort or dissatisfaction in the best way I know how.
- ☐ it helps me get attention.
- ☐ I don't know how to fix my troubles or surrounding environment to work better.

### I excessively cry or display overly dramatic behaviors because...

- ☐ I want to create distractions so the truth isn't seen.
- ☐ someone may "rescue" me.
- ☐ I often feel confusion with a flood of emotions and it needs to come out.
- ☐ I fear not being seen as perfect, not being loved, or not getting my perceived needs met.
- ☐ I feel hopeless in the moment.

As adults, we may have some of the same needs we did as children—to be loved, hugged, listened to, special, and important. But to behave as a child when we're an adult in order to have our needs met, is childishness. After the thorough self-investigation that you'll complete in EMSO Training, followed by practices to support you in becoming the *you* you've never met, childishness won't follow you into your future.

## 3. <u>Jealousy:</u>

### I roll my eyes and "huff" when I notice any attention going away from me because...

- ☐ I'm paranoid of being unimportant or abandoned.
- ☐ I want others to see me and give me attention.
- ☐ I want to be the <u>most</u> special to others.
- ☐ I believe I'm being rejected and I'm resentful.

### I cause a scene because...

- ☐ I'm fearful whenever others seem to be out of my personal control.
- ☐ I want to create a big statement so others will chase me.
- ☐ I have the thought, "I'll abandon you if you're going to abandon me."
- ☐ I have to test others to see if they'll choose me.

### I pick a fight or criticize because...

- ☐ I fear losing a relationship because of my own inadequacy/insecurity.
- ☐ at least I'll get the other party to feel <u>something</u> for me.
- ☐ I want "connection."
- ☐ now the other person's attention has to be on me.

### I yell or become aggressive because...

- ☐ at that moment, I'm certain the other person will choose someone else over me.
- ☐ I've convinced myself that someone else is better than me.
- ☐ I want them to hurt like they hurt me.

### I shame or play emotional games because...

- ☐ I want the other to believe that I have the power in the relationship and that I'm the "catch."
- ☐ I want the other to feel small.

### I threaten to end the relationship because...

- ☐ I want the other person to fear losing me, as it allows me to regain control.
- ☐ it keeps me at the center of their attention by creating the threat of a "take away."

### I destructively compare myself to others because...

- ☐ I'm feeling unaccomplished and insecure.
- ☐ I'm looking to be self-destructive (internally) or gain compliments (externally).
- ☐ I'm keeping myself separate from others.
- ☐ I believe I'm usually in competition with others.
- ☐ I believe that I'm less worthy than others.

### I feel pain when someone else does well or has what I want because...

- ☐ I want to be the best at everything.
- ☐ I want to be the center of attention when others are receiving praise and respect.
- ☐ I often want what someone else has and am dissatisfied with what I have now.
- ☐ I have an attitude of, "Why do they get that and I don't?"
- ☐ I'm entitled and believe that I deserve something more than another person.
- ☐ I believe others are more likely to withhold things from me rather than share them.

These are also leftover reactions from childhood. Now as an adult you display emotions that seem bigger or more dramatic than the situation might call for. After completing this work, jealousy will no longer be a part of your makeup.

## 4. <u>Self-Centeredness:</u>

### I think for others (assume I know what someone else is thinking, feeling, saying, or doing) because...

- ☐ it helps me manipulate situations and people to stay in control.
- ☐ I assume others can't speak or think for themselves.
- ☐ I'm afraid of what they might be thinking, and I need to be ready for what they're about to say or do.

> **COACHING MOMENT**
>
> Thinking for others is one of the most difficult and prominent habits to break. I've sat for hours with people attempting to support them to see where they continue to do this. We cannot know exactly what someone else is thinking! We may think we know based on the history. If we've read their patterns over the years, our level of accuracy may even be high. However, as long as we continue to do this, we'll have the same outcome every time, and we're here to finally change our lives. Thinking for others is a learned behavior. We learn it, we perfect it as a skill, and it becomes an automatic response to survive in our environment.

### I direct others or assign the roles they'll play in my life because...

- ☐ I believe that others are here to be in my movie of life.
- ☐ I want others to behave the way that I want them to behave.
- ☐ I don't want any changes to the "script."
- ☐ I'm guarding and protecting my autonomy—"This is <u>my</u> life, not yours!"

### I passively direct others to get what I want from them because...

- ☐ it allows me to set up a false stage of my life and get what I want.
- ☐ I want to come out "on top" or be in control in relationships.
- ☐ I'm seeking information for evidence under the guise of sincere interest—to "win" my case.

- ☐ I think, "It doesn't matter how this affects or affected you; all that matters is how I feel and what's happening in me."
- ☐ I can't see clearly outside of myself, and I'm the only thing that's real in my world.

**I have expectations of others (demanded or unspoken) because...**

- ☐ of my own past experiences or social brainwashings.
- ☐ I think, "I did this for you, so you should've done that for me!"
- ☐ I obsess about how things affect me and I don't realize that others aren't also thinking about how things affect me.

**I interrupt or talk over others (in argument or general conversation) because...**

- ☐ I've been ignored a lot in the past.
- ☐ I feel impatient or irritable with others' input as I believe I already know what they're going to say and they're wrong.
- ☐ I want to "rule the roost."
- ☐ I'm constantly wondering how I appear to others so I need to make an impression.
- ☐ of the repetitive hysterical thinking in my head.
- ☐ I want others to know I'm important.

**I use gossip or slander (as the participant or initiator) because...**

- ☐ this form of chaos distracts from my own life.
- ☐ it allows me to get attention.
- ☐ I can hide behind a "veil" of chatter.
- ☐ I can keep my own secrets by telling others' secrets, whether real or false.
- ☐ I can connect with others around shared complaints.
- ☐ by engaging in "mutual enemy relationships" (those built around a mutual enemy or group of adversaries), I feel a sense of belonging and increased power.
- ☐ I perceive that I've been rejected or am feeling shame for something I've done.

- ☐ I take embarrassment and turn it into anger while directing the blame or negative attention "over there."
- ☐ the more people I can get on my side the safer I'll be.
- ☐ I can't contain what I believe happened to me.
- ☐ I want my interpretation of others to be heard.

**I use emotional leverage (attempt to impact others' emotional states to get my way) because...**

- ☐ it allows me to generate power over someone.
- ☐ I want to be seen as indispensable to another person.
- ☐ if I show my self-sacrifice, others won't leave me.
- ☐ by using shame or guilt, it increases my ability to maintain a relationship.
- ☐ I easily hold onto anger and blame.

**I get offended or embarrass easily because...**

- ☐ I believe everyone is watching me or talking about me.
- ☐ I chronically analyze others and situations.
- ☐ I'm insecure.
- ☐ I feel entitled to my way even if another person doesn't agree.
- ☐ I see my way as the only way.
- ☐ I'm fairly close-minded in general.
- ☐ I don't often enjoy listening to another's point of view.
- ☐ I think I need to be right.
- ☐ situations are filtered through my thoughts: "What does this have to do with me?" or "What are they thinking of me?" or "Everyone here is as preoccupied with me as I am."

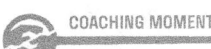
COACHING MOMENT

**Inconsideration is one of the most hidden attitudes and can therefore typically be uncovered only later in our process of fact-finding. This is a great place to check in to see if you're thinking of other people who are guilty of these things or if you're searching only for your own behaviors.**

### I project what I'm "guilty" of onto others because...

- ☐ I often think, "They're doing this to me!" (not me to them).
- ☐ it's the only thing I can see and declare in others because it's the only thing I experience in myself.

### I'm in self-pity/victimization because...

- ☐ I'm establishing myself as someone who needs care, attention, and/or protection.
- ☐ I'm establishing a low baseline—I'm never the one who will be asked for favors; taking the pressure off to contribute/give—"They can't ask me for anything because I'm too _____."
- ☐ I put others on a pedestal; someone else is my hero.
- ☐ I can remain helpless to avoid being perceived as arrogant.
- ☐ it allows soothing compliments to come my way.
- ☐ I'm seeking attention.

These are all often buried tactics, meaning you'll often not even realize you're doing it. These patterns of thought continue for extended periods of time and perhaps a lifetime. Though the subject may change, the consistency and mechanics remain the same. These behaviors are expressions of being stuck in what I call the "Center of Self," and soon you'll be introduced to the "Freedom of Self," as self-centeredness will no longer be a useful tactic for your life.

**COACHING MOMENT**

**Remember that this training is about looking at yourself and yourself alone. If you find yourself thinking about others in your life who display these characteristics, gently set these thoughts aside and come back to yourself.**

5. **Judgmentalism:**
   **HINT: A judgment will always have a negative feeling associated with it, whereas an observation won't.**

   **I'm critical of others because...**

   - ☐ I believe others should live the way I do.
   - ☐ others don't fit my paradigm of good or right— e.g., I resent my child for not sharing my religious beliefs (Exclusionary Criticism).
   - ☐ I think I'll feel safe if I "control" my surroundings by continuously and disrespectfully pointing out flaws in the environment—e.g., "Don't put that there!" or "Why did you do that?" or "Don't stand like that!" (Vacuum Criticism).
   - ☐ I can draw attention away from myself using loud volume so that others' flaws will be seen instead of my own—e.g., "Are you really going to wear that?" or "Why is your floor so dirty?" or "I can't believe you did that!" (Loud Criticism).
   - ☐ it validates my perceived power over them.
   - ☐ I judge others in the same ways I judge myself.

   **I'm critical of myself because...**

   - ☐ I believe I'm lazy.
   - ☐ I believe I'm unlovable, uninteresting, or unimportant.
   - ☐ I won't ever have to be disappointed if I fail.
   - ☐ if I hate myself more than everyone else, no one can reject me.
   - ☐ I can get compliments from others if I criticize myself out loud.
   - ☐ I think there's no need to try if it's not going to be "perfect."

   **I'm avoidant of others who have a different point of view because...**

   - ☐ I don't want to question my upbringing.
   - ☐ I don't want to believe or acknowledge that there's an alternative point of view to my own.
   - ☐ I believe my opinion is not opinion, but fact.
   - ☐ I don't want others to question the way I do things.

### I'm argumentative when another isn't living or thinking as I would because...

- ☐ I'm certain of the way things are.
- ☐ I have a right to decide if someone else's life choices are good/bad or right/wrong.
- ☐ I have little to no consideration of another's point of view.
- ☐ changing my current lifestyle would be too vulnerable and scary; I perceive I'll have no foundation.

### I'm racist/sexist/ageist, etc., because...

- ☐ I feel excessive doubt (especially in my belief system).
- ☐ I've spent my whole life believing what I've believed.
- ☐ I had a difficult experience and now blame the entire group.
- ☐ I was told to be and never changed it (e.g., I may be angered by homosexuality because my parent was vehemently against it).

### I was judgmental of others for being "guilty of that" as I was reading the above statements because...

- ☐ it seems easier to put my focus on others before looking at myself and my patterns.
- ☐ I need to observe and criticize others to feel better about myself.

Each of these ways that judgmentalism appears in your current life has been helpful for maintaining your personal status quo and feeling "good" about yourself. Yet there are levels of <u>really</u> feeling good that you haven't yet experienced in life! Ridding your personality of judgmentalism is another key to that liberation.

## 6. <u>Dishonesty</u>:

### I lie to myself because...

- ☐ I don't like reality and want to convince myself of an alternative.
- ☐ I don't like who I am or what I'm doing.
- ☐ I want to do something that I think is wrong, so I justify my actions with excuses.

### I lie to others (about anything) because...

- ☐ deep down I'm feeling insecure or nervous.
- ☐ I want to be seen a certain way; have a perfect image.
- ☐ I'm ashamed or embarrassed.
- ☐ I want the lie to be the truth.

### I manipulate others by lying to or about them because...

- ☐ I've decided that they don't deserve the truth.
- ☐ I believe that I know better than they do.
- ☐ it makes my stories more interesting.
- ☐ it makes the context fit my agenda/needs.

### I'm sneaky because...

- ☐ I want to have my autonomy, and I believe I'm being controlled.
- ☐ I don't want anyone to know.
- ☐ this is the only thing I have for myself.
- ☐ I feel shame about what I'm doing.

### I omit select information because...

- ☐ I don't want to offer information that may poorly affect my desired outcome.
- ☐ if I'm ever found out, I can claim "forgetfulness."
- ☐ I want to shape a conversation to go my way.
- ☐ I've convinced myself that I'm technically still telling the truth if I tell some of it.

Any area of your life that you feel you need to be dishonest is coming from a lack of self-love or lack of knowing who you really are. Dishonesty has seemed to be an important skill to build in order to get you through life to this point, but it's soon going to be a thing of the past. Get ready for dishonesty to completely work its way out of you.

7. **Secondary Addiction:**

   **I use drugs (marijuana, cocaine, heroin, pills, etc.) because...**

   - ☐ I need to "fill a void" in me.
   - ☐ I need an immediate change in my reality.
   - ☐ it disconnects me from my pain or the mundane.

   **I drink alcohol because...**

   - ☐ I need to "fill a void" in me.
   - ☐ I'm looking to feel something other than what I'm feeling.
   - ☐ I need to "check out" or need "forced" relaxation.
   - ☐ I believe I can't have fun without it.
   - ☐ I'm shy unless I have it.
   - ☐ I believe I'm a better person when I do it.
   - ☐ it's in my lineage.

   **I use nicotine because...**

   - ☐ everyone in my family and/or circle of friends does it.
   - ☐ it calms me down.
   - ☐ it keeps me from eating.
   - ☐ I've done it since I was a kid.

   **I eat food addictively because...**

   - ☐ I need to fill a void in me.
   - ☐ I want to numb my emotions.
   - ☐ I was deprived of this at some point in my life.
   - ☐ I'm "starving" for something.

   **I distract myself using my phone/scrolling/texting/social media because...**

   - ☐ I can't be alone.
   - ☐ I want to see what everyone else has.

- ☐ it keeps me away from reality.
- ☐ I can live in a fantasy or live vicariously.

**I escape by watching T.V./streaming ("binge" watching) because...**

- ☐ I want my life to be like what I see on T.V./movies.
- ☐ I get caught up in the drama/romance/violence that I'm watching.
- ☐ it allows me to not have to communicate.
- ☐ I'm alone and it keeps me company.

**I escape by gaming because...**

- ☐ I like to be in control.
- ☐ I don't know how or who to be in real life.
- ☐ I can drown out my real life.
- ☐ I believe I'm weak, and this makes me feel tough.

**I escape by going on dating sites because...**

- ☐ I get hits of attention and compliments.
- ☐ I like the excitement of getting attention from a new person.
- ☐ I don't have to commit, but am still "dating."

**I escape by chronically entering into new relationships because...**

- ☐ I need the rush of something new.
- ☐ I keep thinking, "The next one will be different."
- ☐ I'm chronically looking for "the one."
- ☐ all of my exes were bad for me.
- ☐ I'm dissatisfied with my life and "the grass is always greener on the other side."
- ☐ I can't be alone.

**I escape into mental fantasies (revenge, romantic, sexual, etc.) because...**

- ☐ I like the gravity of the violence, sex, or emotions.
- ☐ I'm easily bored.

☐ I want to continue my same mental obsession I've had since I was young (e.g., fairytale endings).

### I distract myself with work/hobbies because...

☐ I'm hiding from intimacy.
☐ I believe it's the only way that I have value or add value to the world.
☐ I can't show up anywhere else in life.
☐ I'm obsessed with what I do.

### I distract myself by trading one addiction for another because...

☐ I don't want to miss out.
☐ I'm bored without some type of addiction.
☐ I think that I need something to cope—"at least this is 'healthier.'"

### I behave compulsively through self-injury because...
(e.g., cutting, anorexia, bulimia, extreme exercise or diet, etc.)

☐ I'm restless/impatient.
☐ I can't finish it all or I'm overloaded.
☐ I have to perfect my imperfections.
☐ pain "wakes me up."
☐ I believe I'm ugly/disgusting.
☐ I have to look like others think I should look.
☐ I can't enjoy food and look good at the same time.
☐ I have no value unless I look perfect.
☐ I believe I'm too fat or too skinny.

### I behave compulsively through vanity because...
(e.g., obsession with appearance; taking daily "selfies," posing/posting for attention, excessive plastic surgery, consumed with looking in the mirror, judging my body or looks)

☐ I'm not going to be loved unless I'm attractive.
☐ my body has to be precise.
☐ I want/receive a lot of attention.
☐ no matter what, I can never look good enough.

### I behave compulsively with an inability to be in silence because...
(e.g., repetitive chatter, laughing as a defense mechanism, changing topics to deflect, "scatter bomb")

- ☐ I don't know how to simply be myself.
- ☐ I need the attention to both be on and off of me at the same time.
- ☐ in the silence, someone might have an opportunity to ask me a question or say something that makes me uncomfortable.

### I behave compulsively by isolating, hiding, or rebelling because...

- ☐ I think I need my autonomy and can't get it.
- ☐ I don't want to be observed, judged, or questioned.
- ☐ I don't want to be controlled.
- ☐ I'm afraid of confrontation.
- ☐ I don't want to be seen or have my secrets revealed.
- ☐ life outside is too overwhelming.
- ☐ I like to dwell on things (fantasize, contemplate, or marinate in my current emotional state).
- ☐ I want to be free from captivity.

### I behave compulsively by hoarding because...

- ☐ I'm afraid I'll have nothing if I let things go.
- ☐ I believe that the things I'm keeping might be worth something someday.
- ☐ physical objects keep me safe.
- ☐ I'm never alone when my house is "full."
- ☐ I fear living in lack or poverty.

### I behave compulsively through spending (shopping, gambling, gift-giving) because...

- ☐ I want to have everything!
- ☐ I believe if I buy others something they'll like me.

**I behave compulsively with OCD/repetitive thoughts or actions because...**
(e.g., body tics or twitches, coughing or sneezing fits, excessive cleaning or hand-washing, turning lights on and off, numerical obsession)

- ☐ I don't want to be seen.
- ☐ I need to be seen.
- ☐ I have emotions that I'm shoving down that are trying to come out.
- ☐ it's not safe enough to relax.

**I behave compulsively by engaging in violence because...**
(e.g., bar fights, street violence, violence for entertainment/gaming)

- ☐ my anger has to go somewhere.
- ☐ I can prove how tough I am/"hard to kill."
- ☐ I can establish myself as not being someone to "mess with."
- ☐ I'm safe if others fear me.

**I behave compulsively through voyeurism or stalking because...**

- ☐ I become obsessed with people.
- ☐ I need to know what someone is doing at all times.
- ☐ I fear loss and being alone.
- ☐ I don't have an ability to truly connect.
- ☐ if I'm always there, I won't be forgotten.

**I behave compulsively through sex (excessive pornography, affairs, etc.) because...**

- ☐ it's the only way I can feel anything.
- ☐ I need to know what it would be like.
- ☐ I lack ability for intimacy.

## I behave compulsively by being restless because...
(e.g., not sitting in the same place for long, continuously wanting to move geographically)

- ☐ I'm "running away."
- ☐ I'm afraid to stay in one place.
- ☐ the longer I'm still, the more I have to think about my reality.
- ☐ I need to find someone to protect me.
- ☐ I'm anxious that I'll make the wrong choice.
- ☐ I've never had a choice.
- ☐ I'm confused about how I feel and what I want.

## Are there any additional reasons for your unwanted behaviors?

_____

_____

_____

When we continue justifying our lies, envy, de(fences), and the like to ourselves, all of our ETBs get stronger and stronger. We think we're protecting ourselves, but instead we're making ourselves sicker and sicker.

**COACHING MOMENT**

Great job completing that in-depth look into your ETBs. If you're feeling embarrassed, ashamed, defensive, or angry about what you've learned about yourself at this point, know that all of us are feeling—or have felt—similarly, because we've all discovered very similar things about ourselves. Since every single one of us has experienced trauma in one form or another, and these ETBs are all inspired by these traumas via chemical reactions, you have to identify with only <u>one</u> of these unsober symptoms to meet the criteria of suffering from emotional insobriety.

Remember, <u>you're not to blame</u>. <u>No one is to blame</u>. This is the way humans respond to difficult experiences. But you don't have to continue feeling, thinking, and behaving the same way you always have. Let me guide you forward toward freedom!

Do you now have a better sense of the early childhood dynamics that have informed your current way of being? Are you becoming aware of the beliefs you tell yourself, the filters through which you're viewing life, and the resulting behaviors that don't really feel like "you"? Do you understand that <u>everyone</u> experiences emotional insobriety on some level?

Now let's put it all together...

# 16

# Anatomy of Emotional Insobriety

*When you have an Intoxicated Identity,
you're experiencing emotional insobriety.*

We've now looked at each component of emotional insobriety, and you've likely identified as being somewhere on its spectrum. (Remember, it takes identifying with only <u>one</u> of the behaviors, beliefs, or emotions to benefit from EMSO Training!) Here's what emotional insobriety looks like when we put the pieces together:

**EARLY-AGE TRAUMA**

**INTOXICATED IDENTITY**

**TRAUMA-INFLUENCED SELF-BELIEF**

**EMOTIONALLY-TRIGGERED BEHAVIOR (ETB)**

**TRAUMA FILTER**

**BIOCHEMICAL ADDICTION TO PANE**

1. You experience an Early-Age Trauma at some point in your childhood.

2. You begin forming Trauma-Influenced Self-Beliefs.

3. With repetition, these beliefs form Trauma Filters through which you're now viewing yourself and the world around you. This seemingly helps protect you from re-experiencing the challenging emotions from that trauma, but it actually does the opposite.

4. When triggered, you now experience a biochemical release in your body to hold the memory for your protection/survival. This chemical is a Predominant Accompanying Negative Emotion (PANE) that you feel (resentment, anger, guilt, embarrassment, fear, and sadness). You become addicted to this biochemical with the repetition of remembering, thinking about, and feeling the effects of the trauma.

5. Over time you develop Emotionally-Triggered Behaviors (ETBs), or re-actions to the world around you, due to emotional intoxication or even belligerence.

6. This cycle creates the basis for an Intoxicated Identity—the one you haven't chosen, but now find yourself in.

All of this occurs unconsciously... until now. You're developing self-awareness—or emotional intelligence—around these mechanisms at play in your life and psyche, making you more equipped to change the picture altogether. Now let's look at how this links together in your personal biography.

 TAKE ACTION

**LINK THE DETAILS OF MY INSOBRIETY**
Here's another method we use to find your Trauma-Influenced Self-Beliefs, which is the piece of your anatomy that, when discovered, creates the biggest opportunity for change. These beliefs cause our PANE, which make us react with ETBs.

On the examples provided, circle or highlight the Early-Age Traumas that most closely resemble your personal experience. Use the blank chart at the end for additional entries.

Then circle the subsequent beliefs, filters, and behaviors that you developed because of it. Remember that these were smart strategies that served you well as a child, yet now will only hold you back.

## TRAUMA: SEXUAL ABUSE / MOLESTATION

| Self-Beliefs | Filters | ETBs |
|---|---|---|
| "I'm unworthy" | Unworthiness | Defensiveness |
| "I'm unsafe" | Danger | Childishness |
| "I'll be betrayed" | Betrayal | Jealousy |
| "I'm disgusting" | Unattractiveness | Self-Centeredness |
| "I'm sick" | Distrust | Judgmentalism |
| "I'm only valuable sexually" | Non-Value | Dishonesty |
| "I can't trust" | Victimhood | Secondary Addiction |
| "I'm a bad person" | Unimportance | |
| | Voicelessness | |
| | Choicelessness | |

## TRAUMA: RACISM, SEXISM

| Self-Beliefs | Filters | ETBs |
|---|---|---|
| "I'm unworthy" | Unworthiness | Defensiveness |
| "I'm unsafe" | Lack | Childishness |
| "I'm disgusting" | Danger | Jealousy |
| "I'm hated" | Unattractiveness | Self-Centeredness |
| "I hate _____" | Rejection | Judgmentalism |
| "I'm a victim" | Non-Value | Dishonesty |
| "Everyone hates me" | Victimhood | Secondary Addiction |
| "I'll never make it due to my sex/race" | Unimportance | |
| | Blame | |

## TRAUMA: EXPOSURE TO SUBSTANCE ABUSE IN HOUSEHOLD

| Self-Beliefs | Filters | ETBs |
|---|---|---|
| "I'm going to be just like _____" | Inadequacy | Defensiveness |
| "I'm not as important as their drugs/alcohol" | Danger | Childishness |
| | Distrust | Jealousy |
| "I need drugs/alcohol to cope with my life" | Rejection | Self-Centeredness |
| | Non-Value | Judgmentalism |
| "I can't trust anyone" | Unimportance | Dishonesty |
| "I'm worthless" | Unworthiness | Secondary Addiction |
| "I'll never amount to anything" | | |
| "I have to help others" | | |
| "I have no choice" | | |

### TRAUMA: EMOTIONAL ABUSE

| Self-Beliefs | Filters | ETBs |
|---|---|---|
| "I'm undeserving" | Unlovability | Defensiveness |
| "I'm not smart" | Woundedness | Childishness |
| "I'm unlovable" | Unattractiveness | Jealousy |
| "I'm not good enough" | Non-Value | Self-Centeredness |
| "I can't _____" | Voicelessness | Judgmentalism |
| "I'm a bad person" | Choicelessness | Dishonesty |
| "I don't have a voice" | Distrust | Secondary Addiction |
| "I don't get a choice" | Shamefulness | |
| | Rejection | |
| | Defeatism | |

### TRAUMA: VIOLENCE OR WITNESS OF EXTREME EMOTIONAL REACTIONS

| Self-Beliefs | Filters | ETBs |
|---|---|---|
| "I'm not safe" | Inadequacy | Defensiveness |
| "I can't trust" | Unworthiness | Childishness |
| "I have to be loud to be heard" | Danger | Jealousy |
| "I have to be silent or I'll get hurt" | Fragility | Self-Centeredness |
| "I need to control my environment or I'm going to get hurt" | Defeatism | Judgmentalism |
| | Rejection | Dishonesty |
| | Victimhood | Secondary Addiction |
| "I have to be perfect" | Perfection | |
| | Escapism | |
| | Captivity | |

### TRAUMA: LOSS

| Self-Beliefs | Trauma Filters | ETBs |
|---|---|---|
| "Everyone leaves me" | Obstinance | Defensiveness |
| "If I feel nothing, I'll be safer" | Detachment | Childishness |
| | Unworthiness | Jealousy |
| "I'm often sick like the one I lost" | Danger | Self-Centeredness |
| | Fragility | Judgmentalism |
| "If I appear perfect, no one will leave me" | Defeatism | Dishonesty |
| | Rejection | Secondary Addiction |
| "I can't trust" | Victimhood | |
| | Perfection | |
| | Lack | |
| | Distrust | |

## TRAUMA: LACK OR POVERTY

| Self-Beliefs | Filters | ETBs |
|---|---|---|
| "I never have enough"<br>"I can't get my needs met"<br>"I'm not the kind of person who can have it all"<br>"If I were loved (by others or God), I'd have more"<br>"People who are rich are evil"<br>"I don't want to be like rich people"<br>"If I had more, I'd be worth more to others" | Lack<br>Poverty<br>Unimportance<br>Unworthiness<br>Inadequacy<br>Defeatism<br>Victimhood<br>Danger<br>Escapism<br>Shamefulness<br>Non-Value<br>Obstinance<br>Perfection | Defensiveness<br>Childishness<br>Jealousy<br>Self-Centeredness<br>Judgmentalism<br>Dishonesty<br>Secondary Addiction |

## TRAUMA: DELIVERED TRAUMA (BY YOU)

| Self-Beliefs | Filters | ETBs |
|---|---|---|
| "I'm a bad person"<br>"I should be ashamed"<br>"I'm disgusting"<br>"I'm going to get in trouble"<br>"I'm scared of people knowing what I did"<br>"I don't deserve ___"<br>"It's always my fault"<br>"I can't change" | Unworthiness<br>Unease/dis-ease<br>Danger<br>Distrust<br>Non-Value<br>Unattractiveness<br>Rejection<br>Shamefulness<br>Trouble<br>Unlovability<br>Perfection<br>Obstinance | Defensiveness<br>Childishness<br>Jealousy<br>Self-Centeredness<br>Judgmentalism<br>Dishonesty<br>Secondary Addiction |

## TRAUMA: ABANDONMENT OR NEGLECT

| Self-Beliefs | Filters | ETBs |
|---|---|---|
| "I'm probably going to be left or betrayed" | Unimportance | Defensiveness |
| "I'm of no value" | Perfection | Childishness |
| "I'm unworthy of love" | Unworthiness | Jealousy |
| "I'm inadequate" | Rejection | Self-Centeredness |
| "Something's wrong with me" | Unlovability | Judgmentalism |
| "I'm not important" | Victimhood | Dishonesty |
| "I'll never be loved" | Detachment | Secondary Addiction |
| "If I'm perfect I won't be left" | Inadequacy | |
| "I'm not special" | Shamefulness | |
| | Escapism | |
| | Captivity | |
| | Voicelessness | |
| | Trouble | |
| | Distrust | |

## TRAUMA: DIVORCE OF PARENTS/ SINGLE PARENT

| Self-Beliefs | Filters | ETBs |
|---|---|---|
| "I can't trust" | Unimportance | Defensiveness |
| "If they loved me, they would've stayed together or wouldn't have left me" | Unworthiness | Childishness |
| | Rejection | Jealousy |
| "I'm worthless" | Perfection | Self-Centeredness |
| "I'm no good" | Distrust | Judgmentalism |
| "I have to be perfect" | Danger | Dishonesty |
| "It was my fault" | Inadequacy | Secondary Addiction |
| "I'm unlovable" | Non-Value | |
| | Victimhood | |
| | Fault | |
| | Trouble | |
| | Unlovability | |
| | Invisibility | |
| | Detachment | |
| | Aloneness | |

| TRAUMA: **BETRAYAL** | | |
|---|---|---|
| Self-Beliefs | Filters | ETBs |
| "I'm unimportant"<br>"I'm a joke"<br>"I'm of no value"<br>"I'm always 'ready' to be betrayed"<br>"I can't trust"<br>"I'm unsafe"<br>"I'll be tricked again"<br>"They think I'm stupid" | Unimportance<br>Unworthiness<br>Rejection<br>Distrust<br>Danger<br>Inadequacy<br>Non-Value<br>Victimhood<br>Perfectionism<br>Unintelligence<br>Obstinance | Defensiveness<br>Childishness<br>Jealousy<br>Self-Centeredness<br>Judgmentalism<br>Dishonesty<br>Secondary Addiction |

| TRAUMA: _____ | | |
|---|---|---|
| Self-Beliefs | Filters | ETBs |
|  |  |  |

Are you beginning to see how your ETBs are a reaction to having Trauma-Influenced Self-Beliefs and Trauma Filters in place? Can you see that these stem from your Early-Age Trauma? You're not alone. We're all the same. Everyone experiences this pathway in their lives in some form. The next Take Action is another way of relating the details of your Anatomy of Emotional Insobriety—this time through a writing exercise. This narrative approach will support your growing awareness around who you've been being.

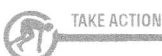
**TAKE ACTION**

**MY TRAUMA PATHWAY**
Use the following set of inquiries as a template to work through several of your Early-Age Traumas. The companion journal includes several blank templates. Remember, right now we're looking only at trauma from around ages 0 to 20.

Early-Age Trauma: _____

- What was said or done to you, or what did you observe, perceive, deliver, or have inflicted upon you? _____
  _____

- What do you now believe about yourself because of this event? What are your Trauma-Influenced Self-Beliefs? _____
  _____

- What Trauma Filters are in place to validate your Trauma-Influenced Self-Beliefs? _____
  _____

- When you believe this, how do you feel, both in your physical body and emotionally speaking (PANEs)? _____
  _____

- What tendencies do you now have due to this trauma? What are your ETBs? _____
  _____

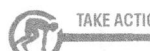 TAKE ACTION

### SNAPSHOT OF MY ANATOMY OF EMOTIONAL INSOBRIETY

You're now more aware of your Anatomy of Emotional Insobriety. Here's an opportunity to consolidate all that you've learned about yourself throughout the EMSO Foundations into one simple design. Write your most impactful Early-Age Trauma(s), then work your way around clockwise. Consolidate what you've learned about yourself regarding each part of your anatomy into one to three total examples. This will become your reference point to remind you what you learned about the *you* you've been being—your Intoxicated Identity.

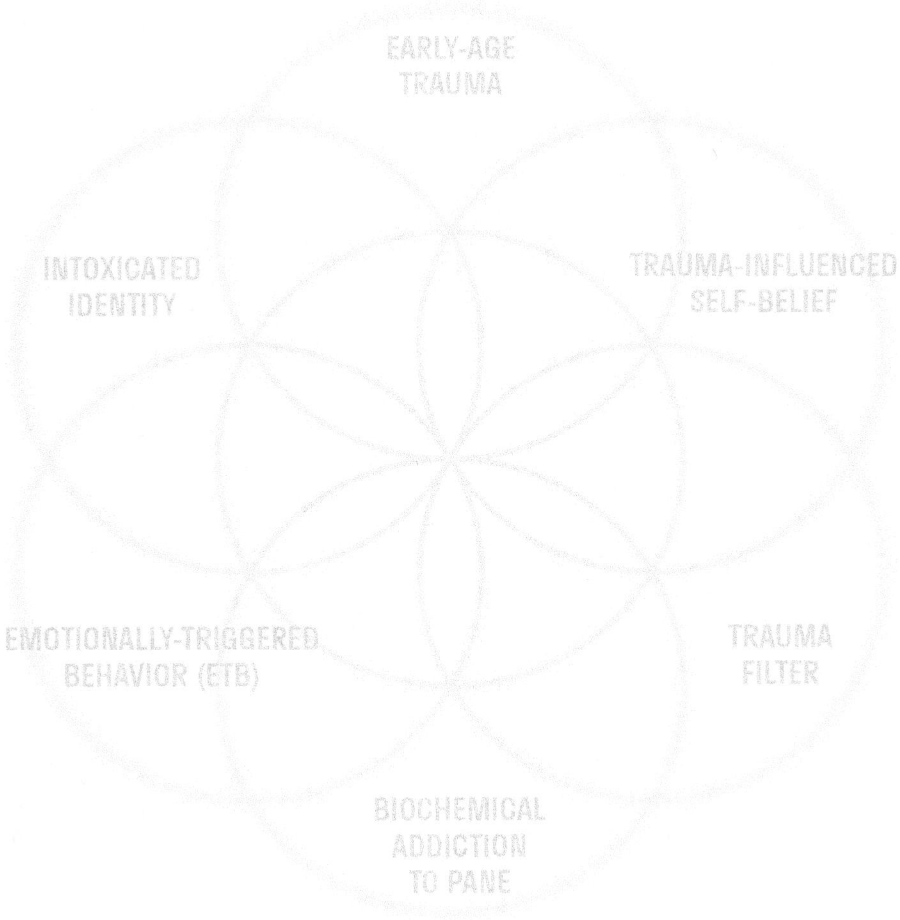

EARLY-AGE TRAUMA

INTOXICATED IDENTITY

TRAUMA-INFLUENCED SELF-BELIEF

EMOTIONALLY-TRIGGERED BEHAVIOR (ETB)

TRAUMA FILTER

BIOCHEMICAL ADDICTION TO PANE

Though this snapshot represents what we might have previously judged as "bad" or "wrong," this now becomes the "seed" of your Emotional Sobriety. The symbol I chose is called the "seed of life," as it will become the thing that births the realization that you aren't only made of the responses to your Early-Age Trauma. You aren't your beliefs, behaviors, or even your emotions.

The next seven chapters will take you through each of the common ETBs, one by one, exploring the initial stages of liberating you from these most obvious symptoms of emotional insobriety. Training away from your ETBs is the next clear step in unwinding your Intoxicated Identity.

## 17

# Remove (De)Fences

*It's easier to walk without the weight of your armor.*

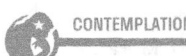  CONTEMPLATION

**RECALL ALL MY REASONS**
Take a moment now to recall the reasons why you're here exploring Emotional Sobriety and attempting change. Hold these reasons with you while continuing to read. I believe it's because you intend to meet the version of *you* that you had never previously thought possible or haven't yet been able to manifest. Perhaps there are so many more reasons. What are you unwilling to lose? What have you already lost? Whatever the reasons, they're important to keep at the forefront as you embark on the next portion of your training.

Now that you've identified your specific symptoms of emotional insobriety—your primary beliefs/filters, emotions, and behaviors—we explore how to further identify your Emotionally-Triggered Behaviors (ETBs). Consider this the beginning of the unraveling of the *you* you've been being.

## Defensiveness

First, I'm guessing that you identified defensiveness as one of your primary ETBs. It would be difficult for me to find someone who didn't have an experience of getting defensive! As I shared, it's often "the strongest force at play." Though many of the invitations to become more aware of yourself in these pages may challenge you, the subject matter in this section may be the most challenging to face. I recommend going in with an open and dynamic mind.

It's only through self-discovery of who you are now that you can then re-create the self, because, you can't edit what you can't see. Let's look again at the current and past version of *you* that you may have not been seeing.

*It is only through self-discovery of who you are now that you can then recreate the self.*

**TAKE ACTION**

**DEFENSIVENESS: OBSERVE MY (DE)FENCES**
Read each statement and fill in the circles next to the ones that sound like you when you think you're being threatened or criticized. Mark all that apply:

- ○ There are secrets I keep for myself or others, and when people pry, I fiercely defend them.
- ○ I feel something come over me and suddenly I'm putting up a "fence" to keep the other person or situation away.
- ○ When people point something out about me, I feel agitated and can't listen.
- ○ When I receive criticism—even if it's constructive—I see the same thing about myself but feel helpless about changing it, and then I get defensive.
- ○ I lie about something surrounding the threatening situation or the other person who's being critical.
- ○ I hide my flaws in an effort to present myself as "perfect" to others.
- ○ I get embarrassed easily. I sense I'm being observed.
- ○ When I feel rejected, instead of saying anything I close down.
- ○ I realize now that it's possible that my defensiveness comes from being emotionally unsober.
- ○ Others: _____

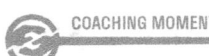
**COACHING MOMENT**

> Great! That can be difficult to do. With self-honesty, you're further getting to know the *you* you may have never even noticed was there. Did you experience any defensive reactions in seeing if there are additional areas where you may be reacting defensively? I know it's a lot to look at, and there may be many feelings that come up when doing this training. Stay the course and do this for you!

We now know that there are beliefs, behaviors, and emotional reactions that were built in at an early age. In fact, these have become an integral part of your personality and formed your Intoxicated Identity. You're so used to being this person, feeling these feelings, and behaving in these ways, that you almost never notice they're there—until you hit a bottom, have a moment of clarity, or have it pointed out to you. Perhaps a trusted friend gently calls your attention to how you seem to lie a lot, or a disgusted partner who's tired of your rage, jealousy, or outbursts, asks for a separation.

It's understandable that noting these things about yourself may create turmoil within you. In my work, I've noticed that there's rarely a calm reception of these communicated observations, rather more of a gripping defensiveness. This is why defensiveness is the first ETB we explore in greater depth, as it is one of the most powerful reactions you likely experience. It's a counter-attack, usually created in order to defend what you perceive is an attack on you. Regardless if someone is offering you useful information about what they see, you often assume it's an attack because it doesn't feel good to hear the negative things about yourself that you haven't yet acknowledged are there; or even the things you already know deep down that you don't like about yourself. So, you react.

You've developed a certain "go to" response to every possible situation. Because of this, you may not be capable of being in a present, reality-based state most of the time. You aren't having authentic, real-time responses. If it's a mechanistic replay of the past, it cannot also be real or genuine in the moment. You're acting out your prescribed roles. These parts may be so ingrained into your subconscious mind that you seem to have no control over them, meaning you don't have control over yourself. Therein lies the issue—not an insurmountable issue, but an issue nonetheless.

*To clearly see who we're being in any circumstance is to reach a genuine level of perfection. We cannot be human and be "perfect," but we can have a "perfect vision of ourselves."*

If you experienced this earlier, you may continue to find yourself wanting to point fingers at someone else for being guilty of these same traits, or even blame another person for your imperfections. It's easy to blame and become defensive due to wanting to be free from responsibility or be seen as "perfect."

I realized early on in my path to Emotional Sobriety that my humility had to be stronger than my compulsion for defensiveness. My "perfection" wasn't going to come from someone's opinion of me, it would come from my ability to see myself truthfully. To clearly see who we're being in any circumstance is to reach a genuine level of perfection. We cannot be human and be "perfect," but we can have a "perfect vision of ourselves."

Again, see defensiveness as your first block to growth. It's an all-emotional outburst—a surge of chemistry and energy—that creates a "safe" divide between you and your "enemy." This ETB is a force that creates an energetic "fence" around you. It doesn't allow you to see beyond the safety of your ego. Ego is stuck in its ways. It's a creature of habit. All it knows how to do is show you what it already knows. It gives you a peek at your future by showing you the past. I think of it simply as:

DEFINITION

**EGO:** the security guard to your status quo.

Ego is not designed for evolution but for competition and survival. Your first skills for freedom will be self-awareness and humility, and sometimes, especially in the beginning, you may need to allow someone else to tell you what they see.

If your body seems to go into a survival reaction when receiving feedback, know that it's doing its job by responding to a past event where you felt rejected or embarrassed, rather than contributory. By producing the same chemicals that match that initial experience, your body creates the same feeling. The physical manifestation of a past memory may feel painful. Being criticized or receiving feedback reminds us that we aren't "perfect." This can be particularly difficult if you've historically struggled with low self-esteem, rejection, or shame. Thus, as absurd as this sounds, our bodies would benefit from taking on a thrilled attitude toward the opportunity to change ourselves and our lives, rather than a defensive one!

Defensiveness is learned as the "best" way to fight for your safety when you feel threatened, even if it's just a simple statement or criticism about you. You have a feeling or thought that you've interpreted based on your Trauma Filter. You also likely saw someone else act in this way and learned to re-enact this same behavior as if it were your own.

DO YOU RELATE?

> John shares: "My best friend let me know that he's bothered by the way that I'm repeatedly a no-show when I promise to meet him at events. He told me that I'm disrespecting him, and I need to change this behavior if we're to remain friends. I told him, 'I'm just fine the way I am!' Maybe he's not really a friend after all if all he can do is criticize me."

Here, John's flooded with emotion and reactively counter-attacks what he believes is an attack on him. Deep down, he really feels sad and embarrassed due to his friend's examination of their friendship—asking for it to be different and more respectful. John's frustrated that his friend doesn't allow for his little mistakes to simply "fall through the cracks." Due to a wave of defensiveness, John shoves the conversation away. When under the influence of his emotions, his friend's wishes can't matter to him. By not accepting the feedback from his friend—and thereby learning more about himself—not only does this leave John without the friendship, but his friend was likely left dejected by the separating tactics of defensiveness.

*Defensiveness keeps others out and also keeps you stuck within.*

The ETB of defensiveness is damaging to you and others because this "(de)fence" you've habitually created keeps others out, and also keeps you stuck within. There are many seemingly understandable reasons why you put up a fight with someone who points out your flaws or "mistakes." Do you get defensive when you're keeping a secret or when you know you're telling a "little white lie" for someone else's benefit? Perhaps you're concerned, like John, that the other person is going to find out you're not "perfect" and that in reality, you're struggling with something? Or, perhaps deep down you know what they say is true, but you have no idea how to change it; thus, it becomes easier to simply defend it? There are countless reasons to put up this fence.

As you begin to know yourself in the present, you create the opportunity to determine what you intend to keep and what you'd like to remodel in yourself. That's what this process is designed to do, and the depth of the remodel requires attention to the entire process. Removing the "fence" that blocks you from looking is a positive and very courageous first step.

In particular, many people are taken aback when they're asked if it's possible that they have an Intoxicated—or traumatized—Identity, and that's why they get defensive. Through these pages, have you heard a voice in your head asking, "How can I not have an identity? I know who I am!" If so, you wouldn't be the first. I can imagine how simply being asked this question may create confusion (or defensiveness!). For those of us who are defensive, we tend to be very set in our ways... certain of things. We are, after all, "creatures of habit."

However, the real you is not a creature of habit; your Intoxicated Identity is. But you no longer need to succumb to this. The EMSO Essentials are of upmost importance as they invite you to separate from your set ways and look at what's really true about yourself. Only then can you engage in the remodel.

**COACHING MOMENT**

At this point in the reading and writing, it's understandable if you're needing rest. It's up to you to know what's true for you. Are you tired from the work so far? If so, know that you're likely experiencing fatigue because your brain doesn't desire these changes. This fatigue is an expected and normal response to what you've begun to do.

Remind your brain and body again and again that it's exciting to get access to things you've never seen before about yourself, and that any changes you make in the future will be in the best interest of all of you—your brain and body included. Now, take some rest if needed, and then get right back to work.

**TAKE ACTION**

**DEFENSIVENESS: REACTING TO NEGATIVE FEEDBACK**
PART 1: First, note any challenging behaviors or traits you demonstrate that have been brought to your attention by a friend, family member, co-worker, or partner:

_____

_____

PART 2: Next, you'll need to call or meet with a trusted friend, parent, or romantic partner. Ask this person to read the list above out loud to you in this way: "You do _____, and you are _____."

Or, they may know you well and be able to share their own feedback without using the list. After they offer this feedback, think about what they shared and respond to the questions on the following page.

This is here to help you get a sense of how you respond or react to feedback or perceived criticism.

> **WARNING:** *If you're unsure you can remain calm after hearing their feedback, simply imagine them giving you feedback without inviting the meeting, and then write about it.*

- How do I feel in my physical body and emotions (PANEs) right now?

- Does their feedback feel true to me? If not, why?

Like all ETBs, defensiveness is caused by a surge of chemically-induced emotion within your body, created by believing a Trauma-Influenced Self-Belief. You may immediately assume the other party is wrong and go into denial of the part you're playing in the discord. You may furiously justify your position or attempt to criticize the criticizer.

If this is what you feel and how you think at the time of possible threat, use it as an opportunity to look at what you're compulsively drawn toward saying or doing in that moment. Even if you feel too heated to change your behavior, simply observe without changing your behavior and become both the student and the observer of the student. <u>Observe</u> what you're doing and feeling, while at the same time, feel whatever you're feeling and do whatever you're doing. Take time to watch and learn about yourself in these moments.

The desired outcome of EMSO Training is to deliver a version of ourselves who doesn't make the chemicals that produce our defensive behaviors. For example, when someone calls attention to something about you and you're emotionally sober, you'll calmly be able to relay your truth about it. You'll know whether or not it's true, have the humility to acknowledge it, and there won't be any discord or harsh energy from the feedback. If the feedback is untrue, you'll calmly relay that and simply move forward. When you practice accepting feedback as a gift, you'll have a rare ability. This creates a freer, more emotionally sober life.

*When you practice accepting feedback as a gift, you'll have a rare ability.*

# 18

# Outgrow Childishness

*Age doesn't promise maturity.*

**Childishness**

The sounds of a laughing baby can be heartwarming. The endless curiosity of a child is astonishing. Even the little one's outbursts are something of a spectacle. Yet you'll probably agree with me that the tantrum thrown by a grown-up is extremely unattractive.

Our duty as parents, to the best of our ability, is to raise our children not to be "good little boys and girls," but to be good adults. ("Good" in this case meaning, cooperative, helpful, kind, considerate, free of self-centeredness, self-responsible, honest, and mentally/emotionally fit.) Children are designed to grow up into adults. They don't have to be strict or boring adults. When we build an identity that retains our child<u>like</u> wonder while leaving the child<u>ish</u> parts behind us, we create a great platform for success in life.

---

*Our duty as parents is to raise our children not to be "good little boys and girls," but to be good adults.*

---

We've learned that we've developed survival techniques as children; and perhaps they worked when we were children. We got the cookie that we cried for (I'm certainly guilty of this!), we got the attention that we screamed for, and we got the new toy that we created guilt to get. However, these tools won't work to get the things we desire as adults. In fact, acting like a child to get something we desire as an adult usually gets us the opposite (if we happen to be surrounded by healthy adults, that is!). If we're surrounded with co-dependent, enabling, or emotionally unsober adults, then we may get everything we're asking for by behaving this way. However, if you're reading this, you're likely not seeking—or no longer wish to engage in—unhealthy, co-dependent relationships; so, let's explore how to outgrow the ETB of childishness.

*If we continue to behave like children, we won't be satisfied as adults.*

We seem to compulsively return to our childhood when we're flooded with emotions, using unconscious survival techniques that we naturally retrieve in moments of crisis. If we continue to behave like children, we won't be satisfied as adults. For example, shaming someone into doing something for you is a destructive habit in relationships, romantic or otherwise. As with all of the ETBs, shaming doesn't produce the result we may want it to. It won't make anyone see our side in a clearer way. It won't make us more powerful in the relationship. Because a great majority of us have experienced some form of feeling shame as children, we use it as a go-to tactic as adults. It isn't as outwardly childish in the same way that slamming doors may be, but it's something that goes hand-in-hand with us expressing our childhood in a survival setting. The issue is that we often don't believe we could be behaving like a child because we look in the mirror and at our lives and see a grown-up. In some cases, we're going to high-level jobs, running businesses, and even parenting children of our own.

Given the lengthy list of behaviors you explored around childishness (the longest of any of the ETBs, in fact!), it may be apparent to you, as it was for me, that childish behavior is a primary go-to when we're emotionally triggered. It seems childishness is the easiest to slide into because it shows up in so many different ways, and because your Early-Age Trauma shapes your reactions when you are literally a child!

It's widely understood that we developmentally freeze after Early-Age Trauma,[12] especially emotionally. You don't advance far beyond that point until you do the work of awareness, and process that trauma as an adult. So how do you outgrow, or grow up, these childish parts of yourself? The same way you change anything: You begin to take action. Here's how:

 TAKE ACTION

**CHILDISHNESS: MY "FIVE-YEAR-OLD" SELF**
Read each statement and fill in the circle next to the statement that sounds like you, and take note throughout the next few days when you're expressing childish behavior. Mark all that apply:

*HINT: You may be very surprised to see your resemblance to your "five-year-old" self (in thinking, feeling, and behaving) when you encounter even mildly stressful situations.*

- ○ When I cry, I expect people to come to my rescue.
- ○ I believe that if I want something or someone, I should be able to have it or them, whenever I want.
- ○ I've hit or slapped someone in the past, or continue to do this presently.
- ○ When I fear that I might get in trouble, I create little white lies to ensure that others don't catch me.
- ○ If I don't get my way, I make a fuss about it until I do.
- ○ I avoid conflict or uncomfortable situations even if I'm responsible for them.
- ○ I often feel powerless to fix things.
- ○ I don't communicate, even when it's important, in order to "prove a point," gain control, make others upset, or because I'm too scared to have a voice.
- ○ When I'm asked to respond, I often don't know what to say or what the outcome may be, so I hide out and avoid.
- ○ I believe that if I'm asked to communicate, it means I'm being controlled.
- ○ Other childish behaviors I'm expressing: _____

Now that you're more aware of what might trigger you to unconsciously slip into childish behaviors, let's note that this ETB most often follows the thought or belief that you're not getting your needs met.

*In this work of self-knowledge you will actively delineate between your conscious wants and your unmet childhood needs that are still masquerading as wants.*

First, let's look at our true basic human needs: food, water, shelter, and warmth, as well as community, connection, physical touch, and a sense of purpose.[13] You'll most likely never be rid of those fundamental needs in your life; so, I'm not talking about outgrowing these types of needs. As adults, we really don't have any true <u>needs</u> other than these. We may think that we need something outside of this list, or even add to this list saying that it's our "love language" or what we expect from our relationships. In reality, what we think we want in relationships, or out of life, may actually be a childhood need that has carried over to adulthood, directly connected to a traumatic experience where we were afraid or went unnoticed or unheard. In some cases these include things you were told you <u>should</u> need, such as receiving gifts on special days, getting married, having a certain career, or even having children. In this work of self-knowledge, you'll actively delineate between your conscious wants and your unmet childhood needs that are still masquerading as wants.

Wants are preferences based on what you know about your lifestyle—likes and dislikes. When these wants aren't obtained, there's not a severity in disappointment but perhaps a choice to make a new decision next time or recreate your environment so that the specific preference is obtained. A want comes from a place of balance and peace and causes no outburst if it isn't received.

Childhood needs are the attachment to unmet needs from childhood and declaring them as a must-have in your adult life. It's simple to tell if something is a childhood need that you've carried over into adulthood by the way you react to its not being delivered. As an adult, a childhood need can absolutely feel like a survival need when it isn't being met. It can create turmoil inside you, disrupt your relationships, and cause you concern that you aren't loved, and you may compulsively act out due to disappointment.

If you behave as you did when you were a child when you didn't get your way, then it's a childhood need, not a <u>conscious</u> desire/want. A childhood need that was not met will often create a child<u>ish</u> reaction.

TAKE ACTION

**CHILDISHNESS: CHILDHOOD NEEDS**
What needs have followed you into adulthood? Look at some examples of childhood needs here and fill in the circle next to the ones that apply to you. Mark all that apply.

*HINT: Think of the needs that might match your Trauma Filters. They'll be most obvious when you can look at where your ETB of Childishness is expressed due to not getting them met.*

*For example, when do you throw a tantrum? Excessively cry? Believe you've been defeated? Feel shame? Have a sense you're rejected?*

I often need to...
- O  be the most important person in the room.
- O  have most of others' spare time spent with me.
- O  have things done for me.
- O  have everything go my way, or the way I believe it should.
- O  be right.
- O  receive gifts on special days.
- O  receive approval.
- O  receive verbal validation.
- O  explain myself, even without others asking.
- O  be understood, even if it doesn't seem possible that I could explain myself correctly.
- O  have others make decisions for me.
- O  Any other childhood needs coming to mind? _____

How do I begin to outgrow these childish tendencies and childhood needs? If you still have any of these "needs" as an adult, it doesn't mean that you're defective or wrong. You may be unnecessarily held back if they're creating challenges in your life such as disagreements in relationships. To reiterate, these needs were not met in childhood, so you carried them with you within your Intoxicated Identity, and they are now attached to your Trauma-Influenced Self-Beliefs. Can you see that any of your wants are actually childhood needs?

 DO YOU RELATE?

> Robert is about to go meet his mother for dinner. He struggles with what to talk about, what to wear, and how to act, because he wants to appear a certain way for her approval. Wanting her to be happy to see him and to be proud that he's her child is a normal response to seeing one's mother. But would her being disheartened by a choice he's made destroy the evening? The production of preparing for such an event would be much more relaxed if his <u>wants</u> weren't translated by him as <u>needs</u> for approval and attention.

For example, do you need your partner to tell you that you're good-looking every day, or do you even believe them if they say it? Can you know that you're attractive to them without their continuous validation? Once you feel secure in yourself, you won't need external validation. You might have a preference for it, but it won't be a detriment when you don't get it. Then, when you do receive it, it will be an added gift!

When we outgrow childishness, everything positive that happens is a "cherry on top" of our happiness, which we ourselves sustain. Before we move on, let's explore a few healthy ways of working with and transforming certain childhood tendencies.

- When you notice that you're giving someone the "silent treatment": When you feel the need to separate from someone (for reasons other than violence or extreme situations), instead of avoiding or "ghosting them," be clear in your communication that it's a separation and that you'll no longer be speaking to them.

- When you realize you're lying to avoid "getting in trouble": Notice when the fear of getting caught comes into your body or thinking, and choose not to follow through with the behavior that might have gotten you "in trouble" in the first place. Then, coming up with a lie to cover it up will be unnecessary!

Do you see how you <u>will</u> outgrow your childhood needs? I know you will!

## 19

# Escape Jealousy

*Love feels like freedom. Jealousy feels like captivity.*

### Romantic Jealousy

Does your heart drop when you see your partner <u>seemingly</u> interested in another? Have you ever felt the pangs of fear leading to jealousy? This is the belief of loss before the imaginary event has even taken place. Or maybe it's a memory of a real loss or betrayal. Regardless of the reason, it's important to note that jealousy is fear. Specifically, it's the stress chemical we feel when we see, hear, or think something is about to be "taken from us."

To make it simple, romantic jealousy is fear of rejection, not being good enough, not being in control, not being attractive enough, and not being "picked for the team." When you're jealous, you're fearing not being the most special person to this particular person. In your mind, this may seem to guarantee your security with them.

*Jealousy is fear.*

The attack of fear can be sudden, and even masquerade as anger, often coming from a mental obsession, or pattern of thinking, similar to playing a role of detective. For example, you may continuously look for ways that your partner may be dishonest, tricking you, or attracted elsewhere. You find something that validates your self-beliefs that you're unsafe, unattractive, unimportant, or unworthy. You're flooded with intoxicating chemistry and stumble over all things that look like betrayal. You can't see straight as your vision is blurred. You may begin to hyperventilate and your sentences may not be as coherent as they would if you weren't feeling fear and anger.

If you're making a stress chemical, your body believes you're in danger—that you're not secure. When it's in full force, jealousy may even seem as though it could kill you. It will often feel like the end of your world. In some cases is can present as Emotional Belligerence. With a flood of emotions like this, you can expect something destructive to follow. Enter: the Emotionally-Triggered Behavior (ETB) of jealousy.

TAKE ACTION

**ROMANTIC JEALOUSY: FACE MY JEALOUS NATURE**
Describe the last experience you had of expressing romantic jealousy toward someone in your life using these questions.

- What did you say to the other person(s), or how did you behave?

- What did you feel before you behaved jealously?

- How did they respond?

- What were you thinking about yourself?

- If you'd come from a place of security instead of insecurity, what might you have asked them or done instead?

With unjustified jealousy, you're harming your partner. Yet does "justified jealousy" really exist? If there's reason that you can't trust your partner, perhaps a different solution would be to not be with them. For this case, let's imagine that you're not jealous for "rightful" or "justified" reasons regarding your current partner or a close person in your life. When you attack with jealousy, you're harming them. You're creating discord in their day, taking away their sense of freedom and peace, devaluing their character, and not allowing the real them be a part of the relationship. You're holding them captive.

*Jealousy is a sign that you aren't paying attention to your unresolved pains.*

Jealousy is a sign that you aren't paying attention to your unresolved pains. You're sweeping them under the rug, sometimes not even knowing they exist. You're getting into relationships without doing the necessary prerequisite work to become mature. When you start relationships without Emotional Sobriety, you're unconsciously asking another person to fill in for your lack of worthiness and value. You seek meaning in everything they do and say. You likely offer yourself completely to them (physically) in order to leverage more stability and implied commitment from them.

You're giving <u>them</u> the job of changing <u>your</u> Trauma-Influenced Self-Beliefs into the belief in your wholeness. This is <u>your</u> job.

If you're compulsively jealous, consider that you may not yet be cultivated enough to be in an adult romantic relationship. If you don't trust your partner, are you faking a love relationship? If you feel you need to protect yourself, is this the partner for you? If you continue to harm this person, are you the appropriate partner for them?

CONTEMPLATION

**ROMANTIC JEALOUSY: ENTERING WITH EXPECTATIONS**
More often than not, a jealous partner entered into the relationship with the assumption that they were going to get their expectations met. They were going to be the most important thing in their partner's life, no one else would exist to them, and no one would ever be interesting to them. Do you think a relationship that begins this way will fall apart when the newness wears off?

With underlying Trauma Filters from our past ruling our kingdom, we don't stand much of a chance when jealousy rears its head. When you experience jealousy in a romantic relationship, there's a part of you that doesn't feel adequate, and a part of you that doesn't trust that you won't be betrayed, or both. You're so unsure of your worthiness that you may even believe you're not enough for your partner. Jealousy will deny you the possibility to build trust in your partner, create drama, and stifle love and connection. Your filters are denying you the opportunity to notice your self-beliefs in the moment that jealousy strongly flares up. No matter the reason for its invocation, jealousy must be overcome.

*There are people who are jealous because in actuality, they themselves aren't trustworthy.*

I've alluded to another predisposing factor for romantic jealousy: the untrustworthy jealous type. These are the people who are jealous because in actuality, they themselves aren't trustworthy.

It may not be obvious to you, but perhaps you're seeking attention elsewhere, subconsciously looking for a new partner, or self-centered enough to hypocritically deny your partner's freedom, all the while holding onto your own with an iron grip. You may become angry when you think you know the indecent motivation of your partner, even if there's little in reality that resembles error. Whether it's something they're wearing, a place they want to go, a phone call they have to take—all of this is misconstrued into what you <u>think</u> your partner's doing, rather than what they are <u>actually</u> doing. Then, your behaviors become based on what a jealous person would be motivated by. This doesn't mean that you—as an untrustworthy jealous person—don't fear rejection; it means that you aren't okay being the one who's being rejected.

It's important to know that rejection is an illusion based on your expectation that you should be chosen. The choice that someone else makes to not date you is not about you—it's their life choice. The true essence of loving another person is granting them the freedom to live their life's choices.

*The true essence of loving another person is granting them the freedom to live their life's choices.*

Love and partnership are a mutual choice... always. If one doesn't choose the other, then it isn't a personal attack; it's their life choice! And there really isn't a bigger choice than a life partner.

You'll either be inspired by them or held back. You'll care for each other or abuse each other. You'll add light to one another's lives or deplete it. You'll bring a massive amount of energy to one another or give it away to compensate for what may be lacking. If you suffer with the ETB of jealousy, you'll experience this in all your relationships until you consciously shift into a new *you*. Otherwise, you will react in the same ways. You may change partners and find yourself engaging the same jealous behaviors because you haven't become the one who's trusting as well as trustworthy.

Relationship struggles are common when you choose a partner while under the influence of your emotional insobriety. You create a contained environment, sustained by belligerence, until there's a breaking point. ETBs such as jealousy will destroy trust in your relationships. They'll cause separation and pain. They'll deny you the very thing you're attempting to achieve by using them. With jealousy, you're most likely embodying traits including abuse, control, and manipulation, and not offering real love to your partner. Partnership cannot thrive when you're looking only at your own pain. Partners in a strong-willed and committed relationship can make necessary changes together to make it work long-term. When both individuals are respectful of themselves and the other, they can work together to create huge growth without codependency—they become co-partners. Yet, there must be work!

Real love is freedom, choice, and connection. Where there's a forced union, there will never be a flourishing one. When you attain Emotional Sobriety, you won't make decisions based on compulsive and unrealistic attachments. You won't be side-swiped by emotion. You won't be belligerent. You won't be reaching for something that the real you wouldn't choose. EMSO Training will allow you to clearly notice yourself being hypocritical, attention-seeking, feeling embarrassed, or reacting based on your embedded self-beliefs. Your romantic relationships will change, because you will change.

*Relationship struggles are common when we choose a partner while under the influence of our emotional insobriety.*

## Comparison Jealousy

Like romantic jealousy, comparison jealousy is most commonly derived from fear. It flares up when you're brainwashed into believing you're supposed to feel, think, or do things a certain way. You're jealous because you think that others have something that you want. You may think that you want a certain quality that they have, to articulate things the way that they do, or achieve or receive what they do.

Are you jealous when you meet someone who exemplifies your standards—this "supposed to" way of being? Jealousy is a reaction, not reality. It isn't that you truly want to be this other person. You don't really want to do what they're doing, think what they're thinking, or feel what they're feeling. You don't really want to look and speak like them. What you're really seeking is acceptance. This is what you see in them—that they're accepted for how they're being or what they're doing.

Comparison jealousy is also contagious. When you're in a shared context with others, you think you're accessing who they are and getting to know them, but you're actually comparing yourself to them and evaluating where you don't measure up (or where they don't measure up to you). I've seen friends jealous of friends, lovers jealous of their lovers, sisters and brothers jealous of their siblings... it's a very common ETB.

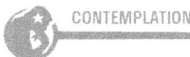
CONTEMPLATION

**COMPARISON JEALOUSY: ME VS. YOU**
Do you ever feel that you're competing or comparing yourself with your partner, friends, or co-workers in an unhealthy way? Do you feel you haven't achieved enough in your life, so you feel threatened by those who seemingly have?

The people with whom you experience the ETB of comparison jealousy are merely an embodiment of your own potential. You can begin to change your jealousy right now first by bringing honest awareness and taking an interest in others rather practicing more jealousy. Know that when you feel the fear that precedes jealousy toward others, it's most likely a signal that you may want to go toward the path they're on. Let that lead you. Perhaps they're humorous, skilled, articulate, assertive, strong, talented, or ambitious. You can befriend them and learn, instead of resenting, shaming, or being angry with them. You can choose to make them your greatest teachers. Ask them questions and find out how you can add value to their life. With EMSO Training, there's no more feeling "small" when you're around them. Instead, get "bigger" and develop your own confidence by listening and achieving more!

Confidence is knowing what you can do based on your past successes. By completing something for yourself, you can begin to gain the confidence needed to overcome your jealous disposition.

*Remember, love is freedom for you, and for everyone else.*
*Jealousy is captivity, for you and for everyone else.*

TAKE ACTION

**COMPARISON JEALOUSY: CHALLENGE MY TRIGGERS**
Think of the last time you were emotionally triggered by a jealous thought toward another person, such as:

- "I want what they have."
- "I want to be like them, and I never will be."
- "They have such a great relationship, and I'll never have that."
- "Why can't I...?"

Write down the qualities you see in this person or in this person's life:

_____

_____

Now imagine that these qualities are describing you or your life. In what ways are you the same? What's one step you can take to embody one quality from this list?

_____

_____

# 20

# Free the Self

*It's self-centeredness that creates separation, angst, and pain.*

**Self-Centeredness**

After our Early-Age Trauma, we're left to heal with no understanding about what happened or why, and usually with no tools to heal.

We realize that something has happened <u>to</u> us and we believe, possibly subconsciously, <u>because</u> of us, and we can't reason through it. Most of us weren't taught the fundamentals of healing and certainly not ways to facilitate feeling our emotions through communication. So, after trauma we're alone with the memories (biochemical and beliefs) of our trauma within us.

Neuroscientific research suggests that our subconscious mind doesn't know the difference between memory and reality.[14] If this is true, our feelings and memories may serve as repetitive traumas. We know that along with a memory of a stressful experience, we'll make and feel the same chemistry we did at the time of the trauma, even if it's been days, years, or decades since the event. We can sometimes feel it as if it were the first time. As you learned in Chapter 10—"Biochemical Addiction to PANE"—because of this chemistry being made over and over again, we become addicted to the biochemistry ignited during our traumatic experience.

Let's go back for a moment to the initial trauma. Once the trauma is experienced, we often retreat and hide, confining ourselves within the safety of our own self. This is where our Trauma-Influenced Self-Beliefs about the incident and Trauma Filters are affixed. This is where we first become a "victim"—seemingly trapped and alone, we experience the ETB of self-centeredness.

The word "self-centered" seems to have a bad reputation. People often react defensively to being characterized as self-centered due to the fact that they believe they're being called "selfish." To be clear, self-centeredness is not the same as selfishness.

Let's look at the difference:

DEFINITIONS

**SELFISHNESS:** when you believe that most things are <u>for</u> you.
**SELF-CENTEREDNESS:** when you believe that most things are <u>about</u> you.

When everything is <u>about</u> you, you create suffering. When you experience the ETB of self-centeredness, you wonder what everyone else is thinking about you, how you appear to them, and what they say about you. Self-centeredness is what pushes you to be dishonest in order to present yourself a certain way once you decide what everyone else would like you to be. When you're self-centered, you cannot be aware of what's <u>truly</u> happening within or around you because you're hiding behind your Trauma Filters.

Self-centeredness requires constant care and maintenance even though you're rarely aware that it even exists in your life. Self-centeredness is another way to describe your relationship with what is often referred to as your "ego mind." Much of your energy is used to keep up with its imaginary needs. Are you constantly thinking of who you need to be? You may be using up much of your creative energy making sure others are aware of you, thereby having little leftover for self-awareness. This self-centeredness handcuffs you out of <u>choosing</u> your own thoughts, feelings, and behaviors, and participating genuinely in your life. You become a caricature of someone else—someone you think you're supposed to present to the world, all while the real you remains buried beneath the surface.

The "dirty work" of your insobriety happens inside of self-centeredness, with the ego reminding you to be on the watch in preparation of your worst fears. You'll mistranslate the words of others and create more chaos—either matching your anxiety or protecting yourself. It reminds you to think for others when you choose not to take them at face value. It encourages you to control everything that may not go your way.

It's also where you have pre-planned conceptions about how others should behave around you—what they should say and what they should think. It stirs your frustration and impatience and reminds you that everything should be done your way, on your timeline, and with your level of accuracy. More important, it helps "prove" your Trauma-Influenced Self-Beliefs.

*The ego reminds you that everything should be done your way, on your timeline, and with your level of accuracy.*

Because self-centeredness is an unconscious "wall," it's hidden even to the person behind it—you. Your ego will sing inside your mind in a little sweet tempting voice: "Without me, you'll die. You'll never survive. You'll be hurt. Don't trust them. Don't do that or say that because then they'll do this or think this about you!" It's one-sided inside your wall of self-centeredness—an uninterrupted, militant planning of how your life will turn out. It uses strategic action to control outcomes and repeated patterns of thought that keep you out of the real world happening both inside and outside of you.

 **TAKE ACTION**

**SELF-CENTEREDNESS: LOOKING CLEARLY AROUND ME**
Review your day today. Write down 5 moments when you were self-centered.

When were you attention-seeking?

When did you easily take offense?

When did you experience concern that others were talking about you or thinking badly of you?

**When did you interpret others' actions or words to mean something about you?**

**If none of this occurred for you today, choose a recent experience where you were self-centered and describe it here:**

1. _____

2. _____

3. _____

4. _____

5. _____

Like every ETB, being self-centered doesn't make you a bad person; it simply means you're in a stifled place. You're in what I call the "center of self," as opposed to the "freedom of self." I think of them as rooms or spaces. When you're stuck in the center of self, you're self-absorbed, obsessed with how you appear, what others think of you, who's judging you, and you're filtering your experiences through these insecurities. You're trapped, hurt, and hiding. In this isolated space, you're attempting to heal your confusion and PANEs without the appropriate tools or support to do so. Since you can't actually heal while in the center of self, you continue the same behaviors again and again, expecting a new outcome.

In the space of freedom of self, you're without self-absorption, self-consciousness and self-deprecation. You aren't holding expectations of others, nor ascribing to to your self-beliefs resulting from trauma. You've rid your body of its habitual creation of PANE. You've done the work, emotionally speaking, to be able to walk safely and confidently through the world without hiding and hurting. You're open, present, and truly free. The following two Take Actions require that you first listen to a recorded visualization. Visit your member page, or read them to yourself from the written version provided.

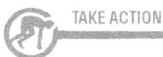

TAKE ACTION

### HOUSE OF MIRRORS VISUALIZATION (Part 1)
Imagine you're inside a very small room. You travel everywhere you'd normally go in life while remaining contained within this room. It's well-lit, and there's nothing around you but mirrors. The mirrored walls are transparent so you can still see where you're going, and you can interact with other people. But as you're walking, working, talking, and even resting, you always see yourself <u>first</u> in these mirrors. Your first thoughts, feelings, and concerns are about you. You assume that everyone else looking through the mirrored walls also sees you the way that you're seeing you.

Now revisit your entire day yesterday, beginning when you first woke up... brushed your teeth, went to the bathroom, ate breakfast... each activity until you lay your head back on your pillow that night... the entire time stuck in your house of mirrors.

### SELF-CENTEREDNESS: CENTER OF SELF
Recall that while you were inside your house of mirrors, you likely experienced a variety of thoughts, feelings, and behaviors. When you imagined being trapped inside that room for the entire day, which of the following occurred? Mark all that apply:

- ○ I felt afraid and wanted to "make it stop!"
- ○ I started judging what was right and wrong about myself.
- ○ I imagined a worst-case scenario.
- ○ It felt secure... "I know best and don't trust anyone anyway!"
- ○ I was easily offended.
- ○ I felt alone and realized I was isolated from everyone.
- ○ I felt sad.
- ○ I was quick to anger at various moments.
- ○ I envied the people outside the room.
- ○ I felt self-conscious about what others might be seeing.
- ○ I kept myself distracted by staying busy to avoid feeling.
- ○ I couldn't give genuine attention to anyone or anything outside of the room.
- ○ I wanted payback from someone.
- ○ I felt like a victim and blamed someone— "You did this to me!" or "This is your fault!" or "Can't you see me?!"
- ○ I couldn't be vulnerable or let my guard down.
- ○ I was irritated.
- ○ Other: _____

It may sound ugly, but realize that <u>all</u> of us have some aspect of the ETB of self-centeredness. It needs to be recognized, and we need to learn how to climb out of it so that we're rarely, if ever, stuck there again. And when we <u>do</u> find ourselves back in the house of mirrors, we don't linger.

**TAKE ACTION**

**HOUSE OF MIRRORS VISUALIZATION (Part 2)**
Now imagine you're outside on a beautiful day. Think of the type of weather and a setting you most enjoy, and go there now in your mind.

A door appears within your Center of Self and you're able to walk out of the tiny, mirrored room and into this place. Once outside, you see the world more clearly. The words of others aren't clouded over by your own thoughts and filtered interpretations. The view of the scenery is more distinct and attractive. You appreciate the smells, sounds, and air. You have no fear, anxiety, or compulsive reactions to anything. Your heart feels like it's grown inside your chest, and your mind is quiet. There are no stories being told about who does or doesn't like you, or about what you did or the shame you feel. You have no anger heating up your room to the point of explosion. You're aware of your surroundings because there's nothing blocking your view. There are no distractions keeping you from connecting to your source of power. You feel peace. You're finally free.

Now revisit yesterday's activities, thoughts, and behaviors, imagining that you were <u>outside</u> your house of mirrors for the entire day in this open and spacious place.

**SELF-CENTEREDNESS: FREEDOM OF SELF**
When you explored life <u>outside</u> your house of mirrors, you likely experienced a different set of thoughts, feelings, and behaviors.

When you imagined being in your beautiful place for the entire day, which of the following occurred? Mark all that apply:

- ○ I laughed at my "mistakes."
- ○ I didn't worry about others' "mistakes."
- ○ I related with others.
- ○ I felt confident but not cocky.
- ○ I didn't compare myself to others.
- ○ I was open to sharing time and space with others—"You can come to me and I can see you clearly," or "My space is yours."

- ○ I found ways to help others.
- ○ I felt happy.
- ○ I wasn't guarded or "needing space."
- ○ I didn't really have any problems.
- ○ I shared myself vulnerably.
- ○ I was relaxed.
- ○ If I did feel something (fear, sadness, anger, etc.), it didn't last long before I came back to a sense of freedom.
- ○ Other: _____

Self-centeredness makes us attempt to control and predict outcomes to keep us safe. This ETB supports us in keeping the people we think we most need around us, even if they're miserable; or let's face it, even if we ourselves are miserable! Maintaining the status quo seems to be what makes us feel safe; and because we must keep people in our lives and keep control of those who might get away, we may play a specific role to manage their perception of us. We lie to make them want to be near us. We tell them what they want to hear or what we think they should want to hear based on our assumptions. We'll be different people, play different roles, and act different parts out in front of all different kinds of individuals. This "role-playing" can become a huge problem over time because it means we aren't living with integrity, which means we're lacking a real identity. We're in our Intoxicated Identity.

**COACHING MOMENT**

I know that I'm repetitive! This is intentional. We learn through repetition not only with our practices, but with our education. I'm continuing to repeat the biggest contributors of emotional insobriety to make sure that this becomes basic knowledge for you and is so recognizable in your daily life that you'll never miss the opportunity to change it. I intend for all Emotional Sobriety students to know and practice EMSO Training so well that they couldn't possibly keep it to themselves, and thereby become an inspiration for others!

In most of the cases I've witnessed, when we're chronically suffering with emotional challenges, we're in self-centeredness. If our personality and behaviors exist <u>primarily</u> for the control and management of others, we aren't coming from a place of personal power and confidence. We're coming from a place of falseness, fear, and lack. Because self-centeredness keeps us from cultivating our own identity, it also keeps us from knowing real, loving relationships. Self-centeredness creates a strong pull toward merely <u>surviving</u>, which is keeping us from freely <u>living</u> as our real selves.

*When we're chronically suffering with emotional challenges, we're in self-centeredness.*

When you're focused on what everyone else is doing <u>to</u> you—the harms you think you're experiencing, the maintenance of others' perceptions of you, and the drama you create and allow in your life—you have much less capacity to be useful.

Our level of usefulness is a large contributor to our happiness. When we're feeling useful, we have a purpose. We're connected and cooperative. When we contribute to others, to life, or to our community, we have a greater level of purpose. Since we're more useful when we're in the Freedom of Self, our level of contribution serves a good gauge of our ETB of self-centeredness.

 CONTEMPLATION

**MY USEFULNESS**
Examine your day yesterday, as well as a typical day in your life, and ask yourself: "How useful was I to the world around me? How happy and satisfied do I feel with my contribution to life?" I'm not talking about how clean the house is or how much money you made. I'm asking you to consider, "How did I connect with others in the most genuine way? Did I show up and cooperate with presence, or did my Trauma Filters dictate how I behaved?"

If you're unhappy or dissatisfied in your life, you're most likely suffering in self-centeredness, and therefore, not reaching the potential of your incredible usefulness. When self-centeredness is eliminated, you instantly become more useful, as you aren't wasting energy on protecting yourself or managing others.

When you exit the Center of Self and enter the Freedom of Self, you'll become more emotionally sober—instantly.

 **COACHING MOMENT**

> What if that thing that bothered you so much wasn't even about you? Do you sense that if you were rid of the habits of fear, anxiety, blame, and constant thinking about how to control others and your life, that you may be more open, present, and genuine? And by experiencing all of life without this barrier, can you see that you would have more opportunity for remarkable happiness?

## Practice Rep #1: "Get Over Yourself"

By completing the Take Actions thus far, you've begun the essential process of exiting your Center of Self, which allows you to live in the Freedom of Self. But how do you continue to practice this? You need to "get over yourself!" Has anyone ever said this to you? It's a statement that most would consider a criticism or a put-down. Previous to reframing it, I never felt good hearing this. When we think about the statement from an EMSO Training perspective, it's actually a simple and realistic truth. In order to change any part of ourselves, our life or our problems, we must get <u>over</u> ourselves for a better view.

In other words, we must go <u>above</u> ourselves—outside ourselves—and look down from a "balcony." We go up—beyond our problems—and look at the parts of our personality that sustain those problems. We must get over ourselves to remove the version of us that created those behaviors which cause our suffering. We must remove ourselves from the mirrored room containing our self-beliefs and filters.

When I'm suffering, frustrated, or in pain, I know that I'm in the Center of Self. When I become aware of this, I get over myself and the problems disappear. "Get over yourself" is a primary practice rep that I teach throughout EMSO Training. You're going to get over yourself. You'll get over your hindering beliefs, frustrations, fears, and guilt. You'll get over your expectations of others and your excessive needs and judgments. You'll attempt to get over the self and the installed filters and beliefs that brought you here. This is where the power of this transformative prerequisite work lies. It's a process that requires action to help you look in, around, through, and finally <u>over</u> yourself. When you accomplish this, your ears and heart will prepare you for new teachings, and your courage will make you the benefactor of a blissful life.

*In EMSO Training you're going to "get over yourself."*

Going forward, when you hear "get over yourself," this is what I mean: you don't need sympathy or attention for your problems—you go above the problem and see that you're the solution. You rise above yourself, your filters, and your dishonesty, and you rise above all of your problems for a better view.

When you're constantly attempting to get others to love you, see you, understand you, or give you attention, it takes most of your day. When you stack those days together, it may use up an entire lifetime. If you're easily offended or sensitive to the actions or inactions of others, then you're not yet in the Freedom of Self.

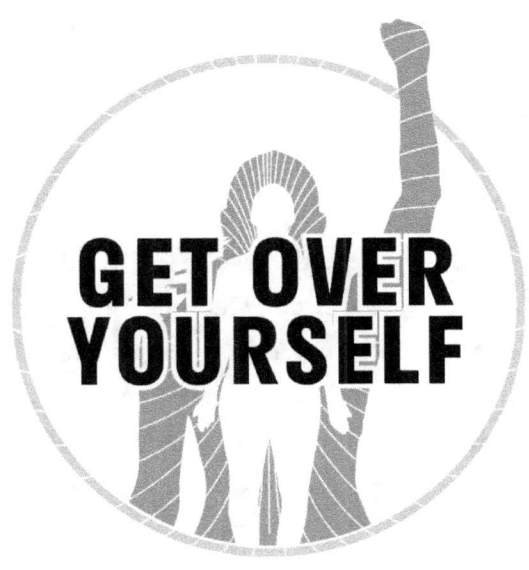

# 21

# Release the Critic

*Nothing positive happens with a closed heart.*

Judgment is an interpretation that follows a preconceived assumption leading to strong negative emotions. This makes it an Emotionally-Triggered Behavior (ETB). A good rule is that judgments contain Predominant Accompany Negative Emotions (PANEs). Judgment is brought to the surface when we have thoughts, beliefs, or behaviors that are different from another person's, and we disapprove of them. A judgment is apparent when we're hypercritical of others, lack allowance for another point of view, feel angry, disgusted, intolerant, or even afraid when someone else thinks, feels, or chooses differently from how we would.

*Judgments contain PANEs.*

So, what brings about these emotions which lead to judgment? You've been influenced by your society, your family, and your friendships for your entire life. You've been a part of a circle of certain beliefs and prejudices that fall naturally into your psyche. You may be under the impression that your way is not only the right way, but the only way. And you react based only on what you know.

Judgment is an ETB based on self-righteous beliefs, self-belief preservation, or self-importance. It happens when you assume another's life should match what you would choose for your own. Again, you may become flooded with emotion, bringing judgment with it. Conversely, an observation (without judgment) is shared without emotion. This means you simply observe what's actually happening without any personal emotional reaction to it.

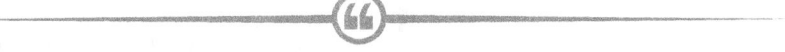

*An observation (without judgment) is shared without emotion.*

For example, a judgment may look like: "I don't trust/like my uncle's new girlfriend because she's [insert race here]. When I see them, I feel scared and anxious, and think I need to be protected based on my past history with someone who looks like them." Whereas an observation would be: "My uncle's new girlfriend is of _____ descent." It's an unemotional observation, not a quality or value-assessment. Saying what someone's race is isn't racism; it's observation. You're not judging them based on their race, you're simply observing what their heritage is and noting that.

Just as judgment can harm those you are judging, judgment can create suffering within the judge as well. To be a judge is to close off your heart and deny yourself and others the opportunity for love. Your judgment is caused by your assumption that your way is the right way, your adamancy on how something should turn out, or your expectation that someone should behave a certain way or believe what you believe. I've seen that some judgmental suffering comes from lack of faith in what you live by—when there's something or someone outside of you that lives in a different way than you do, and it creates a shock to your sense of normalcy.

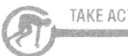 TAKE ACTION

**JUDGMENTALISM: MEET MY INNER CRITIC**
Take a moment to review the list of Common Traits of an Emotionally Sober Person (found on page 46) regarding who you want to become.

List those that you circled:

Answer each of these questions about yourself and see if you get to meet the judge within you.

- When you consider who you want to become, do any inner criticisms come up?

- What are your top three "I can't…" stories when you consider adding these traits to your life?

- Notice when you're judging yourself and write it here (e.g., you caught yourself judging others 15 times today, so you start judging yourself for judging them!)

 TAKE ACTION

**JUDGMENTALISM: DIFFERENT FROM ME**
Think of someone in your life who acts, believes, or thinks differently from you. Then answer these questions:

- What do you feel in your body (e.g., tension, numbness, burning, etc.)?

- What PANEs (emotions) do you feel?

- How do you typically behave around them (ETBs)?

With the ETB of judgmentalism, you feel run over by automatic, extreme emotions—becoming offended, angry, irritated, or hateful, all of which are invading and painful. Via these emotions, you might act out aggressively—whether passive or outwardly—and attempt to right the "wrong" of what's in front of you. You attempt to punish the person you're judging by manipulating them. You may do this to ensure they feel what you're feeling, question their own beliefs, feel shame, or even experience the rejection that you perceive you're experiencing due to their living differently.

We're all people, but we have different viewpoints because we're each looking at the world from unique perspectives—literal different points of view. We're each looking at the world from our own individual set of eyes. We have different parents. We live in different households. We practice different religions. We have different family habits. We have different styles of communicating. We have different experiences in love and relationships. We eat different foods. What we see everyday is either a different subject or from a different angle. Simply think about all the differences... even in the variety of what we read, what we witness, what we value, what we've been taught, and what languages we speak! Every single person has had a very different life... even those who live within the same community, family, or even two people in the same relationship. There may be some overlap in interests, experiences, feelings, spiritual beliefs, or physical attributes, but we're each truly vastly different.

Initially, when you learn to judge, it's typically related to judging the more obvious, radical differences. Later, you may judge the subtle differences more. For example, some religions have nearly identical theories and traditions but may have one or two elements that differentiate them. There may be offense taken or even an urge to push someone to follow your religion. "You're so close to believing what I believe, why don't you just get all the way on board?" Conversely, it may be easier to separate and respect the religious beliefs of someone who's vastly different than yours, even in some cases exclaiming, "Well, they haven't yet been exposed to the truth, so it's not their fault."

You're still believing that your way is better, or the "right" way. For example, if you've ever argued loudly, shunned, or acted in an unloving way toward someone for not believing the same religion as you, you may think you're defending your God. If you sense yourself closely the next time this occurs, you'll realize your Emotional Belligerence is ruling your behaviors as you defend your long-term beliefs. Of all the religions I've studied, I've never sensed a God that needs defending. Our egos, however, are a different story! As you learned in Chapter 17—"Remove (De)Fences"—our egos are constantly serving as our defenders.

Intolerance of a religious or lifestyle preference, racism, sexism, ageism, and the like are all forms of judgment, which I think of as:

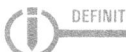

DEFINITION

**EXCLUSIONARY CRITICISM:** any 'ism or social phobia; to deny opportunity to someone based on race or color, religion or creed, gender or lifestyle preference; judgments that exclude other people due to different beliefs, statuses, cultures, or being born the "wrong kind of person."

Exclusionary criticism is lumping an entire group of people into a classification due to what you've learned or experienced from individuals or smaller groups of this same variety.

Sexism is another form of exclusionary criticism worth exploring due to its prevalence in most cultures—"Men should be this way and women that way." All genders are judged in some respect. When we're still brewing the emotions of learned righteousness, anywhere there's contrast there will be judgment.

*When we're still brewing the emotions of learned righteousness, anywhere there's contrast there will be judgment.*

You'll fight to protect your beliefs and values without considering the other person as an individual who also has reasons for believing and valuing what they do. Making space for each other to be ourselves takes the charge out of any situation, and everyone can think more clearly without the drunken effects of our judgment-causing emotions.

Being hyper-critical of others is quite popular, but so is criticism of the self. You may judge yourself for not being who you "should be by now." Perhaps you hear familiar voices in your head, such as "Why aren't you married yet?" "How many times have you been divorced?" "When are you having kids?" "You should lose some weight." "You're just not good at making friends." You may saturate yourself with the judgments of others. You may judge yourself as you assume others are judging you. You may judge yourself as you assume others are judging others. Or, you may judge yourself as you judge others.

The voices you hear in your head judging yourself are the voices you then mimic in your judgment of others. This creates a sense of control. This is what I've termed:

DEFINITION

**VACUUM CRITICISM:** this form of judgment appears as "controlling" your environment by continuously and disrespectfully pointing out flaws in the environment.

Vacuum criticism is usually done in hushed or passive tones. You learn this by watching and experiencing it, and thus it becomes a skill. Another learned skill is what I refer to as:

DEFINITION

**LOUD CRITICISM:** an outward declaration of your judgments.

Loud criticism is demonstrated by judging yourself or judging others elicit the same emotion and sometimes even the same behaviors. Thus, it's essential to continue deeply exploring where self-criticism as well as judgment of others and of outside circumstances is ruling your life.

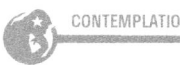

CONTEMPLATION

**AM I CRITICAL?**
Where in your past or present have you been guided to be intolerant of any group specifically? When, if at all, have you personally felt destructive emotional reactions when talking to, or seeing someone of a different group or lifestyle? Can you see where it created a barrier between you and someone else? Where have you passively criticized others? Where have you been loud with your criticism? Where have you been criticizing or judging yourself?

Think about what it would mean to live your own life—to be free. You start by freeing everyone else. Like escaping jealousy, releasing the critic begins when faced with someone thinking, believing, or behaving differently than you would, you allow them to be freely themselves. If they ask for any advice, opinion, or education on how you do things, you can freely give it to them, without expecting them to jump on board with you. With no expectations of another and acknowledging their freedom, you're now without the extreme emotions that create judgment.

An effective way to sober up, emotionally speaking, is to approach everything with neutrality. Not having a strong emotional response makes you a much better listener who makes clearer decisions. This is why we do this training! When you're not bombarded by homemade biochemicals that lead to judgment, you can come from a more open and genuine place, allowing for more usefulness, opportunity, and love. For everyone.

In the same way, you'll continue to have moments of being defensive, acting childishly, and expressing jealousy, and you'll find yourself inside your house of mirrors at some point. You'll also likely judge someone again. You haven't yet managed the biochemicals in your body. So, what will you do in the meantime?

Try this: Observe the judge within. When you initially begin to look at all of your areas of judgment, you may be stunned that you've spent so much of your internal time and energy attempting to observe while making assumptions or judgments about others or their lifestyles.

TAKE ACTION

### JUDGMENTALISM: OBSERVE THE JUDGE

This is an exercise of both self-observation and journaling.

How often are you analyzing others with feelings of resentment, disgust, anger, or even embarrassment on their behalf?

At this point, this exercise is for you to only observe <u>yourself</u> and <u>your</u> habits in thinking and judging—not to share your judgments with the people you're judging.

Share the inner workings of your thought patterns, and you'll begin to look at yourself from different angles.

- Check your inner dialogue and feelings that arise when you witness another living different from how you would. Observe yourself and what you're noticing around your habit of judgment. Share how you feel when you're judging.

- Recognize what you feel when you're judging versus when you're not. How much freer do you feel when you're coming from an open mind versus a judging mind?

- Acknowledge when you've been judged in the past and how that felt. What do you wish the other person would have noticed about your choices? How do you wish they would have responded to you?

Remember, you <u>re</u>act based only on what you know. Once you know differently, you realize that you have a choice to change. This will grant you back so much energy!

22

# Get Real

*We're free to lie, but when we lie we're never free.*

In our human anatomy, we have a spinal column. Within this column, our spinal cord is housed and sends information between the body and the brain, and back again. In order for these messages to flow freely, there must be space for these structural cords to run through. However, there are cases where these spaces may become intruded upon. You can see this decrease in space occur in injuries such as disc herniations ("slipped discs") in the spine, or even tumors or arthritis, all of which occupy space in an area that needs to remain open. For this reason, these structural abnormalities are called space-occupying lesions. They're lesions or malformations that take up space, block blood flow, disrupt nerve impulses, and decrease accuracy of neurological information. In this chapter, we'll discuss the common Emotionally-Triggered Behavior (ETB) of dishonesty. I consider lies to be "space-occupying lesions" in your life.

Space is required for something to be received, put within, or even to simply create something new. This applies to anything. Space allows for endless opportunity. If space provides potential, then lies are in the way of this potential. In addition to our space, they're also taking up our energy, merely by requiring it to keep them. We're continuously—and sometimes unconsciously—juggling our dishonest past and present in order to maintain a status quo in our lives. They get in the way of our ability to pay attention and to receive messages and epiphanies, and they block our connection to others.

A lie is a sign that we aren't completely satisfied with who we've become or our current reality. This is predominantly why we lie. Maybe we're unsure of what and how to say something, or we so desperately want our lie to be true that we think just saying it will make it true. We cannot fully embrace who we are, because we aren't yet in touch with our real self.

*A lie is a sign that we aren't completely satisfied with who we've become or our current reality.*

Oftentimes when working with students and talking to friends I hear, "I don't lie," or "I don't lie to deliberately trick people." When people are courageous enough to realize and admit that they do lie, they tell me that they're sometimes a little dishonest in order to protect others' feelings or manage their perceptions, or that they don't even know the truth themselves. They're attempting to control outcomes and believe that by saying things that aren't true, other people will think more of them or they'll get their way.

Most people who lie daily do so compulsively—not living from a real foundation of truth. They're acting in the "movie" of their lives, and their "lines" and tendencies are of the utmost importance to them. Lies are proof of either self-ignorance (not having an individual identity) or deliberate trickery of others (manipulation/control).

If you react with the ETB of dishonesty, you likely maintain the people in your life with falsities in order to keep things the way you'd like to keep them. You're persuaded by your Intoxicated Identity to outwardly project an imaginary perception of something you actually lack or have yet to develop. You inflate your personality. Or perhaps you're in relationships and lie about seemingly mundane things to not engage an argument. You're still lying.

Correspondingly, when you lie, you deny others their rights within the context of your relationship. Those to whom you lie are stripped of their opportunity to know you, and to respond realistically to what you are in their lives. For example, lying about your feelings in a romantic relationship denies your partner the chance to decide if he/she wants to remain in the relationship. Or, if you're addicted to drugs or another secondary dependency and haven't shared the reality of your addiction with your partner, then you deny them the opportunity to really know who you're being, and who they're with. Similar to lying about <u>who</u> you're being, lying about <u>what</u> you like or dislike to make someone else more attracted to you is denying them the reality of the relationship.

*Those to whom you lie are stripped of their opportunity to know you, and to respond realistically to what you are in their life.*

Dishonesty strips the other person of knowing the real you and therefore denies them the opportunity to decide if you're the one he/she wants to spend their time with. There can be no real relationship where there are lies, because lies are fake. It's surprising how much of others' time you may be wasting without any consideration of them and their lives, just to play out a charade and get them to do what you <u>think</u> you want them to do.

As children, you weren't taught to be honest; you were simply inherently honest. You were taught to lie. To teach yourself to be honest again you must first observe where you lie. Now is a great time to further incorporate the Self-Honesty Checkpoint practice. Mark your "X" below on the line again—somewhere between lie and truth. Feel free to keep this image in your mind and do this practice internally with an imaginary meter before each Take Action:

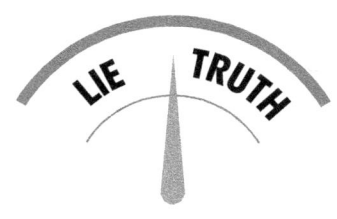

### TAKE ACTION

**DISHONESTY: UNCOVER MY UNCONSCIOUS LIES**

For the entire day tomorrow, take this book or the companion journal with you, or use a voice memo or note in your phone and write down each time you lie to someone else, think about lying, or lie to yourself. Then, respond to these inquiries:

- How might you presently be wasting someone else's time by telling them what you think they want to hear, rather than the truth?

- When have you done so in the past?

- Write about an experience when you were dishonest to make it seem to others that you were more attractive/kind/special:

- What may you be lying about in order to "not get in trouble?":

---

*There can be no real relationship where there are lies.*

I can remember lying about things that didn't really seem to matter to me at the time. Upon reflection, I now know that it surely mattered to the person whose time I was wasting! I would lie to keep my real self further and further hidden away, and to manage other people's perceptions of me. I didn't really know who I was, or wasn't. Most of the time, I wouldn't have even known I was lying, or even thought of the truth behind the lie at the time of telling it. I believe it was learning to tell small lies at a young age that became a habitual character defect into my young adulthood. I'd like to reiterate that half-truths, white lies, and small lies, are still lies. When you add them all up, you have an entire life created of falseness.

What would your life look like after obtaining the rare and special skill of total and complete honesty? I encourage you to do so. Being real is the only way you can be truly free. In fact, if you're struggling with internal angst like stomach aches, anxiety, or overwhelm, there are most likely areas of your life within which you're being dishonest with yourself, others, or both. You may not realize it, but dishonesty is most often the primary culprit for your suffering. And as we know, where you find a lack of integrity, you'll almost always find the Intoxicated Identity of someone who's emotionally unsober.

When we find both the courage and capacity to remove the lies, to eradicate the ETB of dishonesty, we reopen the space that this lesion occupied for more creative endeavors! We can speak, live, and be free.

*Half-truths, white lies, or small lies are still lies. And eventually you have an entire life created of falseness.*

### Practice Rep #2: Get Real

How do we know when we're lying, if it's not conscious? How do we know what lies we've told in the past, or are still telling? Early on in my effort to achieve Emotional Sobriety, I had an honest friend who said that I would be better off if I just focused on being real. They'd say, "Just be real, I just want to see the real you." I defensively conveyed that I was always real. After those conversations, I would isolate and ask myself, "What did they mean by being real?"

Presently—many, many years into my Emotional Sobriety—I thankfully have the clarity to share exactly what's meant by being "real." This is something I wish I'd been taught this simply back then.

Let's do what I call "get real."

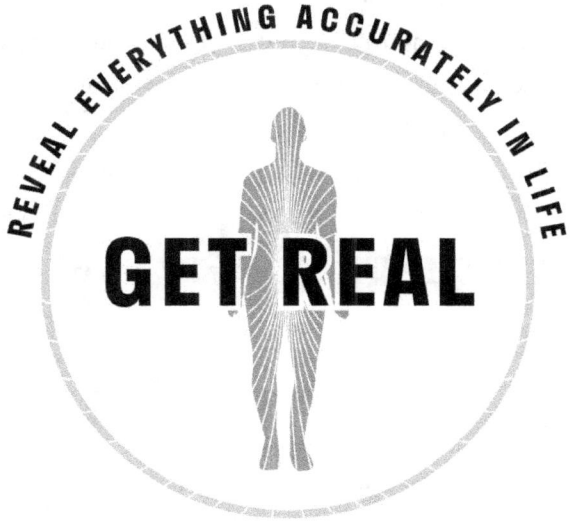

Being honest means revealing everything accurately in life... yes, even if it isn't what you'd like to be true. I couldn't be R.E.A.L. earlier in my life because I didn't want most of what was true at the time to be true. I got into a very bad habit of telling lies and created a false life. I planted untruths in my life and wondered why my harvest tasted so bitter and rotten.

Getting real is where the love is. As one of my dearest friends so gracefully puts it: "Lies and love cannot co-exist." If you're lying, don't expect to feel love. Love and honesty create the sweetest harvest of life.

I now know that to be real means that in any situation or when asked a question, I can take a moment and ask myself honestly and realistically: What is actually existing in this moment (not imagined)? What are my genuine feelings (not the feelings I think I'm supposed to be feeling)? What am I actually intending/my actual motivation (not what I wish I were intending)? What is the accuracy of this (not something I'm making up to fit my agenda)?

Self-honesty is the first step in ridding your whole life of the ETB of dishonesty. A valuable assist in finding your honesty is learning to get in touch with why you have lied or are currently lying, which we explored in great depth in the Take Action "Reasons for My ETBs" in Chapter 15. Coming up soon, you'll learn about Checking Motive and get even more specific about your unique "why's" behind all of your ETBs. What was your motivation behind this lie? Discovering this motive will teach you to talk to yourself more honestly and vulnerably. It will begin the process of honest thinking and will eventually work its way to the outside world. You'll develop honesty within yourself and then once you learn to trust in yourself, you can be honest with those around you.

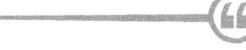

*Self-honesty is the first step in ridding your whole life of the ETB of dishonesty.*

Getting real is also about witnessing what's really being spoken, felt, or experienced. It isn't about what you'd <u>like</u> it to be or what you think it <u>should</u> be. It isn't about what the person in front of you wants it to be or how you think they want it to be. It isn't about anything else but what is actually occurring, or has really occurred.

These are new ways of being that will be so deeply embedded in your psyche that you won't be able to go back to your old habits. In this case, we look at the habituated ETB of dishonesty and how to practice transforming it by getting real.

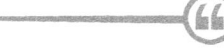

*When you're emotionally sober, what's real will be the only thing that interests you.*

To lie, or to not be real, is to forget all the power you have. If you're lying to get what you want as an adult, you haven't established yourself into adulthood. You most likely haven't chosen your own identity or made contact with your own courage and self-reliance, and your emotional stamina is simply not yet strong enough. Lying because you want the lie to be the truth doesn't make it real or validate that lie. Take action and create what I like to call a R.E.A.Life, and you'll no longer be tempted to lie. When you're emotionally sober, what's real will be the only thing that interests you.

If you're lying in your life, or stuck in a pattern of displaying ETBs, know that it's merely something that you once learned, repeated, perfected, and made a skill. All the things you've learned can be replaced with a new skill of your choosing. If there's something you no longer wish to have in your reality, such as dishonesty, you can learn something else, another behavior in its place. You can repeat that new behavior, honesty, until it becomes a new skill. Practice it. Then you'll have a new way of being!

DO YOU RELATE?

**UNREALITY**: James is on his way to meet his friend, Greg, for a football game. Janet, his wife, asks him where he's going. He tells her, and she responds with a grimace of disdain and shaming. James, now flooded with the emotion of fear, says, "I was thinking you'd be busy tonight, and, uh... it's Greg's birthday." Janet, now feeling relief, exclaims, "Oh, I'm home tonight, and I wanted to watch our show together." James now calls Greg and thinks he has to lie again. "My wife has a really bad headache, so I'm going to stay in and help her out. Might have to go to the ER if it doesn't let up, I'll keep you posted." Or he may make some crass comment about how his wife is being needy (as usual) and he has to stay in.

James lied first to Janet about it being Greg's birthday (due to the PANE of fear and a self-belief of "I don't have a choice") in order to spare the pangs of living with an angry and hurt wife, which then means likely living for the next week or more in an "unsafe environment." He then lies to Greg (due to the PANE of embarrassment and self-belief again of "I don't have a choice"), covering up his true identity and desire. Now, he lugs the lies and the emotional shame around for both people he has lied to. Through this, he's also lying to himself.

**REALITY**: Instead of lying, James could tell his wife: "Janet, I really want some time with my friend tonight... to take some pressure off from work, I'd like to laugh with my buddy." Or he could call his friend and say: "Hey, Greg, I decided that I'm going to spend my evening with Janet. I would like some time with you next weekend if you're available."

Do you see how simple this can be? Simply say what's <u>real</u>. James can choose whatever he desires and tell the truth about it. Lies are in place as excuses, fears of loss, fears of change, or entanglements of other lies. Dishonesty clearly is an ETB. We're triggered to lie via our ego's survival and our biochemistry. In this case, James is thinking for both his wife and his friend, deciding what it is he thinks they want or need to hear, as well as what their reaction would be to his real truth and feelings.

You may be wondering if by telling the truth, you're then stuck with the reaction you were trying to avoid—the anger or the embarrassment? Simply keep telling the truth and feeling what you're feeling. That's the real you.

 TAKE ACTION

**DISHONESTY: REALITY CHECKPOINTS**
To grow your honesty muscle, practice asking the following throughout your day tomorrow: What's real in this moment? (Am I revealing everything accurately in life <u>right</u> <u>now</u>?). To deepen this practice, try pausing three times (perhaps after each meal) and asking yourself these four questions honestly, realistically, and slowly:

| REALITY CHECKPOINTS | | | |
| --- | --- | --- | --- |
| | MORNING | AFTERNOON | EVENING |
| What's <u>actually</u> happening in this moment? (not imagined) | | | |
| What are my <u>genuine</u> feelings? (not the feelings I think I'm supposed to be feeling) | | | |
| What am I <u>actually</u> intending? (not what I wish I were intending) | | | |
| What's the <u>accuracy</u> of this? (not something I'm making up to fit my agenda) | | | |

## 23

## Remove the Reach

*Secondary addiction is the manifestation
of a different issue altogether.*

The final and most common Emotionally-Triggered Behavior (ETB) we'll cover is what I call secondary addiction. You've already noted whether or not you believe you have this ETB and the possible reasons for it being in your life. This ETB is distinctive from the first six that mainly pollute your personality (defensiveness, childishness, jealousy, self-centeredness, judgmentalism, and dishonesty). You can think of secondary addiction as anything you reach for compulsively, outside of what may be considered healthy: dependencies, coping mechanisms, distractors, and more. They're most often demonstrated when you grasp for something outside of you with the hope of changing something on the inside.

In the same way we're looking to initiate an internal chemical state change when we get defensive, behave childishly, or act in jealousy, we may compulsively reach for something. This state change is not only reached for in the form of exogenous chemicals such as drugs and alcohol, but also through secondary distractions and compulsions, which become secondary addictions. This includes things such as reliance on social media, "binge" watching T.V., dating sites or flirting, nail biting, creating drama or starting fights, compulsively entering new relationships, pornography, hoarding, overspending, and more. These are all examples of secondary addiction.

Secondary addiction, like all ETBs, may be hidden from the people in your life, or in some instances, even from yourself. Maybe you don't yet know how desperately you're reliant on exogenous chemicals. Or, with a compulsion or distraction, perhaps you've thought, "I've got that habit beat, I have a handle on it," or conversely, "It's different for me... I really need it." Whatever it is, it takes a very open mind, real honesty, and a searching attitude to find areas of your life where you're still at risk of falling toward, or still experiencing, secondary addiction. Our exogenous secondary addiction is the dependency on things such as pharmaceuticals, booze, street drugs, cigarettes, excessive amounts of food, and more. Though the first six ETBs that change our personality take away our potential for optimal living, our secondary addiction can literally take our lives. Drugs, alcohol, meds, and more can actually kill our physical body.

Uncovering these secondary dependencies is important, but it's also important to realize that they aren't the primary problem. As mentioned earlier, I believe that our secondary addiction is just that: secondary. To me, the primary problem is why we use them in the first place. The primary problem is our emotional insobriety.

Those who have acknowledged their secondary addiction (which most think of as their primary addiction) and have completed rehab, or after they believe they've gone through adequate recovery, will almost certainly experience the return of their secondary addiction if the emotional addiction (or primary addiction) is not solved. Or they may transfer one addiction for another that's less life-threatening.

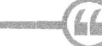

*The primary problem is our emotional insobriety.*

This topic is especially important to me, and quite personal. This phenomenon was one of my primary reasons for developing this training. It was at the forefront of my motive in launching and creating this movement, having seen someone very dear to me lose his life after seemingly recovering from an exogenous chemical addiction; someone who not only focused on not using these chemicals anymore, but also on being the best person he could be in recovery. Yet his pain and suffering, guilt, resentment, and frustration (and who knows what other emotions), Trauma-Influenced Self-Beliefs, and Trauma Filters were still in place. He didn't have the missing element of Emotional Sobriety, and even by avoiding and working diligently to decrease the likelihood of falling back toward their secondary addiction, the overall push and pull of emotional insobriety finally pulled him back and took his life.

Many other and I still miss this person tremendously. Yet I could also sense this person supporting me through my process of creating EMSO Training. In my searching for the "why" behind his death, even after "recovery," many of the answers came to me.

---

*They didn't have the missing element of Emotional Sobriety.*

---

It became so clear to me that when it comes to secondary addiction, replacing the harmful coping mechanism with a healthy one is a good way to create distance from the habit, but it's not a permanent solution. Eventually, their emotional addiction and life circumstance will be too much to bear. The pull toward their past survival mechanisms will become too strong to resist, and this is why the secondary coping mechanisms return.

If you're an addict, a few days after becoming "clean" again, you may be shocked that you're taken "all the way back" to this place of no longer having the power of choice, belligerent on both emotion and on alcohol or drugs. You may be confused as to how you got there, as it didn't match who you thought you were being. You may be confused because you got sideswiped by your emotions. You didn't know that your secondary addiction was really a symptom of you primary, emotional addiction.

This is an incredibly important concept to be understood, whether you're a secondary addict or not, as this can otherwise be a lifelong battle. The primary addiction must be addressed and overcome through EMSO Training in order to alleviate the biochemically-induced behaviors. When we've attained a level of emotional sobriety, our compulsions and addictions will no longer have a place in our lives anymore; there won't be any use for them. We'll have a much more efficient release of true physical dependency on things such as drugs, alcohol, or sugar when we aren't also held at "gunpoint" by our deep-seated emotional belligerence.

Through EMSO Training we'll build our self-reliance, trust in ourselves, know our wholeness and our worthiness, develop the courage to go into the unknown, and become okay with being temporarily uncomfortable. With this knowledge, we can promise ourselves that we'll no longer be a doormat to our chemistry—whether internal or external.

Remember this work is to uncover who you've been being and give you the opportunity to see the *you* you've never noticed. This isn't a judgment against who you've become or what you use to cope with your stress, PANEs, traumas, and more. This is the invitation to look and decide. Do I do this? Does this addiction or compulsion have control over me? Do I want to change this about myself but feel that I can't? I intend on offering you the inspiration that it's not only possible to overcome what's currently controlling you, but a realistic option with the right intention and work. So many people have changed things like you'd like to change. Please delete the shame here; just create awareness. Open your mind, and let this be easy.

We're all the same. We're all right here with you.

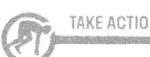
TAKE ACTION

**SECONDARY ADDICTION: WHAT THEY SAY ABOUT ME**
Have others mentioned that you may have an unhealthy addiction. For example, "You drink too much!" or "Why are you such a loner?" or "Can I help you quit smoking?" or "You're on your phone all the time!"

*HINT: These are things that you may do without even knowing you're doing them, but others have tried to bring them to your attention.*

List the secondary addiction(s) that others have accused you of having, even if you don't agree:

_____

_____

**TAKE ACTION**

**SECONDARY ADDICTION: THE THOUGHTS IN MY HEAD**
These are the things you may think to yourself and/or excuses you make regarding your secondary addiction. Mark all that apply to you:

- O Just one more.
- O I need this to fill a void.
- O No one needs to know.
- O I deserve something "bad."
- O I wasn't allowed to have this before; now I want all of it.
- O I need to feel something else.
- O I can't have fun without it.
- O This is the only way I can relax.
- O It's in my lineage.
- O I need this for my pain.
- O I have to do this, or I'll go crazy.
- O I have this under control.
- O I can quit anytime.
- O I don't want to miss out.

**TAKE ACTION**

**SECONDARY ADDICTION: ADMIT TO MYSELF**
Review what you wrote in the previous two Take Actions and what you know to be true about yourself. Using one or two of your secondary addictions, fill in the following statements.

If you'd like to add more, continue on a separate piece of paper.

Remember, this is only for <u>you</u>. Can you get real with yourself right now? You're not alone, as everyone has experienced or currently experiences at least one secondary addiction.

**HINT: I define an "unhealthy amount" as follows:**

- *Damaging my body*
- *Interfering with my self-care*
- *Disturbing my relationships or work*
- *Having a negative impact on children*

1. When I'm honest with myself, I know that I _____ _____ in an unhealthy amount.
2. I tend to do this in order to _____.
3. The reason I do this specifically is that it makes me feel _____.
4. The first time I did this was because _____.
5. What harm has this caused me or others? _____.
6. I've been doing this for _____ years.
7. I've tried quitting, but (if applicable) _____.
8. When I look honestly, I see that I'm addicted to _____.

Remember, only when we work on our weaknesses do we become strong. So don't be afraid to look for your temporary weaknesses, no matter how much shame, regret, or embarrassment may come up with their discovery. This discovery, when looked at honestly and trained away from will remove your need to reach and can save your life. You're worth saving!

You may be starting to notice that many of the exercises thus far address more than one ETB. Getting real, for example, will also help you remove judgment as you're merely <u>observing</u> rather than <u>interpreting</u> reality.

---

*A mistake is an opportunity to give your psyche some deeper lessons.*

You're just beginning the process of being able to see—in the moment—when you're stuck in self-centeredness, lying, or not living in a way you may be intending. Now that you've implemented this awareness of examining what is R.E.A.L, you can implement self-honesty more and more in your life.

Get excited when you notice a "mistake!" A mistake is an opportunity to give your psyche some deeper lessons. With the introduction of self-honesty, you'll be able to redirect yourself from clinging to old behaviors and make a new decision in the moment. When you master awareness in these moments you'll make fewer and fewer mistakes. When you make fewer mistakes, you'll begin to build confidence. When you exhibit new behaviors, you're beginning to practice and express as a different person. Remove the reach by removing the reason for the reach.

24

# Check Motive!

*Knowing your real "why" behind what you think, believe, and do, deepens your self-honesty.*

Knowing your motive behind what you're thinking and doing deepens your self-honesty and exposes where you stand (and once stood) in your Emotional Sobriety.

You have a sounder grasp of the seven most common Emotionally-Triggered Behaviors (ETBs) at this point, and you may even be thinking "I finally know why I act the way I do!" Even though you may be intelligent about your emotions and self-beliefs, and how they puppet you, you need to look at the underlying motives that your Intoxicated Identity has in all areas of life.

## Practice Rep #3: Check Motive

Checking motive becomes a moment-to-moment practice of getting accurate about your reasons for speaking, thinking, and acting a certain way. By seeking your unsober motives, you can catch your dishonesty... and more. There's a layering effect regarding motive that comes with insobriety. This comes from those of us who are continuously unconsciously managing our environment so our Trauma-Influenced Self-Beliefs won't be validated. Even those who believe they're shy or avoidant are still managing their world. Checking, or finding, an unsober motive means to discover the real reasons behind the sneaky things we do, the decisions we make, and the steps we take in order to manage our surroundings and the thoughts, feelings, and behaviors of others.

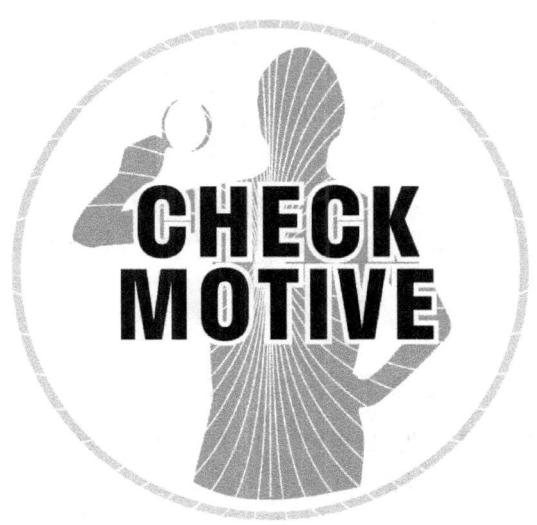

An unsober motive is yet another aspect of the trauma response that's rarely known by the people who wield it—that is, until they search for more truth about what they're really thinking and doing, moment to moment. Looking at our motive shows us exactly where we're being manipulative and controlling something or someone, where we're stuck in our insecurities and still unable to come to the table as our authentic self. If we have a dishonest, manipulative motive, we aren't yet (or aren't currently demonstrating) as emotionally sober. We can look back on past behaviors and feel through to find what our motive was then, revealing how emotionally sober we were.

Our patterns of thinking are developed over our lifetime. The generations before us handed down their "survival skills" to us as well. We've practiced our mental cycles of fear, anxiety, anger, and sadness so diligently that now our pattern of thinking and behaving has become something we just do naturally.

We must become aware of our motivation (our thought process) behind every decision or action. This may sound tedious, but it's non-negotiable. To earn your trust, you have to <u>earn</u> your trust. That doesn't come with one or two exercises. By becoming aware of your ETBs and Trauma Filters, you can see why you became emotionally unsober. Being aware of your underlying motives allows you to see where you stand in your level of Emotional Sobriety as you do the work to get there! You'll discover if you're still reacting based on previous feelings and thoughts. Let me give an example of why it's important to know what you're really thinking and doing in order to know what motivation is behind your decisions and actions. This is detected by searching your innermost thoughts while you are about to make or have just made a decision or take action.

DO YOU RELATE?

> Joe is discontent in his relationship. He thinks about other people and even attempts to get other people interested in him romantically. He even complains to his friends how dissatisfied he is with his partner's work schedule, her daily habits, and that his needs aren't being met. He says, "She's not paying enough attention to me." Although he's disconnected from the relationship, he discusses getting engaged and having children with her. He's still committed to the <u>idea</u> of being in a long-term relationship.
>
> He's magnificently surprised when she ends the relationship. He can't believe she would break up with him and immediately finds all the things wrong with her reasoning for the breakup. <u>She</u> was obviously the problem—she wasn't on the same page as him, maybe she was cheating on him, or she was scared of how wonderful he was. Even though he wouldn't have considered this before, now he proclaims she was his "soulmate" and questions what he'll do without her.
>
> He's compelled to get her back. She's all he can think about. He cries himself to sleep. He starts drinking too much, calling her parents for support, and even begins to show up at her workplace. To Joe, it's a complete mystery that she could have been unhappy in the relationship with him. He filters every word and action she makes through his Trauma Filter of rejection.

His pain isn't about losing this particular woman, it's about not being chosen. His filter is rejection, the fear of not being the most special, the most important. When he really searched for his motive behind his compulsive thinking and actions, he realized he really wanted her to say, "I love you, I only have eyes for you, I'll never leave you, you're the most special and important part of my life." He could now see that his motive in the moment had been derived from a need for attention due to emotional overwhelm of rejection and embarrassment. He attempted to control—he stalked, called, texted, and pleaded to have her fill his deficit made by the filter of rejection, instead of first healing his deficit individually. By witnessing his actions, he was able to stop himself mid-ETB and find his real motive. Now he's less likely to do this again.

The next time he engages in any compulsive behavior, he'll be able to ask "What's my motivation here?"

I use Joe's story, as it is such a common experience. And within this commonality is always the pain of the break up. Knowing your motives, filters, and emotional deficits is imperative in romantic relationships. Otherwise, you can be unhappy in a relationship, complain about it, even be unfaithful and still feel immense pain of rejection if you aren't the one who ends the relationship.

I've seen people who seemingly could have been relieved by their partner leaving them, but the attachment to the meaning behind them leaving, and the way it felt against their Trauma Filters and Self-beliefs, was too exposing. They still clung to control of the individual, rekindling their original infatuation due to their needing to be validated, appreciated, and important. This is damaging to both parties.

Take a moment and ponder the following to continue clarifying the "why" behind your actions.

CONTEMPLATION

**MOTIVATING FACTORS**
Recall the last time you may have been motivated by fear to act a certain way, or manipulated a situation without really being aware of your motivation behind it. For example, am I "doing everything" for everyone else so that others will think I'm irreplaceable? Am I giving up a part of myself to someone else so that they will love me? Why did I give them my phone number? Why did I buy that car? Why did I say that to her? Am I supporting them just so that they'll support me later? Use the graphic on the following page to support you in beginning to know which underlying motives you are using.

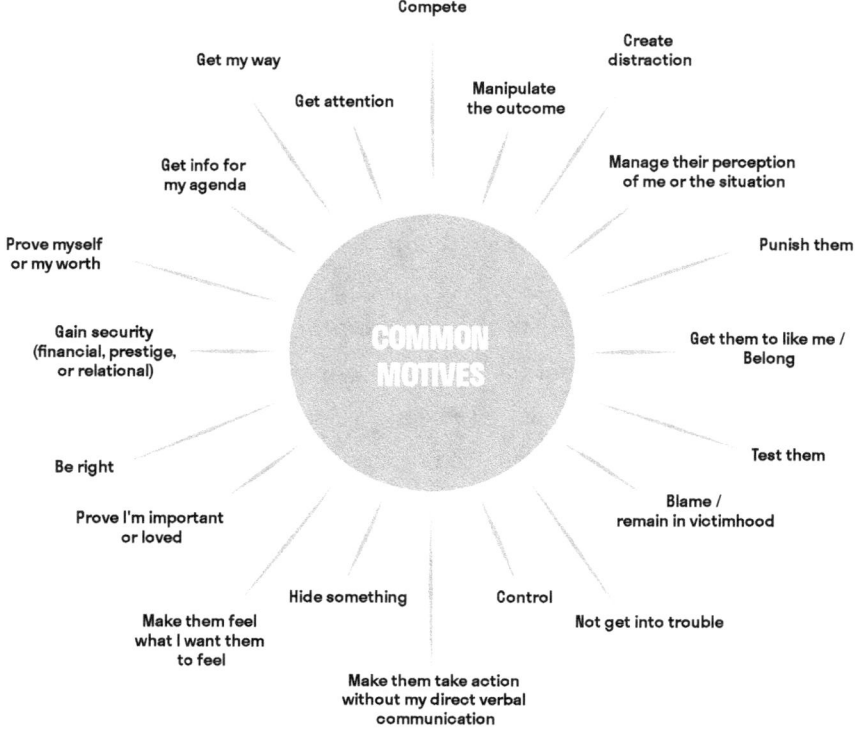

(Add any you experience by drawing more lines out on the graphic above.)

In terms of motivating factors for dishonesty, lying to manage the perception of others is a predominant, recurring theme that I see with my students. Because the development of an Intoxicated Identity is so common, we live in a society that lies and places pressure on people to lie (or at least we think we have to lie). Lying is an extremely manipulative and hidden skill that even the liar is sometimes unaware they're participating in.

Knowing and continuously checking your motive are foundational for getting real, and required to build your Emotional Sobriety.

TAKE ACTION

### CHECK MY MOTIVE

After having explored each of the seven most common ETBs, it's important to begin to develop a new level of maturity before moving on to the EMSO Investigations. We do this by growing the capacity to do the practice rep: "Check Motive." This is one of the foundations of EMSO Training. Think of the last time you used each of the common ETBs and write in the motive, meaning:

- What was I hoping to accomplish by behaving this way?
- Why did I behave in this way?

1. I was defensive so that _____.
2. I was childish so that _____.
3. I was jealous so that _____.
4. I was self-centered so that _____.
5. I was judgmental so that _____.
6. I was dishonest so that _____.
7. I used a secondary addiction so that _____.
8. Additional examples: _____

Checking motive can expose your manipulation. It shows your insobriety as clear as day. Most people are shocked when they first see it. The secret here is that to build the capacity to check your motive, you're taking the reins of your thoughts and intentions, perhaps for the first time. You're cornering your ego and saying, "I see you and I know what you're doing!"

Now you're beginning an even greater journey of awareness and becoming your own best resource for finding out who you've been being.

# 25

# Case Studies: PANEs & Motives

Throughout the development of this curriculum, we've witnessed countless people unravel their own Anatomy of Emotional Insobriety. We've observed various students' stories and experiences through the lens of their Early-Age Trauma, Trauma-Influenced Self-Beliefs, Trauma Filters, and Emotionally-Triggered Behaviors (ETBs). These have become the case studies for this movement of Emotional Sobriety. Now, I invite you to look for similarities in dysfunction and mechanistic reasoning for the <u>emotions</u> themselves to be there. While reading the following stories, see if you notice the underlying reasons that a particular emotion makes an appearance

In each of these cases, consider the following: Why are these chemicals produced during each individual situation? Are they situationally different, yet the same mechanisms are in place (emotional insobriety)? Are we seeking our next hit of biochemistry using a new audience or scenario as our "dealer"?

You may begin to see how all of our insobriety is an emotional, biochemical addiction. Study the why and the how around who they're each being, what they're doing, and why. What are they feeling, and why? In these cases, notice how once their beliefs are validated through their Trauma Filters, the flood of emotions is released in liberal amounts, causing intoxication or belligerence. This intoxication allows for their unchosen behaviors (ETBs) to come out under the guise of protection.

## Case Study #1: Fear

*A man who had massive emotional charge and ETBs when his wife would talk to other men.*

After checking his motive and deepest conversations with himself, he realized that he didn't trust his wife with fidelity because he <u>himself</u> was not trustworthy. That was a hard one to get to the bottom of—think of how he must have had to be fearless and honest when looking for his feelings here! Once he did, he felt relieved and worked on making himself more trustworthy (shifting his ETB of dishonesty). By looking at and changing himself, his marriage was positively affected. Now that he has strong integrity and trust in himself, he isn't threatened when his wife is around other men (another ETB shifted: jealousy). This has allowed him to create real and lasting friendships with men without fear of something happening with them and his wife.

## Case Study #2: Anger

*"I'm so angry with my son for not calling me back!"*

She senses an anger response due to the hurt from her son not calling her back, but is there another reason for this hurt? When asked if she was hurt, she initially reacts, "No, I'm angry!"

She was advised to look at the PANE graphic and see if anything stuck out to her. I asked her to be really honest with herself. She quickly came to realize that she's not angry, rather she's suspicious. Here was her response, with my insertions of the various EMSO components:

"I'm embarrassed to say this, but I realize that I'm angry with my son because I believe when he doesn't call me that he's up to no good (her assumption). I'm so used to controlling every detail of his life. I realize I don't trust him because I've always done everything for him. I'm afraid that he thinks he can do things without me (her insecurity). I also realize that I've continued to do everything for him as a young adult because I want to solidify my position in his life (her motive). I now realize that because he's capable of living without me, I'm insecure. So I'm not angry, I'm in fear (her real PANE). I've always felt important to my son, and I don't want it to go away now that he doesn't need me. I believe I'm unimportant and that he's going to leave me (Trauma Filters). What I thought was anger is really fear (PANE), and that caused me to act out defensively (ETB)."

She did so great on this one! We know that most of our initial responses are not what's really going on inside of us. Had she acted out that anger with her son when he finally called, that could have gone very badly as it had in the past. Instead, she was able to calmly use her new clarity to speak to her son. She chose to be honest and vulnerable and let him know that at first she was angry and then realized that she had put a lot of pressure on him to make her feel needed. She apologized and told him that she would like it if he could call her every week, but understood if he was too busy, because she'd prefer he be driven by his own truth rather than pressure from her. She was able to release her grasp on him, realizing he was an individual and a grown man who was going to have his own life; and now, she could too.

## Case Study #3: Sadness

*Here we witness how someone got over themselves to see what they were actually feeling, and why (motive).*

What are you feeling? *I'm upset with my husband.*

Why? *Well, because he doesn't do the chores around the house.*

What does that mean to you when he doesn't do the chores? *He doesn't care about the house or what I ask. All he thinks about is himself.*

What does that mean? *That he doesn't care about me.*

And what does that mean? *That he must not love me.*

How do you <u>feel</u> about him not loving you? *It makes me sad and scared that if he doesn't love me, he's just using me.*

What does that mean? *That I'm replaceable and not important.*

Do <u>you</u> believe you're important? *Not really.*

Why do you believe you're unimportant? *Probably because my dad abandoned me when I was five.*

Did your dad leave <u>you</u> when you were five or did he leave your <u>mom</u>? *My mom and me.*

Have you ever left a romantic relationship that you felt you couldn't stay in anymore? *Yes*

Can you see that your dad—although it did affect you—departed as a reaction to feeling emotional overwhelm that he obviously didn't have the capacity for or the tools to fix? Can you see that maybe after he left, he was too scared, ashamed, or embarrassed to come back? *Yes, I can see that.*

Do you see that there's a possibility that he may <u>not</u> have thought any of this through? Perhaps it wasn't in his mind to decide if he should stay because of you or leave for himself? It was a knee-jerk reaction or a compulsion to disappear. *I guess so, yes. It may have not been about me at all, in fact, it couldn't have been because it was <u>only</u> about him at that time.*

Now that you're an adult, can you see that sometimes relationships end, even when children are involved? *Yes, I see that everywhere. Two of my friends chose to leave their spouses and are raising the kids. I've always assumed that my dad's departure was about me. I never even considered that he's his own person and made choices he thought he needed to make for himself.*

It's normal for your child-self to have come to the conclusion that your dad left <u>you</u> and that meant you weren't important to him. But you seemingly not being important to your father, doesn't mean you aren't important to your husband. *Yes, I can definitely see this.*

What are you noticing now? *Wow, I guess I put a lot of pressure on my husband to show me that I'm important, even in the most mundane ways. I notice that I even jump to the conclusion that if he doesn't do the dishes, it means he'll probably leave me.*

How do you behave, or what ETBs do you display, when you feel unimportant? *I create a scene to make him see what I'm feeling and often yell or cry hysterically.* Yes, the ETB of childishness.

Can you find the underlying motive for this? *I want him to feel sorry for me and show me attention and affection. Then I would know I'm important.*

## Case Study #4: Embarrassment

*"My partner didn't call to tell me he was going to be late. For several hours I was worried about him. This makes me really mad when he does this."*

When I asked her why she was "mad," she looked deeper and said it was because it meant he didn't respect her and she wasn't valued. "I cook every night just like my mom did for my dad, and when my dad was late, it upset her. She'd always say, 'Men are inconsiderate!'"

She then realized that her belief that he didn't respect her or that she wasn't valuable meant that she, and the gift of her dinner, was being rejected.

She began to see that she wasn't actually angry, she was embarrassed.

"I cook him dinner so he knows that he's important to me, so when he doesn't call me, I feel that I'm not respected or important and that makes me embarrassed because I feel rejected. I think my mom getting angry may have been her way of handling having a filter of rejection as well."

This particular woman may have a better time communicating how she feels to her husband when she tells him the real emotion she's experiencing. Reacting in anger when she really felt embarrassed made it more difficult for him to be around her, as well as more difficult for her to hear his perspective on things. Also, if he doesn't know the real feeling she's struggling with, reconciliation is blocked. This also causes distress within the relationship that may make the husband not want to be home in time for dinner and creates a cycle of him fearing coming home to criticism, and the wife feeling embarrassment with the illusion of her and her gift of dinner being rejected.

What about looking at her own behaviors? Does she feel she must make dinner for him every night because that's what her mother did? Then she realizes her real motive for cooking every night was for herself—so he would see her in a certain way, thereby establishing the role she thought she had to play to keep him and be accepted and loved.

*Each person had a moment in which they recognized who they'd been being—how they'd been behaving, thinking, and what they'd been believing.*

Were these people all suffering from Intoxicated Identities due to emotional insobriety? I believe that the <u>why</u> behind our suffering is the same for every person on Earth: emotional insobriety.

Real, honest emotional awareness, and understanding the real reason we do things are important for this area of self-discovery. When each of these individuals were asked to get over themselves, identify their actual feeling tone and name it more accurately (get real), and then check motive, they were able to then calmly communicate them outwardly.

They each had a moment of awareness during which they recognized who they'd been being—how they'd been behaving, what they were actually feeling, and what they'd been believing about themselves. They explored their underlying motive for acting, feeling, and thinking in these ways. This is the foundation of attaining Emotional Sobriety: awareness of our emotional insobriety. Revisit the snapshot of your Anatomy of Emotional Insobriety on page 153 before proceeding to EMSO Investigations.

# EMSO INVESTIGATIONS

THE *YOU* YOU'VE NEVER NOTICED

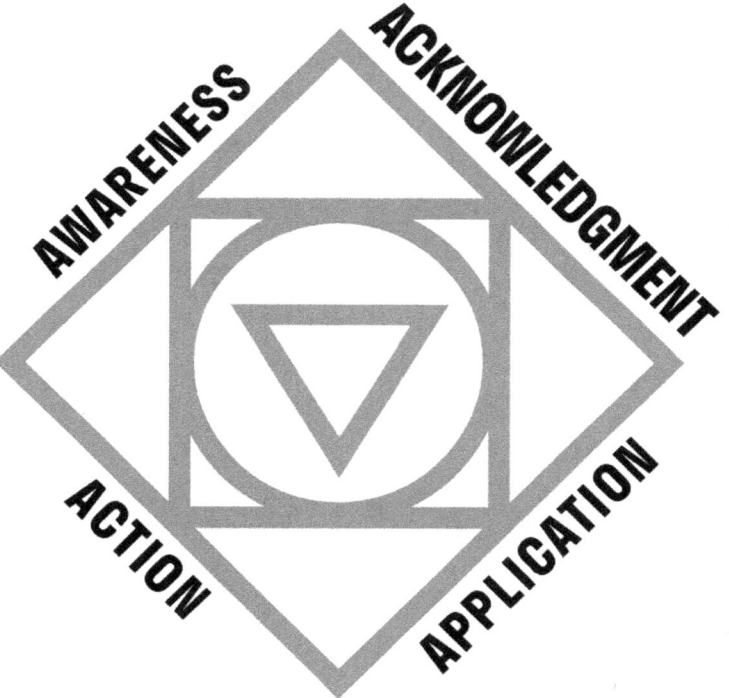

**26**

## Desire, Intention, Action

*Your intentions for change cannot be turned into reality until you take action. And nothing happens without sustained desire.*

If you turned the page and decided to continue your EMSO Training, welcome to the next stage of your transformation!

You've now completed the first EMSO Essential: **Foundations**. This has allowed you to begin developing the first A in The 4A Formula: <u>awareness</u>. This includes awareness of the seeds of your Early-Age Trauma and the subsequent Trauma-Influenced Self-Beliefs and Trauma Filters you formed. You know your egoic and biochemical intelligence which created an addiction to various Predominant Accompanying Negative Emotions (PANEs) as a means of survival. And you're aware of the most obvious symptom of your insobriety—your Emotionally-Triggered Behaviors (ETBs), all of which make up your current Intoxicated Identity.

Now you begin the second EMSO Essential: **Investigations**, where you'll learn and practice the next A: <u>acknowledgment</u>—recognizing the part that you've played in perpetuating your patterns. Each Take Action in this section supports you in deconstructing your emotional insobriety, giving you space to construct Emotional Sobriety in its place.

While some students find this part of the curriculum difficult, others greatly enjoy it, as they respect the grand opportunity that it offers. If you're someone who gets excited about the concept of change, this will likely be a gratifying experience for you. Acknowledgment allows you to deeply accept who you've really been being over your lifetime. First, you deserve a little "exhale" afer the challenging topics you've faced thus far in your EMSO Foundations.

 TAKE ACTION

**THE REAL ME, PART 2:**
**WHAT I (ALREADY) LIKE ABOUT ME**
In "The Real Me, Part 1" on page 46, you considered which emotionally sober traits you wished to attain in the future. Next, list five (or more) things you already like about yourself, what others like about you, or things that you intend to keep as part of your chosen identity going forward.

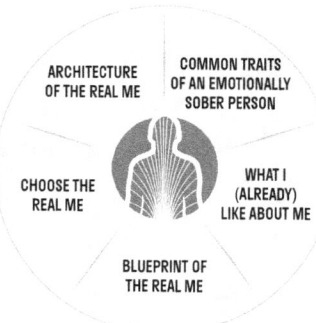

1. 
2. 
3. 
4. 
5. 

Now... ready, aim, fire!

After being introduced to motive and the specifics of your insobriety, is there a spark in you that's ready for change? If so, you now have one of the three essential ingredients for change—you have desire! I know I wouldn't have become the person that I am today without three ingredients:

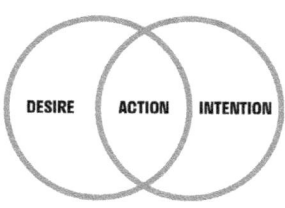

1. <u>Desire</u> to change
2. Witnessing the contrast of who I was versus who I <u>intend</u> to become
3. Taking the necessary <u>actions</u> to change

Once my desire was turned on, I began to see the contrast described here, which gave me the rare ability to course-correct. By becoming aware of my Anatomy of Emotinoal Insobriety, I had a map of where I was, and could compare it to where I desired to be. I desired to become the ruler of my thoughts, emotions, and behaviors, to have whole, healthy relationships, and to be unconditionally loving. In moments when I felt my old patterns grab at me as I progressed on the path of change, I would vividly recall where those paths had led me in the past, and acknowledge that they didn't match where I intended to go in the future. Though not always easy to see, it was because of this contrast that I was inspired to take new action.

In EMSO Investigations, you'll take the action to look at the real impact of all of your ETBs— how your dishonesty and self-centeredness have kept you isolated, how your judgments and jealousy have affected your life and the lives of others, the losses that your defensiveness and childish actions have yielded, and the affects of your secondary addiction on you and others... all of it. Parts of the path that you're currently walking are reversible, and all of it is transformable. You'll be astounded to see the possibility of living a drama- and problem-free life. New and aligned opportunities will fall into your life. You'll feel smarter. Your communication will improve. This is a massive gift for yourself and for those around you. You'll become safe and others will feel safe in your presence.

Success in any task is created through desire, intention, and action. This includes the task of change—changing simple habits or drastically transforming who we're being. The energy of desire, the energy of intention, and the energy of action are already within you. Some people will read a book or seek teachers or coaches to be given something that they don't have. My job isn't to give you this power, rather I'm here to remind you that you already have it, and the training supports you in uncovering it.

Remember, your compulsive behaviors don't make you wrong or bad; you can now simply choose something different for yourself.

Your desire will expedite your success. To me, desire simply means:

DEFINITION

**DESIRE:** a strong, energetic drive for something to occur.

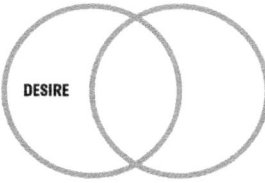

When desire is true, it's relentless. It always wins when it's fed with intention and action. There's nothing that can replace desire, and nothing that can get in its way.

Recall that your ego, body, and parts of your brain will want you to stay the same. Any addict in rehab who doesn't have the desire for change is going to be looking for the next escape to avoid the work toward betterment, due to the level of discomfort it entails. Even if you have massive desire and have committed to change, you'll still be uncomfortable. Yet you'll acknowledge that being uncomfortable is a good sign that you're heading toward change. If you feel the same way you've always felt during this investigation, then you aren't doing anything differently. You must use your desire for change to inspire you to think differently, more honestly, and look at everything from a fresh angle.

*Being uncomfortable is a good sign that you're heading toward change.*

In my teaching, I don't create the desire for change in my students; they do. They do the honest searching for the truth about themselves. They do it with the aid of their desire, decision, and commitment, and with their authentic desire to transcend who they've been being. They do it with the power that's within them and all around them. I simply hold them accountable to their decision. I alert them if I feel withholding or dishonesty and help them to become whole-heartedly aware of their patterns. Once they're aware of who they've been being, they have a decision to make, just as you will. They ask themselves: "Do I choose to remain the same or do I desire change?"

CONTEMPLATION

**DO I DESIRE?**
Ask yourself now: Do I choose to remain the same, or do I desire to change? What's my decision? Am I committed to this next step? What's my level of desire?

DEFINITION

**INTENTION:** the planning and aim toward your desired outcome.

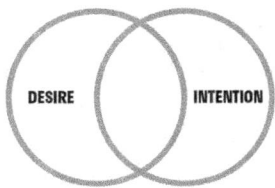

Once you have your desire, you already <u>are</u> the future you... in <u>intention</u>. To reach your desired destination, you then have to do the things that the future version of you has already done. Let me repeat that: you'll now have to do what the future you has already done in order to reach your destination.

*Your "in-tension" is the applied force of your decision to become the new you every single day. It's a re-deciding every single day.*

Think of intention as not only what you're intending to do, but what has already occurred and you've already succeeded at. It's what you're putting in place in front of you to be able to move toward. I like to think of this as a tightrope. If one end is attached to the future you desire, then you must have consistent "tension" on the rope to cross over. Your "in-tension" will be the consistent force you apply through thought and determination. This will hold you up along your journey. Your intention, therefore, is the applied force of your decision to become the real you every single day. This requires re-deciding every single day.

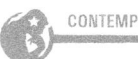
CONTEMPLATION

**A PEEK AHEAD**
Picture yourself easily knowing how to deal with the problems that arise in your environment. Imagine you're calm, peaceful, and levelheaded. Witness the possibility of knowing your emotions won't be a hindrance to maintaining this, and that you're able to stay effective and engaged, even during discord or arguments. Ask yourself now: What do I imagine I've already succeeded at in my future? What does my future hold? This is your intention.

DEFINITION

**ACTION**: the doing part of life—the movement or work to achieve your desired intention.

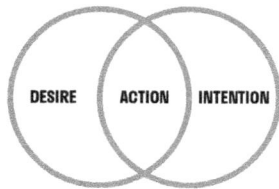

If you're reading this book and you've accomplished the task of uncovering your unique Anatomy of Emotional Insobriety, you already know something about taking action. Completing your first EMSO Essential in your training required much of it! Perhaps you weren't as aware of your desire or intention, but something drew you to receive this curriculum and take some initial steps. Now imagine how effective the subsequent action steps in your training will be with your desire and intention behind them!

CONTEMPLATION

**NECESSARY ACTIONS**
Ask yourself: Am I ready to take the necessary actions to achieve my desired future?

Keep this desire, intention, and action-based mindset with you throughout this self-investigation and beyond. As the building blocks for a meaningful life, may each of these ingredients serve your change process, and be useful tools to return to again and again.

If you now have the desire to move forward, and the clear intention to meet the *you* you've never met, how do you know if you're ready for action?

# 27

# Readiness for Change

*Making real change requires a huge leap.*

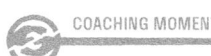
**COACHING MOMENT**

**In the Take Actions we're about to do in your EMSO Investigations, I want to be clear and remind you that I'm not here to be your judge, nor shall you judge yourself! A deep examination of your life is required to see which behaviors create resistance for you, and determine if you are ready to courageously remove them.**

Can you see any areas of your life where your emotions, thought patterns, or behaviors may have played a role in your problems? Can you see how changing these behaviors or emotional patterns may change your entire life for the better? There's power in knowing that your problems are your own responsibility. Let's discover your power together. This chapter offers a re-invocation of your choice: Are you ready for change?

Indecision keeps you right where you are. So, the only chance you have to begin, persevere, and succeed at finishing anything is in the moment you decide. When I work with my students on the transformation of their lives, I observe many signals during our first meeting—signals that give clues to where they are in their readiness for change. I observe and listen for an important qualifier: Are they here for attention, or are they here for guidance? The truth of this cannot be discovered until they are asked to not only become aware of their patterns, but to then acknowledge their part in them and take action to change.

Sustained change seems to be a challenge for everyone. Even if it's not difficult to <u>realize</u> that you need to change something about yourself or your life, some believe that to take action on this change requires an admission that how you're currently behaving or who you're being is wrong. Let's look at this differently. You're not wrong! You've done the best you could up to this point!

DO YOU RELATE?

**Paolo has played piano for most of his life. He decides one day to take a class to bring his skill to the next level.**

Deciding he's ready to take a new class doesn't suggest that Paolo's current level of development as a pianist is wrong. It simply shows his interest in learning more—in growing.

The decision to change here in EMSO Training is only advancing your skill level as a human in relationship to yourself, others, and the world you live in. You educate yourself to develop new capacities, possibilities, and opportunities to advance to the real version of yourself. Although there may be immediate change in your thoughts and behaviors, acquiring new skills and making them permanent takes time. Just as earning a doctorate may take an additional four to eight years of postgraduate study, mastering your Emotional Sobriety requires effort and time as well. Time is going to go by anyway. It's up to you to decide who you intend to be when that time elapses. In four years, you can be four years older, or four years greater. It's all about who you commit to becoming between now and then.

*Time is going to go by anyway. It's up to you to decide who you intend to be when that time elapses.*

Committing to unveiling the real version of yourself is like investing in yourself. It requires consistent action and patience with the ups and downs. When you're faced with a "down," you'll need to restate your desire and intention, reinforce more of the new into your life, and reapply the work on the "up."

Acceptance of the severity of the impact of your insobriety on yourself and others allows you to deepen your desire for solutions. You're likely to reach out for help when you realize that you haven't been able to help yourself up. Acknowledging that you need help teaches you to get real and accept where you really are.

In this process, ask these questions again and again using your three Practice Reps:

1. **Get Over Yourself:** Can I "go to the balcony" for a clearer view?

2. **Get Real:** Who am I really being? What am I really thinking? Feeling? How am I really behaving?

3. **Check Motive:** What did I hope to accomplish by thinking, feeling, behaving in this way?

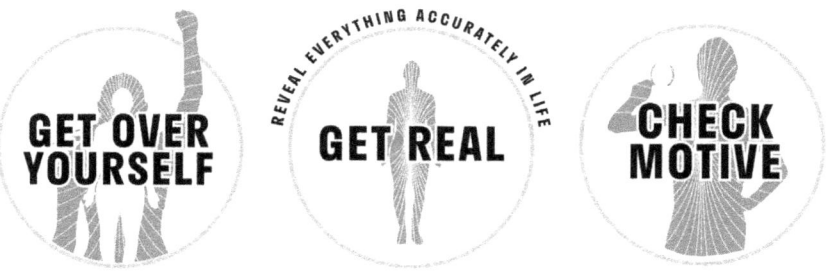

While living in the problem, you drown in the unreality of your own life. You're taking on water. Once you can see that nothing this version of you tries to do ever fixes your problems, you throw your arms up and surrender. You confess that you can no longer continue the same way and expect a different experience. I like to think of this as a moment of realization that you need support. This is the moment you finally see that you've lost our legs and have been trying to walk alone.

A universal way to get beyond the Intoxicated Identity is to connect with something bigger than it, something that can thrust you outside of your self-centeredness. A "higher" or "greater" energy that you can access for assistance in recreating your life. Let's explore that energy or power that's going to help you solve all of your problems. This higher energy or power could be called God, spirit, universal intelligence, the divine, energy... whatever it is that feels true for you.

The concept of higher power can be understood only by you, as it's unique to each person. We each have different beliefs and understandings regarding spirituality, science, and religion. When you're not told where to look or what to look at as your higher power, you can genuinely cultivate your own spiritual connection. If you're atheist, pure scientist, or agnostic, think of this power as the electricity that lights your home.

Perhaps this power could be named "The Real You," inviting itself to be revealed and in the driver's seat of your life.

This is the energy that's inside of and surrounding each and every one of us. It's the ocean we're all swimming in together. This power is what makes your heart beat with neither your consent or demand, and what gives you life without your will or command. When you realize that you have this power surrounding you and inside of you, you can understand that it's a power that your personality cannot outsmart nor overturn. It's there for you to rely on for your betterment. This training doesn't change due to what religion you were born into, or even what religion you have or haven't chosen as an individual ideal. Your higher power that you tap into during this training is your choice. Start paying attention to it and acknowledging its presence. In my experience, it doesn't seem to matter what we call it, as long as we call upon it. The recognition of a transformative and creative power will be what pushes you alongside your own will and eagerness and energizes you through this training.

*This energy is the paint, the canvas, and the brush with which you'll create your new life.*

Do you think this energy that heals your wounds and moves the planets is capable of being powerful enough to help you through this change?

It's my understanding that the energy that runs through me and loves me is the same energy that runs through and loves you. When you really search for its feeling, you begin to recognize that it's always with you. That you have a power that is far greater than your current problems. When you first meet it consciously, it can startle your norm and your ego may reflex with stubborn resistance. But we cannot deny its existence. Our power comes from this power. This energy is the paint, the canvas, and the brush with which you'll create your new life.

Read this intention quietly to yourself first, and then say it aloud if you agree with it. For each of the intention-setting moments here, you may also change the wording to most accurately match your personal experience:

 INTENTION-SETTING MOMENT

> "The current version of me hasn't been able to fix my problems. I say I'll do better next time, but that hasn't worked. I remain unchanged, and my problems continue. I feel an emptiness that this version of me cannot fill, and nothing outside of me can either. I desire change and I truly seek it now."

Now read the following aloud while feeling the words in your heart:

 INTENTION-SETTING MOMENT

> "I choose to feel the energy that made and keeps me. I choose to feel it around me and within me. I believe this power will inspire me toward clarity. It will help remove from my life what I haven't been able to remove by myself."

Allow these to sink in. If there's no change without our changing, then we must make different choices, do different things, and be different people to have the change we're searching for in our lives. In these intention-setting moments, you're recognizing there may be a solution for your problems other than your old ways.

There was a point when I realized why I hadn't done well trying to change my own life. I hadn't even been aware of what was happening within me—my thoughts, feelings, and emotions. I hadn't noticed my behaviors or the impact they had on others. And I hadn't been listening to what was happening around me. I was trapped inside of myself—in the Center of Self. I'd had many things happen in my life, but hadn't even yet lived.

> *This training bridges the you you've been being, with the you you've never met.*

Emotionally sober people can modify their lives in an instant with their beliefs, thoughts, and intentions. Those who cannot are missing a fundamental component of life that's remained absent. They haven't achieved self-awareness or a level of consciousness that would allow them the capacity to initiate and create sustained change in their lives.

EMSO Training fills the gaps in the story of your development. This training bridges the *you* you've been being, with the *you* you've never met. The sooner you finish all of the components of EMSO Training, the sooner you'll have a shift into what's real for you. Then you'll be able to create your life as you desire it. The next step is leaning forward with a strong decision to change from where you currently stand.

> *You'll be able to create your life exactly as you desire it.*

If you've made this decision and are ready to move forward, read the words on the following page aloud, and feel your intention behind it:

### INTENTION-SETTING MOMENT

> "I decide to make changes in my life. I understand I cannot use my old ways of thinking, believing, or behaving to have a different life. I'm ready to uncover the real me and am committed to grow with both eagerness and joy. Where it feels difficult, I'll bring more focus. Where I may want to quit, I'll ask myself for love, my higher power for energy, and continue the process of change. I deserve a new life, no matter what I've done or has been done to me in the past. I deserve a freer life of pure happiness and health."

To attain Emotional Sobriety with willingness and readiness, the process I've outlined in the next chapter could expose you to having a big shift toward more clarity, and quickly! When I deeply surrendered to the self-investigation part of my process, I was so impressed by the immediate changes that I was experiencing that I wanted to spread it to everyone in my life! I had to tell them that I'd had this incredible reboot, and that it felt like a huge weight had been lifted off of me. I was becoming someone that I never even thought possible. I would describe it by saying, "It's as if I met myself for the first time. There were always glimpses of her, but she's finally here."

Doing the investigatory work of EMSO Training can contribute to what other teachings may consider an "awakening"... a stunning moment of clarity, a clearing, or a sudden shift into greater awareness. This can be a grounded, powerful shift that can stay with you indefinitely. This is the moment where we see who we've been being so clearly in front of us, and we see our patterns and pain as something we never need to experience again. I call this a moment of sobering up, emotionally speaking.

A big observation as I became awakened during my investigation was that what was real wasn't about what I wanted it to be, or thought it should be. It wasn't a screenplay or a scripted version of reality. What was real was what was <u>actually</u> happening—without projected beliefs, perceptions, or false wishes regarding what I was begging for it to look like. Once I saw reality, I couldn't claim ignorance anymore, and it would no longer be acceptable. Once I was offered the gift of real eyes, I couldn't deny their power to change me.

I've now seen this happen numerous times with various EMSO students—where the investigation alone shifts something within, causing a fundamental change that ripples to many corners of the person's life. I've heard things said such as: "I'll never be that person again," or "I know I'm different now," or "Everything seems so simple now!" They weren't completely emotionally sober, but were inspired to better themselves even further due to how much freer they already felt. My personal process resembles this. While the initial shift into sobriety came nearly immediately, there were many ongoing practices I used to refine and eliminate the more subtle filters that affected my biochemistry.

If after completing the EMSO Investigations you don't experience a similar "instant" awakening, it doesn't mean you're not going to get there. Together, we'll uncover the real you.

*Once I saw reality, I couldn't claim ignorance anymore. Nor would it have been acceptable. Once I was offered the gift of real eyes, I couldn't deny their power to change me.*

After my personal transformation, I became more helpful and useful to the world. I was no longer hiding underneath layers of my past. I wasn't lying to manage someone else or to avoid exposing parts of myself. I ended the cycle of addiction to my emotions. Think of all the energy I was saving! I was free.

And I wish this for every single person.

Do you now wish this for yourself?

You've leaned into the concept of change. You're more self-aware than you've ever been. Next, you leap.

# R.E.A.Life Investigation

*We bury our secrets until they bury us.*

This chapter continues your EMSO Training by moving toward deep and honest acknowledgment of your life experiences, or what we can now call your R.E.A.Life—the life where everything is accurately revealed to yourself in honesty. It also gives you the opportunity to have an "out of body" experience in order to see yourself from a new angle... to truly get over yourself—perhaps for the first time in your life.

 COACHING MOMENT

> As you begin this part of the process, know that you're loved. You're wonderful and special beyond anything you can conceive. You've made it this far in life as the current and many other versions of you, and each version has pieces of your uniqueness that no one else can claim as their own. You have something to give the world that only you can offer. This process supports you in keeping and expanding upon these essential pieces of you, while assessing and eliminating the parts that are non-viable or destructive for your life.

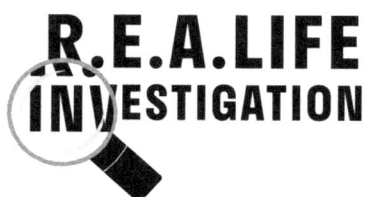

This is my favorite part of the process of change, for many reasons. One is that it requires the most transformative character trait: self-honesty! As you know by now, this is an area I once grappled with because I had no real grasp on what was real in my life. It was once such a huge struggle for me that I decided to make it my <u>most</u> exercised chosen trait. I intended on becoming an honest person, knowing that a weakness is waiting to become a greatest strength. I became a superhero for myself and an aid to others when I took on this new way of being. It profoundly shaped who I became, and who I am today.

So now you can try on your heroic cape of honesty. Charge yourself up and become fearless in your attempts to acknowledge who you've <u>really</u> been being.

*A weakness is waiting to become a greatest strength.*

The second reason this is my favorite part of the process is that it separates the doers from the pretenders. It not only requires your honesty, but also humility and honor. You'll regard yourself with great respect as you begin to demonstrate a deep desire to solve the problems in your life. This is where you can declare your right for a sober life of physical, mental, emotional, and spiritual health and peace.

There's a long tradition of searching within ourselves for truth. A multitude of programs and practices, whether religious or psychological, including twelve-step programs, have exercised the concept of doing a self-investigation as part of the process of healing ourselves. I'm not introducing a new concept to the world by advocating for this investigation. It's long-standing and proven to be a massive catalyst for human metamorphosis.

I began my inner investigation when I completed an Al-Anon twelve-step program. This was fundamental in helping me achieve greater self-awareness, as it allowed me to become subtly unblocked. However, it didn't allow the depth of peace, clarity, and levelheadedness that I now have. As you know, this is one of the reason I've written this book (the one I wished I had!) to take you as deep as possible for a chance at real Emotional Sobriety. This is what I hope for you—that you wholeheartedly and seriously engage in this carefully guided R.E.A.Life Investigation, and then advance far beyond in your continued EMSO Training.

This may seem like "too much work." In fact, I've witnessed many people struggle as they go through this process, while others do only a portion of the work and stop. The latter never took the time or endured the angst of its therapeutic result and thus inevitably failed to overcome their problems. No matter how tedious, deep, or uncomfortable this gets for you, I assure you it's <u>required</u> to attain Emotional Sobriety.

I wouldn't have become the woman I am today without this drastic life "house cleaning." I left some things out in the beginning of my process to save face, thinking "This will be enough, I don't have to write it all down," or "I'll save that for another time." You may be tempted to distract yourself while doing these exercises. For example, when asked a question about writing down your past struggles, you may experience an urge to blame someone else—"Well yeah, this happened, but it was my ex's fault. Even if I had a part in it, it wasn't really my doing." You've already been introduced to and have some practice with the concept of removing (de)fences, judgment, and a host of other behaviors that may be triggered in this process. Now is the time to continue getting over yourself, getting real, and checking motive. Step out of blame and into a curious exploration of your life.

*Trauma is not yours to keep, return, or extend to someone else.*
*It's actually the seed of your Emotional Sobriety.*
*It's for you to overcome.*

If you want to experience all of your true power, you must first shed the idea that your problems, beliefs, behaviors, or thoughts are someone's fault. There is no productive reason to blame someone else, or yourself for that matter! Right now, remember that you and everyone in your life has experienced trauma. You now know that your trauma is not for you to continue to relive again and again in different forms. Trauma is not yours to keep, return, or extend to someone else. It's actually the seed of—or the thing that births—your Emotional Sobriety. It's for you to overcome. It's a gift from which to launch off and teaches you to become the strongest version of you, the empowered version of you, the *you* you've never met.

Empowerment isn't about marches, arguments, sounding intelligent, or being strong enough to hurt someone else. The way I define it is:

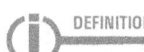

DEFINITION

**EMPOWERMENT:** the experience of having once been a victim and now choosing to become victorious; to remember your power.

It's to remember or recognize that you have always had the power within you. That you're inherently a whole being already. It's the remembrance or decided utilization of this inherent power. Once you've done this, it will seem that nothing can harm you. Nothing happens to you anymore. You happen… for the world.

This investigation is a cleanup. It isn't only about looking at your patterns, but also about clearing out your secrets. Of all the ETBs, we've probably discussed dishonesty the most due to its powerful and destructive effect on you. With shame and its associated biochemicals holding down the lies, it seems they're too heavy to bring forward. You may often feel that you can't lift the weight of the lie, and with that shame and heaviness comes illness, lethargy, confusion, and more lies! You're juggling different scenarios and controlling outcomes by attempting to choose your own "truths" instead of revealing what's real. You can't accept new data or retrieve any past certainty when you're filled to the brim with falseness and destructive biochemicals, which block your real self.

*Nothing happens <u>to</u> you, anymore. You happen… <u>for</u> the world.*

Do you feel nervous when someone asks you a question? Do you keep secrets that are keeping you sick, stuck, or scared? This is the case for most people. If you think you don't have any, you may not be looking closely enough at yourself and the environment around you. Here's your chance.

Do this R.E.A.Life Investigation on your own and remove distractions. If possible, finish this section in one sitting. The sooner this is completed, the faster you'll start to feel yourself changing. I've noticed with students that the thing you think impacted you the <u>least</u> may have actually had the <u>most</u> impact—the Early-Age Trauma that you "don't really care about anymore" tends to be the thing that you end up needing to work through the most. Keep that in mind as you go through this part. I want you to write <u>everything</u> down, even the things you feel you've already overcome.

Can you see that by denying yourself access to the truth of who you've been being, what you've been thinking, what your motives have really been, and what has happened to you, you may be blocking yourself from further growth? Your secrets keep you sick; holding and protecting them for others will as well.

Once you admit you've been deceitful with yourself, you may find yourself at a crossroads: Do I choose honesty and humility, or give up, lie to myself, and remain the same? It takes a massive amount of bravery to do this investigation. Remember that the fear inside of you is your body chemistry doing its job to hold you where you stand, to keep you "surviving." Yet this has become a bio-chemical addiction and you're ready to change.

Take a moment now to reaffirm your oath to complete honesty with yourself while doing this work. How honest are you being with yourself right now? How honest do you <u>intend</u> to be with yourself as you investigate?

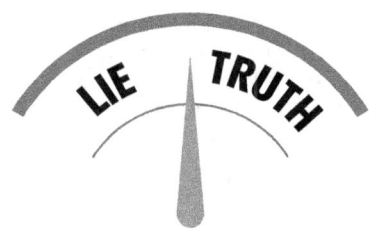

You're going to begin to unravel what your subconscious mind stored for you in your early life by tapping into what you're <u>really</u> feeling when you feel threatened. Take a deep breath... and again...

Please read the following Intention-Setting Moment as many times as you need until you feel an impressive commitment to this task. When you do, pledge your honesty, humility, and thoroughness to receive the assured outcomes of this training. When you feel the feeling of readiness, read it again out loud:

 INTENTION-SETTING MOMENT

> I will detect and describe who I've been being in my past and present. I will leave nothing out to save face. I will disclose all of me, collecting my insobriety so that it may be cleared out. There's nothing in me that must be kept hidden, for it's these things that are keeping me here, where my life isn't what I desire it to be.

Now, become an excellent detective and hold nothing back. Let's begin with a journey through time. Either continue reading below, or visit your member page at **liftedacademy.com/tyynm** to listen to a recorded version.

 TAKE ACTION

### MY LIFE MOVIE
Listen to the recording (recommended) or read through the following visualization a few times. Then, close your eyes, take a few deep breaths, and settle into a comfortable seat to rest inside the visualization for as long as you need.

**VISUALIZATION:** Imagine that you're sitting with all of your family members, friends, co-workers, coaches, teachers, romantic interests, etc. You're all in a movie theater and you're holding a remote control with a "stop" button. When everyone is settled in, a movie begins to play. Very quickly you realize that this is the movie of your life. Of course, you're the big star. Moving forward you notice that <u>every single moment</u> of your life is included in this film and that <u>every single person</u> you've ever known is sitting in this theater watching this film. They're watching the story of your life until the present day.

Write the first five stopping places.

*HINTS:*

- *Your stopping places are the ones you wish no one (including you) would ever have to see again.*
- *Write down your first five right away. Get them out now, as these are your biggest blocks.*
- *These moments may either be in the distant or recent past, and they usually involve the moments where your actions hurt others or yourself, and/or bring embarrassment, regret, or shame.*

Where in the film would I like to hit the stop button so no one will ever see what I see? Whom did I hurt? What did I do? What happened to me?

1. _____
2. _____
3. _____
4. _____
5. _____

Take a break, such as a walk or at minimum a few deep breaths and come back later to write down <u>all</u> of your stopping places.

Write these in list form—only a few words for now—enough for you to know what they mean. You'll use this as you continue your investigation.

---

After you've "watched your movie" for as long as you like, and outlined <u>all</u> of your stopping places, continue reading.

Before considering this, you may not have known that a particular event or memory was so impactful to you. When you put yourself in this scenario of watching your life on screen, the things that jump out at you are most likely the things that you've always known were there, somewhere deep inside. Or perhaps you've often thought about them, yet before today you hadn't consciously conversed with yourself about—or even admitted—them. These are the parts that you most want to be kept from seeing the light of day, desperately digging the hole deeper to stay buried within. You may have even been attempting to lie to yourself—convincing yourself that there's nothing there to bury. Remember these pesky thoughts: "I've already uncovered all of this. I'm fine!" or "But I'm a good person... they just don't understand me."

COACHING MOMENT

> Watching your "life movie" at this new level of detail and honesty will support your transformation. These parts you believe are the most repulsive are the obvious cracks within you, yet usually the most hidden inside of you in your day-to-day life. By thinking you can work around them and clean up all the rest, you'll have left the darker corners of your life untouched.
>
> I promise that keeping these memories, traumas, delivered traumas, acts, or experiences that you may find repulsive, embarrassing, or impossibly unfixable is a huge component of what keeps you sick and stuck with your problems.

If these parts that you don't want anyone to witness aren't looked at and released, you'll be unable to meet the *you* you've never met. That version will remain stuck... buried under the illusion of protective shields. You must promise to leave nothing out to save face and you must not attempt to save someone else's face by harming your own. When we leave the big pieces out, our work is just as incomplete as we feel.

You probably know children who flaunt their ability to tell the truth. Honesty is our natural state. You learned to lie, so what would happen if you now learned to tell the truth again? What if you learned to override your default dishonesty and create change toward self-exploration or even self-actualization?

CONTEMPLATION

**FEELING FLOW CHECK-IN**
Having simply acknowledged these moments, what are you feeling in your body? Your emotions? Any thoughts running the show?

TAKE ACTION

**IF EVERYONE REALLY SAW ME**
Next, fill in the following statement as many times as is necessary to further discover any remaining stopping places in "My Life Movie."

I want to hit the "stop button" when I think about this scene, person, or situation from my past... _____

_____ ,

because if everyone in the "movie theater" saw this, I'd feel _____

_____ .

*Your secrets keep you sick;
holding and protecting them for others will as well.*

In many cases at this point in the process people feel hopeless, lost, and without enough guidance. This is caused by biochemical confusion. I remember feeling this way—lack of faith, not believing I could ever get onto the path, stay on it, or see the other side of it. I felt a mix of self-hate with a flip-side of arrogance that I knew better. I felt unbelievably low self-esteem, yet at the same time stubbornness and refusal to see who I was really being.

Many people decide to enter a change process like this simply to control others and control their circumstances. Sometimes students of this work intend on staying just as they are, even while also being desperate to change, putting off their transformation only due to lack of real desire, courage or know-how.

Now that you've stirred some memories of your life, let's move on to what I call the EMSO Master Chart process. This was developed as I witnessed a clear pattern of where most people get stuck or quit, and where they continue to lie to themselves. I began to admire the people who would think to themselves, "Wow, I realize that I'm lying to myself right now! I feel fear writing that thought or memory down because that means it will be out. Even if I don't share this with anyone else, at least I'm admitting it to myself."

The EMSO Master Chart process contains 10 distinct areas of inquiry into your past and present, which are each clearly outlined (A–J) in this chapter and in the companion journal. You can easily find your copies of the blank chart in the back of the journal, on your free downloads page at **liftedacademy.com/tyynm**, or you can scan this code: Master charting is another non-negotiable for attaining Emotional Sobriety, so be sure to have a clean copy available before you proceed.

Here's what it looks like:

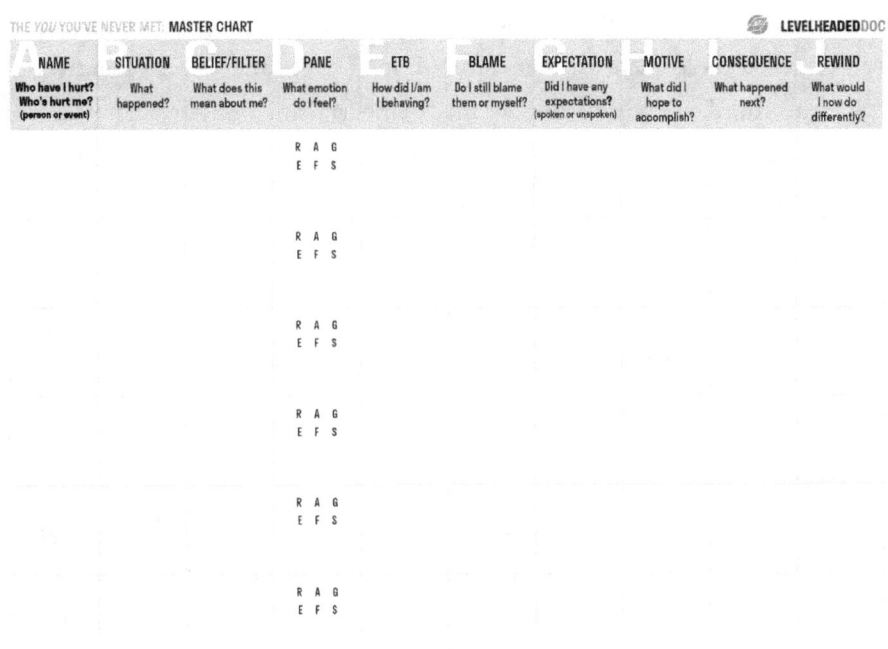

While all of the Take Actions will continue to be provided within the pages of this book, for the EMSO Investigations I highly recommend using "The *You* You've Never Met Companion Journal." This will allow you to keep your charts organized, with easy reference to the EMSO Master Chart Key, the associated Take Actions, and more. If you don't yet have a copy, it's available at **liftedacademy.com/store**.

Before we move on, I wonder if you know how courageous you are? What is courage? It's a power that can be greater than fear if you choose it to be, and it will save your future. I think of it as...

DEFINITION

**COURAGE:** going "all-in."

I find that the people who go "all-in" with this investigation have the greatest and most rapid transformation, and also see more immediate changes in their lives. They are also the kind of people who I want to be around. They are choosers. They are inspirational. They aren't letting their old patterns and traumas hold them back anymore. I don't judge the places within them that they think are wrong, or have made embarrassing or "terrible mistakes." Instead, I'm so proud of what they're choosing now and who they're intending to become. Let's now take our honesty and courage and continue.

*If you don't like who you've been or what you've done, don't be that same person today.*

### Column A: Name & Column B: Situation

Next, we explore the people, groups, and situations in your life that have been challenging, or that have left a lingering "bad taste in your mouth." They could be from your far or recent past. They could be people that you share your life with right now, such as your spouse, children, colleagues, or friends. In addition to the "Stopping Places" Take Action you've just completed, the following series of Take Actions will support you in the deeper discovery of your R.E.A.Life Investigation:

- Acknowledge Whom I've Hurt
- Body Signals
- PANEs by Age
- Institutional PANEs
- The Sex Scenes

Each exercise is carefully designed to support you in discovering who belongs in Column A: Names, and what details belong in Column B: Situation, on your EMSO Master Chart. Follow along one-by-one for clear guidance here, or as they're replicated in the companion journal.

If you don't like who you've been or what you've done, don't be that same person today. The first place we investigate is <u>you</u>: Whom have you harmed? Whom have you hurt?

TAKE ACTION

**ACKNOWLEDGE WHOM I'VE HURT**
Review your stopping places, and use the prompts below to acknowledge whom you've hurt. Did any of your ETBs hurt any of these people in your life?

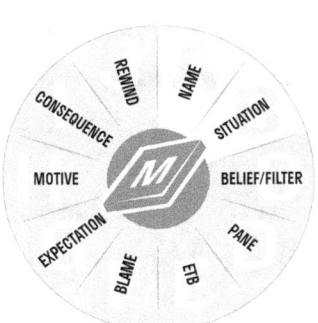

- Romantic interests/Partners
- Family members
- Children
- Friends/Acquaintances
- Co-workers
- Coaches
- Teachers/Mentors
- Strangers

 Now turn to your first blank EMSO MASTER CHART. These are the first people to write in Column A: NAMES. Then, add to Column B: SITUATION by writing what happened in "My Life Movie" with each person. Include yourself on this list, as well as those who've passed away.

REMINDER: Blank copies of the EMSO MASTER CHART are located in the back of the companion journal, downloadable for free at liftedacademy.com/tyynm, or available by scanning this code:

I lied to:

I physically hurt:

I emotionally manipulated:

I neglected, disregarded, or used:

I cheated on:

I bullied:

I stole from:

I hurt:

I'm impressed with your courage. This level of acknowledgment isn't something that most people ever do in their entire lives. The next Take Action is just as powerful, and a little more fun. Let's continue.

A great assistant for revealing the reality of your unsober state is to reflect on how your physical body is affected by your biochemical addiction. You can do this by witnessing its current state. This will give you more information and data that may urge you to move forward. Your emotional health is less obvious to observe. It takes practice to be in tune with your emotional body; however, the general state of your physical body is easier to notice as its messages can literally block your day-to-day life. You know you have blocks in your relationships due to emotional overwhelm, as these feelings, behaviors, and tendencies have been with you for a very long time. Your body is also a great indicator of your emotional state, as it took time for these ailments to show up due to the chronicity of your emotional addiction. By observing the state it's in, your body tells you whether or not you're chronically exposed to more damaging chemistry. It shows you both what you've been through in the past, and what you're still going through. Let's begin this exploration with a contemplation.

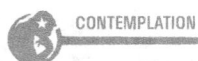

CONTEMPLATION

**MESSAGES FROM THE BODY**
Your body is likely communicating with you about things you may not be looking at. Symptoms within the body present themselves as a message regarding your overall state. Are you experiencing any of the following physical symptoms? Simply contemplate the following and observe the real state of your body, now and in the past.

- Chronic sickness (often catching colds, etc.)
- Recurrent pain in the skeletal muscle, joints (lower back, shoulder, knee, neck, hip, etc.)
- Easily injured
- Cardiovascular disorders (high blood pressure, arrhythmias, etc.)
- Respiratory issues
- Skin problems
- Metabolic or reproductive system dysfunction (thyroid issues, heavy cramping during menstruation, erectile issues, etc.)
- Fatigue
- Frequent headaches
- Excessive cravings
- Slow healing
- Stomach pain or intense digestive issues
- Compulsive bodily reactions (coughing/sneezing fits, etc.)
- Others?

If you struggle with physical ailments, consider them messages that <u>something</u> is hurting within you—and perhaps this "something" isn't the obvious physical pain or disease, but the stored dis-ease from your emotional insobriety. We'll acknowledging and begin to remove this biochemistry as well. I've come to believe that our physical pain, disorders, and diseases are presented to us after long periods of emotional/biochemical overdose.

Are these external disorders merely symptoms of our internal dis-order?

Our emotions don't communicate only through long-term messages such as these chronic symptoms, but also moment to moment through physical changes it presents. I call these short-term messages, "body signals." The following practice can give you many clues as to whom needs to be on your EMSO Master Chart, if you've inadvertently left anyone out in the previous Take Action.

TAKE ACTION

**BODY SIGNALS**
Get out your primary devices (phone, computer, tablet, etc.) and/or address book, and take a moment to slowly look through the names of people in your various contacts lists, inboxes, and friends lists.

As you read each name, pay attention to the changes within your body when you think about that specific person, group, or situation.

Do you feel any strangeness in your body (see list below for example)? This strange feeling indicates an unresolved issue, and that means this NAME must make it onto your EMSO MASTER CHART!

Add them now to Column A: NAMES on your EMSO MASTER CHART, and respond to the question in Column B: SITUATION for each.

Here are some things to feel for:
- Boiling sensation from legs to head (overwhelm)
- Shaking or rumbling in your solar plexus
- Acidity
- Fist clenching
- Jaw tension
- Stomach discomfort
- Tightness around the naval, wrapping around rib cage
- Nausea
- Dizziness
- Tingling

- Anxiety
- Nervousness
- Fatigue
- Squeezing of chest
- Lump or tension in throat
- Rectal changes
- Hunching of shoulders (hiding heart center)
- Becoming smaller
- Other: _____

These symptoms are a clear message. Checking in regularly with your body allows you to know if you have a lingering issue or an unresolved situation with someone or something. Listening allows for the opportunity to take action by alleviating what could be causing the problem.

**DO YOU RELATE?**

**Mary's looking through her phone during her EMSO Training attempting to find any name that she needs to have on her EMSO Master Chart. She sees the name "Tony" in her contacts list. A boiling sensation shoots through her body from head to toe, followed by a feeling of having been punched in the gut. She instantly recalls this situation: "I went on a dinner date with Tony about a year ago. I'd had a crush on him for several months prior. When we were at dinner, I noticed that he wasn't particularly flirty and didn't seem overly interested in me. At the end of the date, he didn't pay. He actually asked if we could split the check! I remember thinking throughout the date if it was even a date at all? But since he didn't say anything I was too nervous to ask. I was disappointed and angry about having to pay for my own dinner, and thought he would notice my disappointment via my huffing and irritation towards him at the table. When we said goodbye, he gave me a quick hug, and never called again. I'm still so angry! I wish I'd never even met him!"**

**On her EMSO MASTER CHART in Column A she writes "Tony" and in Column B: "Bad dinner date."**

We'll continue to follow Mary and Tony's process throughout this chapter, so stay tuned for what she discovers as we progress.

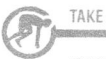
TAKE ACTION

### PANES BY AGE

Next, go a little more slowly, and review your life age by age, looking for any PANE that arises when you consider what was happening to you and around you during each of these time periods.

For each of the following ages, recall the individual people, groups, and situations with whom you were angry during that period of life, anyone you continue to harbor resentment toward, and with whom you feel guilty or embarrassed. Explore your fear and sadness during each age range.

 Then go to your EMSO MASTER CHART and add each new name from this exercise in a box in the Column A: NAME and share what happened in Column B: SITUATION. (The following pages include supportive prompts for completing this exercise.)

| AGE | RESENTMENT I was hurt by: | ANGER I was angry with: | GUILT This person made me feel guilt: | EMBARRASS-MENT This person embarrassed me: | FEAR I felt fear with: | SADNESS I felt sadness with: |
|---|---|---|---|---|---|---|
| 0–5 | | | | | | |
| 6–10 | | | | | | |
| 11–17 | | | | | | |
| 18–21 | | | | | | |
| 22–29 | | | | | | |
| 30–39 | | | | | | |
| 40–59 | | | | | | |
| 60–75 | | | | | | |
| 76+ | | | | | | |

**Age 0–5 (Baby & Toddler)**—Who were your primary caregivers, and who was in your family? What were the dramas, traumas, and frustrations of your childhood? During this period of life, was I embarrassed by anyone? Did anyone hurt me? Who am I currently still holding resentments against? Did anything from this time cause me to feel shame or guilt?

**Age 6–10 (Elementary School)**—Who was I around during this time? Again, who were the caregivers I spent the most time with? Do I recall not liking being around my caregivers? Siblings? Family members? Teachers? Classmates? Did I have enemies? Was I embarrassed by anyone? Did anyone hurt me? What was my family life like? What main events occurred at this time? Did I meet anyone new? Any large milestones that trigger memories of hurt or shame?

**Age 11–17 (Middle and High School)**—Who was I around in this timeline? Who were my best friends? Who were my romantic interests? Did I have enemies? Was I embarrassed by anyone? Did anyone hurt me? What was my family life like? What main events occurred at this time? Did I meet anyone new? Any large milestones that trigger memories of hurt or shame?

*Note: The traumatic experiences that influence who you've been being may not have occurred only at an early age. The following prompts will help you discover the moments when you were flooded with biochemistry and emotion later in life.*

**Age 18-21 (College-Age)**—Who was I around in this timeline? Who were my best friends? Who were my romantic interests? Did I have enemies? Was I embarrassed by anyone? Did anyone hurt me? What was my family life like? What main events occurred at this time? Did I meet anyone new? Any large milestones that trigger memories of guilt or pain?

**Age 22–29 (Early Adulthood)**—Who was I around in this timeline? Who were my closest friends? Who were my romantic interests? Did I have enemies? Was I embarrassed by anyone? Did anyone hurt me? What was my family life like? What main events occurred at this time? Did I meet anyone new? Any large milestones that trigger memories of trauma?

**Age 30–39**—Who was I around in this timeline? Who were my close friends? Who were my romantic interests? Did I have enemies? Was I embarrassed by anyone? Did anyone hurt me? What was my family life like? What main events occurred at this time? Did I meet anyone new? Any large milestones that trigger memories?

**Age 40–59**—Who was I around in this timeline? Who were my best friends? Who were my romantic interests? Did I have enemies? Was I embarrassed by anyone? Did anyone hurt me? What was my family life like? What main events occurred at this time? Did I meet anyone new? Any large milestones that trigger memories of harm?

**Age 60–75**—Who was I around in this timeline? What occurred when I retired from my career? Who were my best friends? Who were my romantic interests? Did I have enemies? Was I embarrassed by anyone? Did anyone hurt me? What was my family life like? What main events occurred at this time? Did I meet anyone new? Any large milestones that trigger memories of harm?

**Age 76 and on**—Who was I around most during this time? Who were my best friends? Who were my romantic interests? Did I have enemies? Was I embarrassed by anyone? Did anyone hurt me? What was my family life like? What main events occurred at this time? Did I meet anyone new? Any large milestones that trigger memories of harm?

In the same way you may experience various forms of PANEs with individuals, you may have had experiences with institutions that trigger your emotional insobriety as well. I've had countless students share with me the long-term effects of attending a religious elementary school or having been on a sports team. For example, perhaps school was an environment within which you experienced repeated struggle. Sometimes it's not a specific individual, but a group or entire institution that has contributed to your challenging biochemical addiction. Let's continue by identifying what these situations have been for you:

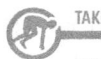
**TAKE ACTION**

**INSTITUTIONAL PANES**
What are the groups or institutions that you've encountered throughout your life for which you feel resentment, anger, guilt, embarrassment, fear, or sadness? These might be organizations, institutions, civic groups, schools, etc. If it helps to spark your memory, go age by age again.

*HINTS:*

- *Review your life experiences with your religion, school, workplace, civic organizations you've been a part of, and more.*

- *This is also where Observed Traumas are often noted. What situation did you observe that left you with PANEs? This could be something you saw or experienced as a first responder, doctor parent, counselor, etc.*

 Transfer the names of these groups and the situations to Column A: NAMES and Column B: SITUATION.

I resent: _____

I'm angry with: _____

I feel guilt around: _____

I'm embarrassed by: _____

I feel fear with: _____

I feel sadness about: _____

Lastly, turn your attention toward your intimate past. Sex is one of the most common ways to connect, yet it's also what you may be the least prepared for. Let's now complete Columns A & B by looking <u>only</u> at your sexual relationships—both romantic and non-romantic.

Why do you look here specifically? It seems to be an area of particular struggle that most exposes ETBs, and is therefore a gateway to your biochemical "hit." It's where you may tend to have fewer boundaries, excessive trauma filtering, and possibly either over-guard or over-give. Here you may notice you're most often attention-seeking, and all of your sickest patterns come most easily into play. Sexual and/or romantic relationships are an area of particular vulnerability that may lead to higher levels of shame and guilt. It's where you often go "backwards" in your growth if you're not on solid ground going in and not completely aware and honest with yourself and others.

We often seek to be loved or get attention, and therefore enter into romantic relationships with anyone who's willing. We do so without the consideration that it may not be the right fit, or it may even be harmful to ourselves or the other person. A real relationship rooted in honesty and vulnerability may be so foreign to us that we don't even know to look for it.

> *Sex is one of the most common ways to connect, yet what we may be the least prepared for.*

Sex is often viewed as a very delicate topic and an area in which people get confused, hurt, or make "mistakes." This is often associated with many negative emotions which have stemmed from shame, resulting all the way from sexual trauma to basic romantic "failures." Know that what most people feel shame for is usually quite normal within the scope of human experience.

Shame is known as the lowest vibration emotion. Our vibration is the energy we emit via our state of being. An example of a high level of vibration would be that of joy, love, and peace… or dare I say levelheadedness! Our lower states of vibration, such as chronic negative biochemical overdosing, can cause physical illness and limit our enjoyment in life. David Hawkins, M.D. shares about the vibration level of shame in his book "Transcending the Levels of Consciousness—The Stairway to Enlightenment." He writes: "Early life experiences such as neglect, or physical, emotional or sexual abuse lead to shame and warp the personality for a lifetime unless these issues are later resolved. It is destructive to emotional and psychological health and in some cases can cause physical illness."[15] This means that shame is harmful to the individual than anger, or even hate. This is why it's so important for us to raise our vibrational frequency away from shame by realizing our past is not so different than everyone else's, and that we can choose to be free of the influences from our past right now.

The most powerful portion of the sexual relationship review is to first become aware and acknowledge that you've hurt others in the past due to your ETBs. Then the work is to disconnect from the beliefs you formed and behaviors with which you unconsciously and habitually re-act in order to move forward with more healthy and genuine relationships. You'll also use this process to relieve yourself from any resentments, anger, or shame you may be carrying due to sexual experiences that have hurt you.

Look at both your romantic and non-romantic sexual contact. Some examples may include pornographic addiction, molestation, rape, incest, affairs, etc. In addition, people who suffer from religious abuse or sexual prejudice may feel shame from youth that is carried into adulthood.

**COACHING MOMENT**

I've known very few people who weren't terrified when sharing their sexual story with me, as they viewed themselves as repulsive, disgusting, or embarrassing. They felt intense levels of shame. While in reality, there has never been a sex discussion that has shocked me; as difficulties in these relationships—like all other parts of our lives—were created through our Trauma Filters. I can so clearly see them in each person, and therefore there could never be judgment of their experiences and actions. I urge you to see and do the same for yourself right now.

**TAKE ACTION**

**THE SEX SCENES**
With whom have you had either romantic or non-romantic sexual relationships? Where in your life movie did you hit the stop button during a sex scene? List them all on the following page, or at the very least, those whom you've hurt or who've hurt you.

*HINTS:*

- *If it helps prompt your memory, go age by age again.*

- *This is completely confidential between you and you right now. Be specific and thorough.*

- *If shame arises, feel it and write it anyway. If the paper gets wet from your tears as you remember past love or difficulties, dry off the page and continue.*

Add these to Column A: NAMES and what happened in Column B: SITUATION on your EMSO MASTER CHART.

Romantic Sexual Partners:

Non-romantic Sexual Partners:

Did you ever have a subtle connection with someone and romanticize it to make it more serious than it was? This would be an example of attention-seeking behavior—an ETB—triggered by neediness, believing you're unimportant, or having low self-esteem. Were you self-centered, jealous, physically abusive (<u>any</u> physical harm), or manipulative in any of your sexual relationships? Did you cheat, steal, or lie to them or yourself? Were you hypocritical (what was okay for you to do but intolerable for them)? As you add each to your EMSO Master Chart, be specific and get real about what happened in each relationship.

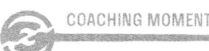 COACHING MOMENT

When you complete the intimate past portion of your cleansing process, it can be difficult to look at. Remember that most of us have the same shame, guilt, trauma, and hurt. We found dishonesty, manipulations, and regrets when we revisited these parts of our past. This is a big part that really begins to open our eyes to who we've been being. You may feel miserable in observing who you've been, but I invite you to instead choose to feel the inevitable freedom from your patterns by first becoming aware of them, and now acknowledging them.

Upon deep reflection and completion of our EMSO Master Charts, some of us were shameful for how we were treated and what we experienced, while others are guilt-ridden for how we treated others. Most were even shocked at how misplaced their anger was toward their exes when they looked at their part in the relationship. Some were able to see where they were contributing drama, lies, arrogance, control, manipulation, and more. Many even exclaimed, "Oh my gosh, I'm such a jerk!" (harsher language usually used here).

If you're like the majority of us who have struggled with emotional insobriety, you may have had many "failed" relationships. By looking closely and realistically at who you've been being in your relationships, you can see that you no longer need to do these things, because these things will bring forth confusion and more "failed" relationships. As you advance in EMSO Training, those behaviors can dissolve and you'll move away from guilt and shame, anger and hate, and into productivity, and eventually, healthy relationships.

Do you now understand that you, like your previous partners, may have been caught up in thoughtless, reactive, and ETBs? You cannot know their traumas completely and what they've seen or experienced. You may not be able to see through their eyes or feel what they feel, but now that you're becoming more consciously aware of yourself, you can choose to make different choices in your relationships and be respectful of others and their pasts.

### Column C: Belief/Filter

As you've probably guessed, what you've now completed in Columns A&B contain the bulk of the work for your R.E.A.Life Investigation. The following three columns should go smoothly if you did the work in your EMSO Foundations to truly get over yourself and get real with what you're *actually* thinking, feeling, and doing. If you know your Anatomy of Emotional Insobriety, this should be a clear process.

I've watched countless people continue to suffer by thinking that if they focus solely on changing their behaviors or feeling the previously unfeelable emotions, that they would change. However, this is a dead end. It's <u>only</u> when we also investigate, question, and eventually replace our Trauma-Influenced Self-Beliefs and the Trauma Filters that we actually become free from our emotional insobriety and Intoxicated Identities.

As I've shared, when you complete this portion of the training, it can offer you an awakening, and I'm delighted you've made it to this point where you're ready to look at what you've bene believing about yourself in relation to each person, group, and situation on your EMSO Master Chart. Now is a good time to review your Anatomy of Emotional Insobriety as well as the common beliefs, as some new ones may pop up as you continue here.

TAKE ACTION

**BELIEF/FILTER: What does this mean about me?**
Use your developing self-awareness from EMSO Foundations to identify the self-belief that this particular person, group, or situation validates about you.

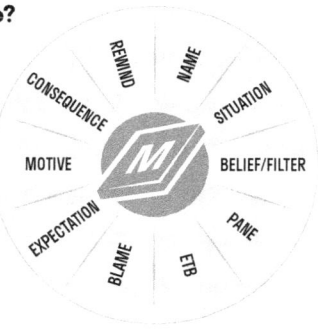

 Fill in Column C: BELIEF/FILTER with the code from the key on page 91 in the companion journal for each line on your EMSO MASTER CHART to identify the appropriate Trauma Filter(s) and/or write out the Trauma-Influenced Self-Belief if that helps you.

This [situation] was difficult because of my Trauma-Influenced Self-Belief(s) of: _____

I may be filtering this person, group, or situation through my Trauma Filter(s) of: _____

_____

DO YOU RELATE?

Revisiting Mary's EMSO Master Chart, after reviewing her date with Tony, she shared, "When I think about what Tony's behavior meant about me, I realize that I believe that I'm unlovable, rejectable, and unimportant. To me, when he asked me to pay, that was proof of my unimportance. When he didn't call me after that night, it was proof of my rejectability and unlovability. In Column C she writes UL (unlovable), UI (unimportant), and RJ (rejection).

## Column D: PANE

If you've made it to this point in your EMSO Training, you're probably aware that you've harnessed some "bad" feelings toward some of your past experiences. I invite the perspective that if there's something in your heart other than love, start cleaning house. In order to clear these pieces out, you first must have awareness, and then acknowledgment. Let's continue the 4A Formula with more acknowledgment of the *you* you'd never noticed.

You recall from developing the awareness of your Anatomy of Emotional Insobriety, that what you're really addicted to is the biochemistry that you associate with your emotions, or what we call PANEs: Predominant Accompanying Negative Emotions. We delved into the six most common: resentment, anger, guilt, embarrassment, fear, and sadness, and you identified your most dominant addictive emotion.

The next step in your EMSO Investigations is to clearly identify which emotions were the most present with each person, group, or situation on your EMSO Master Chart.

Before continuing to work directly on your EMSO Master Chart, let's spend a little more time understanding the Common PANEs, one by one.

DEFINITION

**RESENTMENT:** continued bitterness regarding having been seemingly treated unfairly by someone else.

Resentment often shows up when you have an expectation. You'll know that you had an expectation if you feel disturbed in your body when the thing you thought should happen or that you wanted them to do or say doesn't occur. For example, Mary expected Tony to pay and to show interest in her, thus leaving her with leftover production of resentment.

DEFINITION

**ANGER:** an immense "burning" of pain, directed at someone who was believed to have caused it.

You'll know that anger is present with someone on your EMSO Master Chart when you read their name and feel a rush of "fire" and sometimes hate. You may have a thought that you want to become physically violent, vengeful, or punishing in some way. Even if you haven't actually directed your anger outwardly, you may also be feeling humiliation or resentment, as these often dance together.

DEFINITION

**GUILT:** self-resentment or the feeling of having done something wrong or failed obligation.

Guilt is a by-product of what you've done (often delivered by your own experience with expectation being placed on you). For example, forced obligation of family, societal traditions, and more may invoke guilt. It's often associated with the beliefs "I'm a bad person" and "I should be ashamed."

DEFINITION

**EMBARRASSMENT:** a strong feeling of being exposed, overly-observed, objectified, or made a joke.

Embarrassment is when you feel like you've been or are being judged, overly-observed, or criticized, or you make a mistake that brings attention to yourself. It's most obvious when you look at where you're hiding. You can even ask yourself, "Why am I hiding this?" and "What feeling comes up in me when I think about revealing this out loud?"

Resentment, anger, guilt, and embarrassment are perhaps some of the simplest emotions to identify while getting in touch with your past. These often come with a lot of changes in body chemistry, and therefore access to your memory and attention. However, there may be other emotions behind or alongside these, including fear and sadness. You can discover these by continuing to ask the question: "Do I really feel this way?" again and again until you feel what's <u>actually</u> true for your experience. This part can be difficult for those who have come from families that didn't communicate feelings or primarily communicated through anger or shaming. Or for those who have familial or societal programs of strict religion or lineage influences.

### DEFINITION

**FEAR: a feeling of helplessness.**

When you're trapped in fear, you're demonstrating that you have little to no faith in a power greater than your problems. You're expressing your belief that you're helpless. It comes from a place where you lack trust in others, and also in yourself.

Anger and other more outward emotions often hide the feeling of fear. It's the "big dog" that comes out to defend. Loneliness, depression, and fatigue can all be confused with the outward appearance of anger, even in the person who's experiencing the emotion. An example of anger camouflaging fear would be in the case of betrayal. Often, the feeling of fear within betrayal is really disbelief and confusion as to why an expectation was not met, or anger from the trapped desire for something to have gone differently.

### CONTEMPLATION

**FEELING FEAR**
Look for where in your "life movie" that you've been fearful in the past.
Did what you were fearing actually happen?

Finally, let's get a bit more specific about the nature of sadness.

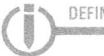
### DEFINITION

**SADNESS**: a feeling of hopelessness.

Sadness is an emotion that we lay over things such as a fight with a friend or bad news about a job interview. However in greater extremes, sadness over a traumatic loss is actually <u>grief</u> and isn't related to your insobriety or something to overcome.

Obviously, there are circumstances that are very tragic and when feeling excessive grief, it's best to be overseen by a healthcare professional and/or ask for help from your immediate community. These are not questions for someone who's grieving the death of a loved one, for example, but it's good to answer these questions realistically for other related experiences that invoke sadness.

### CONTEMPLATION

**SENSING SADNESS**
Where in your life are you currently feeling sadness? Contemplate: When did I come to believe that I was hopeless?

With this deeper exploration into the common PANE, you'll continually seek what's <u>actually</u> there. For example, sadness always has a component of loss. Fear and sadness can be considered "negative" emotions as they deplete your energy, but they can also spark a clearing... an opening up of your future. This is of course only if you work <u>through</u> them instead of sitting <u>within</u> them. Most of the time you may feel sadness and fear together, and it usually falls into the theme of someone or something validating your Trauma-Influenced Self-Beliefs. This "validation" collects both your sadness and fear that it may be true. Sometimes the process of changing your long-standing identity can create a normal level of sadness and fear. You're saying goodbye to who you used to be. You're saying hello to someone you've never met.

Overcoming your biochemical addiction to fear and sadness is more of an Advanced Practice in EMSO Training. Ridding yourself of resentment, anger, guilt, and embarrassment is often simpler than removing fear and sadness because they're usually pushed down within, whereas anger is more often expressed outwardly.

Now that you may have a better grasp on how to search for the real emotion, it's time to identity the dominant PANE on your EMSO Master Chart. Use the following Take Action, as well as all of your continued awareness of emotions to get to what you were really feeling.

COACHING MOMENT

It's common to have difficulty translating all of your challenging emotions into one of these six. Remember to refer to the PANE graphic on page 70 and find the one that most closely resembles what you're feeling. For example, "anxious" usually boils down to fear.

TAKE ACTION

**PANE: What emotion do I feel?**
This is your chance to uncover what you're truly feeling in relation to each person, group, or situation on your EMSO MASTER CHART. It's important to know what you're feeling—not what you or others think you should be feeling, nor what you wish you were feeling.

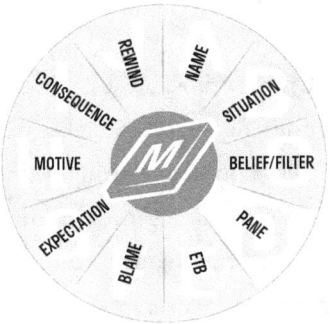

 Fill in Column D: PANE for each line on your EMSO MASTER CHART by circling the letter(s) for the emotion(s) that most closely matches what you feel.

*HINT: It's common to have more than one PANE (emotion).*

Because I've convinced myself that [belief/filter], I now feel: _____
_____.

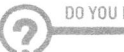
DO YOU RELATE?

Regarding Tony, Mary first identifies anger and resentment as her PANEs. However, after deeper consideration and looking for what she was actually feeling at the time, she states, "I really felt fear and sadness in those moments that my beliefs were validated. These feelings came from when I interpreted his actions (or inactions) to mean that he didn't like me. I felt these feelings because I thought I really wanted a romantic relationship with him. I had a rush of fear as my filter of rejection came up to stand guard. I also felt embarrassment, believing it meant I'm not lovable or important. I can now see that it wasn't anger and resentment, these were simply the feelings that came up to protect me from feeling embarrassment, fear, and sadness."

In Column D, she circles "E" (embarrassment), "F" (fear), and "S"(sadness).

How many experiences in your life might have gone differently had you been levelheaded, patient, and considerate of yourself and others, rather than flooded by emotion and thereby making meaning out of?

These tools aren't for you to blame yourself, but to spark the questions... what if I'd been different? How would my life have been different? What if I become different now? How will my life look different from now on? How will it be more enjoyable, easy and free? The following exercises help you establish that difference and to make your life not merely manageable, but blissful.

Did you successfully acknowledge your PANEs? Then you've completed one of the most essential parts of your path to change. Because this opportunity is yours, you'll be able to add any details that you may have forgotten whenever they arise at a later date. With more training, you'll also become an expert at working through resentment or frustration with people if and when it comes up in your day-to-day life. You've begun to take responsibility for your insobriety. When we take responsibility for the condition of our lives, we're empowered to change it.

Amazing job! By now, you may have quite a comprehensive list of people, groups, and situations that have made an impact on your life in one way or another. And you've identified the self-beliefs and the predominant feelings— PANEs—present with each of them. Now, let's explore what behaviors you demonstrated and may be continuing even today.

## Column E: ETB

We come to the all-important ETBs! These are our most obvious insobriety symptom, and they're the outward expression of our unresolved Trauma-Influenced Self-Beliefs and PANEs. It's highly likely that a person, group, or situation made it onto your EMSO Master Chart because of an ETB that you, they, or both delivered. Given how deeply we explored your ETBs during the EMSO Foundations portion of this work, I imagine this next part will go quite smoothly, so let's dive right into the Take Action:

TAKE ACTION

**ETB: How did I/am I behaving?**
Get specific with which ETB(s) is at play with each person, group, and situation on your EMSO Master Chart.

 Fill in Column E: ETB with the specific behavior(s) you displayed. Use the code(s) from the key on page 91 in the companion journal.

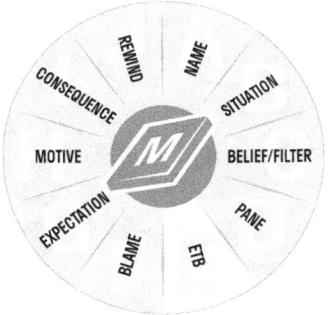

The emotion I felt compelled me to behave in this way with this person, group, or in this situation:

___

DO YOU RELATE?

In Mary's process she shared, "I can completely see my Anatomy of Emotional Insobriety here in my experience with Tony! I was self-centered by making his actions about me and my self-beliefs. I was defensive and judgmental when he didn't buy my dinner. I was dishonest because I didn't tell him how I really felt about him or ask if it could be a date. I was childish for huffing and making a scene at the restaurant."

In Column E, she adds self-centeredness (SC), childishness (CH), judgmentalism (JG), defensiveness (DF), and dishonesty (DH).

## Column F: Blame

Now we look at where you may be blaming the person, group, or situation for your PANEs. Also consider if you may be blaming yourself. You'll know you're blaming because you're still holding them or yourself responsible. There's not yet freedom. Let me give you a taste of freedom!

TAKE ACTION

**BLAME: Do I still blame them or myself?**

Fill in Column F: BLAME, indicating why you blame each person, group, or situation, and/or if you blame yourself for what happened.

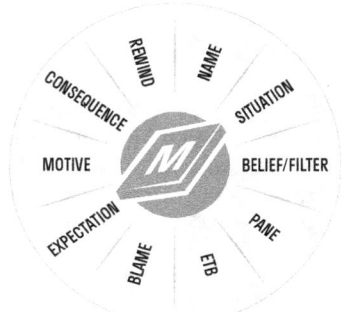

I blame _____

for my PANE because _____ .

DO YOU RELATE?

Mary said, "Initially, I only blamed Tony for the bad date. Now that I look at this from his point of view, I'm horrified with myself! Now I'm carrying self-blame for how I treated him.

In Column F, she writes: "me."

## Column G: Expectation

Expectation appears in this process when you look at the person, group, or situation and feel a disturbance in your body or any destructive emotion following their action or inaction. If you circled "R" (resentment) in Column D, you may want to investigate whether there's an expectation of yours that was not met in this relationship or situation. The Take Action is simple:

TAKE ACTION

**EXPECTATION: Did I have any expectations? (spoken or unspoken)**

 Fill in Column G: EXPECTATION with specifics about what the expectations are or were with each person, group, or situation on your EMSO Master Chart. Indicate if these were spoken or unspoken.

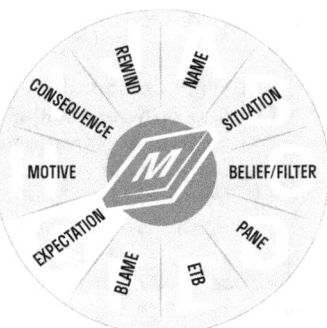

I had/have expectations of _____,

which specifically include _____.

 DO YOU RELATE?

Mary had many expectations of Tony and the date. "I expected Tony to romance me to prove I was lovable and attractive. I expected him to pay for my dinner and to choose me as his girlfriend, or I wouldn't have had bad feelings when he didn't. I expected that he'd call me to find out what he did wrong when I huffed and acted distant at the end of the date.

In Column G, she writes: it was a date, he'd romance me, pay for me, ignore my behavior and still choose me.

## Column H: Motive

We took at deep look into motive in Chapter 24. Here's your chance to see precisely where various motives have come into play in your past and present life through the lens of the EMSO Master Chart. Stop and think authentically about what your motive is or was with each person, group, or situation.

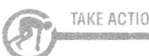 TAKE ACTION

**MOTIVE: What did I hope to accomplish?**

 Fill in Column H: MOTIVE for each line on your EMSO MASTER CHART with an explanation of what you were hoping to accomplish by using the ETBs that you did with each person, group, or situation.

*HINT: Use the Common Motives graphic on page 216 to aid you.*

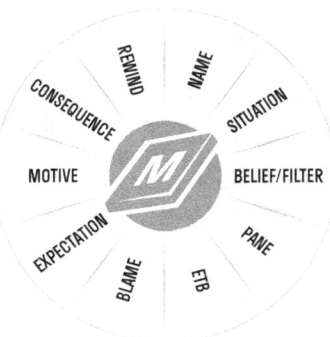

I behaved this way in order to

_____.

After your first past, look at each name/situation a second time and deeply ponder what you were thinking at the time of the event or during the relationship. Why did you truly do what you did? What motivated your behavior?

 DO YOU RELATE?

In the process of charting her experience with Tony, Mary realized "I had underlying motives of wanting to get attention and to be chosen, as well as have control over my life and relay without words that I was the 'catch of his life.' I also now recognize that I wanted to gain security through having this relationship, to prove that I was important or lovable. I had the motive to behave in these ways in order to both test and punish him."

In Column H, she writes: get attention, be important, be lovable, test and punish.

## Column I: Consequence

Sometimes, acknowledging the hurt you've caused can make you fear the consequences. Ignoring it will make you sicker, just as ignoring the hurt you've experienced will. By seemingly guarding yourself from consequence, you're actually stalling your chances at a better life—keeping you in position to relive your past over and over, and making the same "mistakes" again and again. Although we'll go deeper into the nuances around consequence later on, I'd like to shed some light on the topic and use this in the EMSO Master Chart to help you further investigate each person, group, or situation in your life.

Become acquainted with the word <u>consequence</u>. To me, it simply means,

**DEFINITION**

**CONSEQUENCE:** what happens next—after something.

Every day, you make decisions. No matter the nature of the decision, there's always a consequence. There can be painful consequences, or even wonderful consequences following any given decision. Know the power that you have over your life by virtue of your choices. You get to decide who you want to be, how you want to feel, what you're going to think, and what you're going to do.

**TAKE ACTION**

**CONSEQUENCE: What happened next?**

 Fill in Column I: CONSEQUENCE with an explanation of what happened next. Did you lose anything? Did things remain the same?

After my experience with this person, group, or situation, this happened next: _____

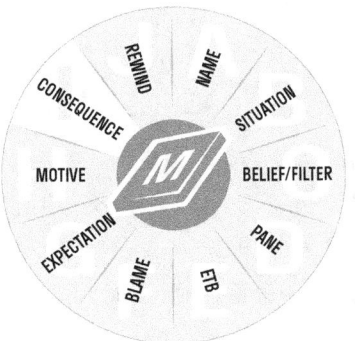

Do you imagine your life would improve, if in the future—before you acted—you ask yourself the simple question: When I make this choice, what might happen next?

I recall asking myself questions such as: "How could a different level of maturity have saved me from being hurt or harming others? If I had made different decisions related to this harm, what different outcomes may I have experienced? How could I have made a different decision and not harmed someone else? How could I have made a different decision and not put myself in a position to feel hurt, angry, embarrassed, or afraid?"

This is another opportunity to decide which behaviors you'll embrace going forward when you've completed this process. Which behaviors will demonstrate your new knowledge of your power, increased maturity, level-headedness, and compassion? How will you now pay attention to yourself and how you think, feel, and behave in new ways?

 DO YOU RELATE?

> Returning once again to our process with Mary and Tony: At this point, Mary's now deeply contemplating her emotional insobriety in the situation and realizes new components to add to her EMSO MASTER CHART: "I was childish because I didn't tell Tony (directly) what I really desired. I was thinking for him when I made assumptions when he didn't pay attention or flirt with me. I'm embarrassed for how I behaved at the restaurant—being huffy and judgmental of him."
>
> In Column I, she writes: Lost opportunity due to ETBs and not being real.

## Column J: Rewind

In "My Life Movie," you identified where you would want to hit the "stop button." But what if you could also rewind, or have a do-over? Your "rewind" helps to clearly identify the moments when you had a part in creating the problem. Let me explain...

One of my favorite quotes by author Richard Bach is: "Argue for your limitations, and sure enough they are yours."[16] What he's saying is that when you argue for your limitations, you get to keep your limitations. An argument is often in the form of an excuse. When you argue for your PANE, you get to keep it.

In this case, by not taking responsibility for your own behaviors, or defending why you should continue to be angry or resentful, you're limiting yourself. By limiting yourself, you get to keep your problems. Did you know that the real you has one of the most attractive trait? It's self-responsibility, and by continuing the EMSO Master Chart process you will discover it within you.

*Self-responsibility develops self-sufficiency
and eliminates outsider influence on our inner peace.*

If you want to be further empowered, here's your opportunity. You're going to have to jump headfirst into a new level of maturity by taking responsibility for yourself, your life, and all of its circumstances. (Yes, I said all.) You'll choose to use the new abilities that you learn here to respond differently to the influence from your past traumas. Your level of willingness to take responsibility is an example of your courage. If you've been abused, your negative behaviors are most likely a product of self-protection, but now you can utilize the impact of your traumas by tapping into your resilience.

Self-responsibility develops self-sufficiency and eliminates outsider influence on our inner peace. It frees us from being enslaved by our resentful emotions and keeps us out of the vibration of victimhood, which eliminates future pain.

How much pain could you have saved yourself and others if you'd always been mature, levelheaded, secure, honest, straightforward, peaceful, and brave? Again, you're not blaming or judging your past self, rather observing who you were. How different would your life have looked if you'd been in charge of all of your thoughts, feelings, and behaviors? If you could've responsibly handled any and every situation, what might be different for you now?

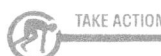
TAKE ACTION

**REWIND: What would I now do differently?**
By answering this question for each person, group, and situation on your EMSO Master Chart, you'll discover what your part was in each situation. This is self-responsibility.

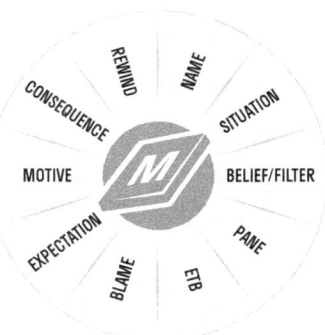

 Fill in Column J: REWIND with the answer to that question for each person, group, and situation on your EMSO MASTER CHART. To support you in better understanding what you would now do differently, read the following examples:

*HINT: This isn't about regret, this is simply about rewinding and practicing making new decisions using old events!*

- I would be honest.
- I would think more about them.
- I wouldn't have expectations.
- I wouldn't judge them or be hypocritical.
- I would communicate more.
- I wouldn't emotionally manipulate.
- I wouldn't follow along with the crowd.
- I would love more openly rather than be so fearful and attached.
- I wouldn't express my anger in that way.
- I wouldn't keep that harmful secret.

DO YOU RELATE?

Mary's rewind looked like this regarding Tony and their "bad date":

"I would have told Tony up front that I would like this to be a date and that I was interested in him. I would have asked him if he intended it to be a date. I would have decided to communicate how I felt instead of waiting for him to do what I was 'secretly' expecting. My expectation created resentment when it didn't go according to what I imagined.

I never attempted to contact him because I thought I was angry. I realize that I was actually fearful and ashamed, and I felt uncomfortable every time I merely thought of him. I missed the opportunity to have something real with him. Therefore, thinking for him and due to my dishonesty, I actually may have hurt both of us.

In Column J, she writes: If I could do it differently, prior to that date I would connect with myself about how I really felt. I'd be clear and communicative with Tony, instead of assuming the date should be what I thought it should be. I would be the real me! The one who's strong and happy, and curious about others. I would have had fun and gotten to know Tony for who he was, not the attention and validation I compulsively believed I needed him to offer me."

Can you see how detailed Mary gets when she looks at the date with Tony from the angle of a "rewind"? She really searched for all the ways she could have been more mature, levelheaded, and considerate of herself and the other person, which could have saved her and him from emotional pain. This included unnecessary resentment, anger, embarrassment, and fear. Working it through to the end ensures it will likely not return. She's now free from her PANEs within this situation. Although this isn't the case for every experience, this one was overcome by seeing who she was <u>actually</u> being at the time, and what she could have done differently. Feel the power in that!

Like Mary, I invite you to pay attention to whether or not embarrassment is playing a role in why you may be holding onto anger and resentment. This is either insecurity or plain embarrassment for doing something you regret. "What could I have done differently?" is an excellent exercise for reprogramming your insecurities and lingering embarrassments.

When you become aware of and acknowledge your "mistakes," you're giving yourself an easy way to reduce the likelihood of making them again. This process is a natural course-correction that allows for a new possibility to take place in the future. Also, by noting what you would now do differently, and by choosing to take responsibility for these moments and your part in them, you may feel as though you've rewritten the past, and in some cases, it presents as if you actually did.

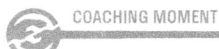
**COACHING MOMENT**

I've made countless "mistakes" and been through this same process. If you're struggling with seeing your part in something that you're angry about, or you feel offended that you're even being asked to do this, that may be an indicator that you're in the perfect moment to be doing this exercise. It's new, it's scary, it's transformational, and no matter what "mistakes" you've made, you absolutely deserve transformation.

If in your EMSO Master Chart process you couldn't think or feel anything, then move forward and maybe you'll be enlightened to something further on in the training and will choose to come back to this process. This challenging but essential investigation into your deepest truth builds a stronger bridge between your current life and the *you* you've never met.

**29**

# A Taste of Freedom

*With freedom comes great responsibility,
but with self-responsibility comes great freedom.*

Now you can move on to the most liberating portions of your EMSO Training. When you can begin training to release your connection to the negative emotions of resentment and anger, and the debilitating constraints of judgments, childish behaviors, and more, they'll no longer have any influence on your life.

As you continue, you'll likely notice that you left some things out on your EMSO Master Chart, and you may want to go back and update with more "real eyes" as you move on. In my experience, the first round is often incomplete—sometimes by choice or by unconscious avoidance. Sometimes, you won't even see the things you most need to write down—especially the part that you played in a challenging situation or relationship. Sometimes, your resentment and anger are there primarily due to the harm that you personally caused in the situation. The negative feelings toward the other may really be the embarrassment you feel for the harm you caused. Or, a fearful feeling that some part of you will be exposed by this person will transfer to feeling resentment toward that person.

---

*If you desire to be someone different in the future,
you must become this person now.*

This is all a subconscious reflex—to not want to <u>do</u> something different, to not want to <u>be</u> something different, or to not have faith that you can. But if you desire to be someone different in the future, you must become this person now—even if just for a moment. Try on the feeling of being super-courageous and search even deeper for the honesty about your past and current thoughts, beliefs, and behaviors. Don't allow your ego to undermine you, or to take charge. The ego gets frightened and pulls us back. Challenge it with love. Talk to your body and let it know that it's okay to change. It will be so much more comfortable and safer for all.

Take a moment to look back at the Common ETBs, or the uncooperative, destructive behaviors that contributed to the creation of stress in your life and the lives of people around you. If you recognize any of these traits in yourself—past or present—they may assist you to recall more details for this next step in your EMSO Training. You can begin to ask yourself:

- What if this problem, or part of it, could be <u>my</u> responsibility?
- What if I had thought, believed, or behaved differently?
- What if this problem could really be over?

Many people struggle with self-responsibility, as it is where we choose victory over victimhood. Choosing to find out what part of any situation might have been your part, is brave.

When you can more clearly see your part in your problems, in who you've hurt, and in your intimate past, you're liberated. You can shift your perspective by realizing that you're not punishing the person you resent as much as you are being punished. You can never hate someone enough to heal. Ask yourself "Who's my suffering helping?" "What's my responsibility? My part?" "If <u>I</u> changed, would <u>this</u> change?" If yes, then this is your part in the situation.

*You can never hate someone enough to heal.*

Destroy your connection to the PANE that holds you back from your happier and freer life. Let's go! You can do this. Remember that you set an intention to be transparently honest with yourself and you desire to change your life! Time for a Self-Honesty Checkpoint:

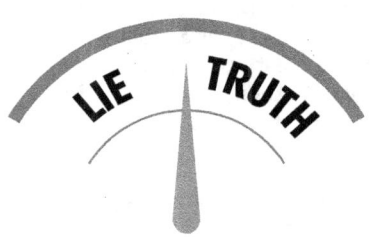

Did finding your part in each situation from your movie via your rewind take you by surprise? Some are reluctant to look at their responsibility in creating (or sustaining) the discord in their life. However, with greater clarity and openness around finding your part in each situation, you'll experience real freedom surrounding it.

 TAKE ACTION

**MY PART = MY RESPONSIBILITY**
Take this opportunity to reflect on the lines on your EMSO MASTER CHART that surprised you the most when you realized that you actually had a part in creating the situation. Take responsibility in a new way and notice the freedom that comes with it. Repeat this with as many people, groups, or situations as needed.

REMEMBER: We're all the same. You're not alone.

I acknowledge that the part I played in the experience with _____

was _____.

I now take responsibility for my part in this.

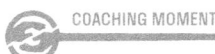 **COACHING MOMENT**

Self-responsibility isn't about blaming yourself, and this exercise is not about looking closely at what the other person has done to you. This is about changing the way you respond to a "harm" done by seeing the situation as a whole and relating to both sides. I'm suggesting that you seek to see your possible similarities in suffering with the person you're blaming or where you could be responsible. I'm not asking you to be friends with people who have harmed you. I'm asking you to be open to the possibility that they may have harmed you as an unconscious response to their own traumatic event.

 **DO YOU RELATE?**

***WARNING:** Please be aware that the following scenario includes a more severe trauma and therefore strangulated resentment. A filter resulting from this may be more challenging to mitigate, but it can also be done, as it was for Abigail!*

Abigail shares: "An adult family friend touched me quite inappropriately when I was seven years old. My part/role/responsibility in this situation is that I was inconsiderate of myself for believing I had to continue to see him every Christmas. I believed I had to be happy and kind to him. I always felt uneasy and fearful around him, even when I grew up. Yet I somehow felt the compulsion to constantly protect this secret by being extra friendly to him, as if to let him think I didn't recall the event. I was really embarrassed every time I was around him or if his name was brought up, and this was followed up with pangs of anger. I realize now that I'm empowered by choice. I have the choice to remove myself from any event where he'll be present, and I have can overcome my anger, embarrassment, and shame."

To truly embody what you've just learned about yoursef, you're going to require a few additional tools, including what you've heard me refer to as "EMSO Advanced Practices." In the beginning of the next section, I offer an introduction to a few of them to support this next step on your journey. Let's take a nice, big exhale and explore these essential principles.

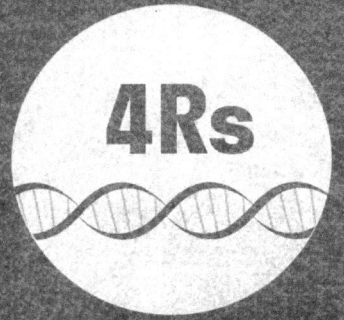

# EMSO REPAIRS
### THE *YOU* YOU'RE REVEALING

## 30

# Choose Freedom

*It's an illusion to think you cannot choose who you are.*

Now, we turn our attention toward the third and final component of the EMSO Essentials, or what we call "EMSO Repairs." For this, I've designed the 4Rs, and the next four chapters will outline each one, leading you to the essential practice of making repairs. I consider this one of the most healing components of EMSO Training.

Before we dive into the 4Rs, let's pause and once again check in with your emerging self—the real you—the one who's always been here but has merely been covered up by your unconscious beliefs and behaviors.

Review the snapshot of your Anatomy of Emotional Insobriety on page 153. Please don't be discouraged by reviewing each component, as they're actually highlighting your potential growth by showing you more precisely where you're beginning, which also helps inform what you intend to change. This will allow you to see objective growth as you continue to engage this process. Your potential is your opportunity. For example, if one of your ETBs is dishonesty, this becomes a gateway for you to choose and train honesty. Your self-centeredness may become your altruism. In EMSO Training, your weakness becomes your greatest strength.

*In EMSO Training, your weakness becomes your greatest strength.*

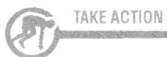

**TAKE ACTION**

### THE REAL ME, PART 3*: BLUEPRINT OF THE REAL ME

In the left-hand column, rewrite the most obvious Trauma-Influenced Self-Beliefs, Trauma Filters, and Emotionally-Triggered Behaviors (ETBs) that have made up your past.

For lack of a better term, these will be looked at as your "past weaknesses."

In the right-hand column, write what you perceive to be the opposite beliefs, filters, and behaviors as "new strengths." These will replace your old ways of being and will become your starting point in training to remember and continuously choose the real you, thus forming your chosen identity.

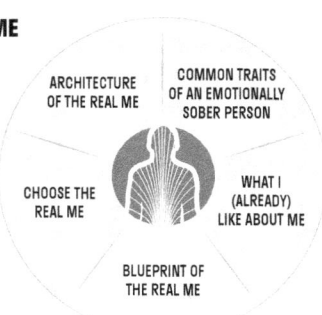

*Note: The Real Me, Parts 4 & 5 are covered in the EMSO Practicum.*

*HINT: Your "weakest" and seemingly most negative traits are actually manifesting on the same plane as their opposites (potential replacements!), meaning these profoundly new and more useful qualities can become your greatest strengths.*

| PAST "WEAKNESSES" (Self-Beliefs, Trauma Filters, ETBs) | NEW STRENGTHS (Replacement Beliefs/Filters/Behaviors) |
|---|---|
|  |  |
|  |  |
|  |  |
|  |  |
|  |  |
|  |  |
|  |  |

Carry this knowing of your new strengths with you through the rest of your EMSO Trainings, and the rest of your life, for that matter! We will use this a lot in the EMSO Practicum, should you choose to advance.

### COACHING MOMENT

**I'd like to take another moment to stand in awe of you... what extraordinary accomplishments you're making. You've done so much work to get to this point. Work that most would turn away from, as it is hard, gritty, earnest, and brave work. I'm excited to see what else you'll do!**

You've become aware of the *you* you've been being and acknowledged the impact of your Intoxicated Identity on yourself and others. You've begun to take the necessary actions to consciously bring forward and choose the real you, again and again. The next section will further all three of these, and invite you into the primary action of conscious choice—actively choosing who you want to be in every moment. To truly live what you've just learned about who you've been being, you're going to require additional tools, including more advanced EMSO practices. I offer an introduction to a few of them here to support this next step on your journey.

So, let's take a break from doing exercises, and learn a little more about the clearest ways to progress your Emotional Sobriety. I call these your EMSO Choices. The first five are introduced in this book:

- Blame vs. Self-responsibility
- PANE vs. Understanding
- Punishment vs. Consequence
- Expectation vs. Acceptance
- Unconditional Attention vs. Unconditional Love

## Blame vs. Self-responsibility

As I shared, real, lasting freedom comes when you take responsibility for your part in creating all of the conditions in your life—especially the situations where you're blaming others. Let's explore introductory self-responsibility to ensure you understand this practice and can apply it to your life.

The responsibility of a problem lies on the person whose life it's happening within. Your life is your responsibility. Self-responsibility is the antithesis of self-centeredness—the behavior in which we're trapped in the Center of Self and we filter everything to be about us and our insecurities. Looking at your EMSO Master Chart, you may have noticed how self-centeredness has played a role in harming your life. If self-responsibility is the antithesis, what would a life built upon it look like? When you blame others, you give them the responsibility for your PANEs, which means they own your feelings. What controls how you feel, controls you! Before, you simply didn't know any better. You didn't know who you were actually being or how you actually felt, but once you become aware, you become responsible.

I use the following example to provide a very basic understanding of self-responsibility: Let's say you haven't brushed your teeth in 30 years. Now your teeth are starting to fall out. Who's responsible? Some may say, "My teeth are falling out because my parents never taught me to brush my teeth. They never even told me that I was supposed to!" That may be true. But at some point, you must have had a symptom in your mouth indicating that there may be a problem with your teeth (bleeding gums, bad breath, severe pain). Perhaps you had some indication that your teeth needed attention to heal. The symptoms were there to indicate that something different needed to happen. Even if you'd never been taught to care for your teeth when you were in your early-age years, you can no longer blame someone else for the symptoms you've been ignoring. You are the owner of those teeth. You're the only one connected to them.

*The symptoms were there to indicate that something different needed to happen.*

The same goes for your ETBs and all emotional addiction. Even if you were never taught levelheadedness, clear and honest communication, or how to build an identity, at some point there were symptoms in your life pointing to those glaring areas of lack. Most likely, those symptoms are what have brought you here!

You may have felt anxious, fearful, resentful, used drugs/alcohol for coping, had an eating disorder or a sex addiction, were compulsively lying, and/or had a slew of unhealthy relationships… and at some point, you had to look at the dysfunctional, repetitive symptoms of your life as things you weren't paying attention to, mastering, maintaining, caring for, or improving on.

These areas of our lives are like the teeth we're not brushing, and it isn't our parent's fault. It isn't our partner's fault, our ex's fault, our friend's fault, or our sibling's fault. It isn't even our dentist's fault. To choose to look for ways to remove blame and take responsibility when it seems so easy to blame someone else, is heroic. I know there can be a temptation to blame those around you for your life circumstances. Self-responsibility isn't self-blame. It's the removal of all blame. It's turning the produced negativity of a situation and cracking it down the middle. If the responsibility lies outside of you, so does your power to change it. You're the one who can change everything you don't love about yourself or your life.

### DO YOU RELATE?

If Mary hadn't looked for her part in her PANEs, or at the perspective of what Tony was going through as well, she never would have been freed. By removing blame from them both, she also freed them both. She would have spent her life re-triggered every time she thought of Tony and the date. Can you see how this situation (and many others in her life) would have remained a problem, keeping her captive to her own insobriety?

By not doing the work of EMSO Training, each situation, person or group has the opportunity to be your "drug dealer." You would always have something in place to practice biochemical addiction via sustained blame and victimhood. The "stories" of what others have done (and what your Trauma Influenced Self-Beliefs have made that to mean about you), allow for another "hit" of the PANE you're addicted to making.

*To take responsibility when it seems so easy to blame, is heroic.*

What will you choose to take with you as you move forward: blame or self-responsibility?

### PANE vs. Understanding

Another effective way to take responsibility for your problems and life is through understanding. In EMSO Training, learning compassion is simplest when I teach people how they're the same, not where they're different. This is where understanding comes into play. Understanding yields compassion. When it seems impossible to overcome your PANE around a specific situation, utilize the opportunity to understand. When you do this, you grant yourself and those around you freedom from your resentment, anger, embarrassment, and more. Understanding requires knowing that in the same way you've made "mistakes" in your life, someone else has made them as well.

Your PANEs, similar to your secrets and lies, will make you sick. Your anger, fear, and resentment can create Emotional Belligerence within you, which means your continued overproduction of biochemistry will put you in a position to make your own, new "mistakes." You now know that <u>everyone</u> had Early-Age Trauma—whether it was extreme or subtle; and the people who contributed to your Early-Age Traumas also had their own. Most hurts aren't caused by someone trying to hurt you. Most hurts are caused by someone trying to protect themselves. This doesn't excuse them for hurting you, just as your getting hurt by them doesn't excuse your hurting others. The point here is that all of us have been hurt, traumatized, or betrayed—every one of us.

One of the ways we demonstrate compassion after trauma is to show understanding to our "enemy." We're not dismissing, allowing, or excusing the behavior of these "perpetrators." To do this would be to become what's often referred to a "doormat" or "enabler"—allowing people to treat us in any way they wish with no retaliation. To be clear, I'm not suggesting that understanding is interchangeable with martyrdom. I'm advocating that you break the cycle of victimhood which may bring about more victims. If anger and hatred are responsible for your traumatic event, having hatred and anger as a result of this at the very least attaches you to the event and diminishes you. If you analyze, judge, or even hate the perpetrator, nothing has been corrected. Under the illusion of powerlessness, we indulge the trauma by hating it, and that loops us back to the problem again.

A simple principle: If you want a joyful life, give up your PANEs. Your negative emotions and subsequent ETBs have gotten you into trouble and only caused more discord and pain. Your insobriety became an unchosen part of your identity. When you're trapped behind the wall of a Trauma Filter such as victimhood—which invokes countless emotions such as resentment, anger, fear, or embarrassment—it's a challenge to remain in the present moment or experience the life around you honestly.

*Most hurts aren't caused by someone trying to hurt you.*
*Most hurts are caused by someone trying to protect themselves.*

Understanding requires desire, intention, and action. You look for the ways in which the person or group which has caused you to feel PANEs is drawing from the same PANEs and self-beliefs that you have. It's work. It can lead to an advanced state of permanent freedom from PANEs. You get to choose: Keep your PANEs, or use the introductory skills to begin understanding.

### Punishment vs. Consequence

By means of the work you've already done, you now recognize that there are consequences to all of your actions and inactions. Again, consequence simply means, "what happens next."

I've experienced negative consequences, and I know what positive consequences feel like as well. By becoming emotionally sober you can shift the probability of the consequences of your actions to being primarily positive.

Consequence and punishment are not the same thing. Making a clear distinction between a consequence and punishment is important because oftentimes people mistake punishment for a natural consequence. This isn't the case.

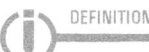
DEFINITIONS

> **CONSEQUENCE:** what happens next—after something.
>
> **PUNISHMENT:** a chosen sentencing with the intention of invoking shame or balancing the suffering that you've experienced; making someone else feel the pain that you feel.

Whereas consequence contains the potential to create wisdom by virtue of experience, punishment is an intentional or hurtful reaction to a behavior you've witnessed. If a consequence is perceived as negative, it may produce very strong personal feelings of temporary guilt for what was done, yet it's also perceived as a natural occurrence that hopefully teaches a lesson.

An example of a consequence would be a breakup of a relationship due to infidelity. If there were an agreement within the relationship that was broken, the consequence to breaking that agreement may be a dissolution of the relationship. Another example would be the loss of trust due to dishonesty or even violence. If someone lies to us or physically harms us, we naturally trust them less. This is a consequence to the reality of their behavior.

Punishment, on the other hand, includes attempting to instill blame, long-lasting negative emotion, or permanent shame in the other person or the self. Our Intoxicated Identity thinks that by hurting the person who hurt us, it will decrease our own PANE. We believe that watching them experience PANE may have the effect of temporarily distracting us from our own by giving us the illusion that we're controlling how they feel. Punishment is often utilized to teach a lesson or change a behavior, but it often comes from a place of creating more pain for both parties involved. Punishment is most easily identified in situations such as physical abuse, shaming, guilting, or "getting even" after experiencing a hurtful act.

If you're tempted to punish or are currently punishing, you may choose instead to allow a natural consequence by expressing new boundaries or discontinuing the relationship. Punishing someone else keeps you from evolving, since much of your creative energy is being poured into the management and perceived control of another.

Natural consequence aligns with your understanding. You can choose to exit a relationship with love and understanding. This is a consequence, not a negatively intended punishment. It may also include leaving situations that don't promote your growth, support your truth, or allow for your safety. These decisions are best made with levelheadedness and honesty, and then be impeccably communicated.

 CONTEMPLATION

**PUNISHMENT OR CONSEQUENCE**
Now that you more clearly understand the difference between these two, revisit your EMSO MASTER CHART and find Column H: CONSEQUENCE. Do you have a greater understanding of the difference between a natural and rational consequence, versus an intentional and harmful punishment? Who do you think is punishing you? Are they really punishing you, or is this perhaps a natural consequence due to something you've done or failed to do? In your list of people you've hurt, do you now see where you had any intended punishments?

Moving forward, will you choose to punish yourself and others for your mistakes, or simply notice the natural consequences and learn from them?

## Expectation vs. Acceptance

In the twelve-step process, it's often stated that expectations are premeditated resentments. Why? When we hold onto expectations we're in unreality; we're thinking for others and/or controlling outcomes without clear communication. This all falls back onto us for not having clarity and levelheadedness within our relationships. From our mail carrier to our spouse, we must be free of expectations—especially unspoken expectations.

DEFINITION

**EXPECTATION:** a premeditated, often unspoken, standard for how someone should speak, behave, or feel.

Expectation creates a slew of unwinnable situations. Firstly, you'll likely feel a PANE yourself (e.g., resentment, anger) when the expected outcome doesn't match up with reality. Even if someone meets your expectations at times, you'll inevitably experience disappointment with them when things don't go as you've planned in your head the next time around. We're often shocked when we notice our expectations, as we realize that most of them were never spoken out loud, leaving others no chance to know—let alone meet—our premeditated "standard."

Instead of expectations, what if we had acceptance of others' actions, beliefs, and feelings exactly as they are? Practicing acceptance requires understanding. We acknowledge where we've been having expectations—and thus PANE—regarding others not being who we think they should be to us.

DEFINITION

**ACCEPTANCE:** a premeditated, often spoken, peacefulness surrounding others' words, behaviors, and feelings.

Acceptance is a choice to understand others, while knowing that our "standards" cannot be expected in them. We find the opportunities to be at peace, regardless of reality, while maintaining clear boundaries.

Acceptance isn't the same as submission or martyrdom. We don't allow people to treat us abusively or with no regard. We simply figure out what it is that we require in terms of our personal preferences and inform those around us—directly—as to what these are. For example, do you prefer when others are on time, kind, respectful, pay their own way, or do their own laundry? Finding your expectations allows for you to narrow down what it is that you actually want and then you can communicate these wants.

Without Emotional Sobriety, we'll have expectations that irritate us to the core. They'll put us in a position of feeling out of control, take us out of our "fairytale" life, and slam us into reality. Notice that expectation does an incredible job at keeping us in PANE—contributing to the biochemical addiction and follow up ETBs that our Intoxicated Identity is more than happy to create for us.

In EMSO Training, you've looked at where you still hold the expectation of each person or group on your EMSO Master Chart to play a part in your Life Movie. Now it's time to practice acceptance by coming to grips with knowing that other people aren't going to speak, behave, and feel in the ways we think they "should." They certainly won't get the lines of our unspoken script correct for the movie we're subversively making for ourselves and everyone around us.

Expectation is deeply rooted in our unawareness that others live, believe, and respond differently than we would. It offers us a sneaky way to test out if we are indeed lovable or important to others if we can control them, making us feel more powerful. The PANE made when our expectation isn't met validates our Trauma-Influenced Self-Beliefs and leads to the ETB of judgmentalism. And with this judgmentalism, we're flung into a repeatable pattern to compulsively attempt to have our next expectation met (proving our importance or lovability). We may sneakily play games or test others. "Maybe this time he'll be on time for dinner. Then I'll know he loves me." "I wonder if I leave this here, if she'll clean it up. Then I'll know I'm important to her." This of course encases us in a loop of PANE and expectation over and over again.

Expectation is to seek your version of perfection in others, while acceptance is to be prepared for imperfection knowing it's a part of reality. In sobriety, your job is to be diligent with your emotional health, to be responsible for yourself, and to be clear of your PANE, leaving you levelheaded. You'll accept others' differences and stand strongly. You won't feel the need for, or have the habit of, holding expectations of others. You'll be freed by trusting your life and by stabilizing yourself to live freely within that life.

The world you live within will become peaceful because the world within you will be peaceful.

### Unconditional Attention vs. Unconditional Love

Now it's time to discern whether you're in healthy loving relationships or those based mostly on getting or giving attention. It's important that you start to understand which relationships contain the "hook of love." These are relationships that initially and/or sporadically give you relief from your Trauma-Influenced Self-Beliefs and also offer a powerful positive biochemical release of dopamine or oxytocin (the bonding chemical). The unconditional attention-based relationships that give you a "hit" of your old biochemical addiction to fear, shame, or anger are often the relationships within which you can also easily demonstrate all of your most challenging ETBs.

You'll learn to feel the nuance in this and make conscious choices to engage in loving relationships that point you closer and closer to the *you* you're now getting to know. Knowing the difference between unconditional attention and unconditional love helps you navigate old and new relationships as they're transforming... another tool to help you get real! A principle for "real-ationships" is understanding that love and attention aren't the same thing.

Our families, friendships, relationships with co-workers, and romantic endeavors all lead us toward what we think is a mutual goal: unconditional love. We're searching for that person, or establishing a familial relationship with someone, who's our source of unconditional understanding, support, and connection. We're hoping for a relationship within which we feel free, while still knowing we can rely on this individual if something dark or difficult would come into our lives. With healthy relationships of all types, there must be a mutual contract; meaning it's a place where both parties feel this freedom and feel that they can rely on each other in the ways they need to be supported.

> *A principle for "real-ationships" is understanding that love and attention aren't the same thing.*

If this isn't the case, then we may find ourselves in a "parasitic," co-dependent, or even one-sided relationship. It may be best to call them "unconditional attention" relationships. Unconditional attention thrives under the guise of unconditional love, but it isn't. One is love- and freedom-based, while the other is attachment-based.

DEFINITION

**UNCONDITIONAL ATTENTION:** the compulsion to give or receive continued attention, regardless of level of trustworthiness, respectful treatment, or mutual interest.

Who are the people you call during your emotionally unsober episodes? If they contribute to or sit back and allow you to stay within this cycle, validating your dishonesty or hysteria, then these are the people with whom you have an unconditional attention relationship. This doesn't mean there's no love or care in this relationship. There's simply not yet the skill of Emotional Sobriety in this relationship. To be crystal clear, it's not an act of unconditional love when someone allows you to vent to them over and over again. You're certainly not taking love away if you choose to stop participating in others' emotional outbursts.

Unconditional attention agreements appear in a variety of ways. For example, perhaps you can verbally abuse a friend or partner one day and expect them to show up to your party the next day (or guilt and anger will be laid upon them!). Or you call a friend to complain about the same problem over and over and continue to rely on them for advice without any real push toward a solution (or vice versa).

Each of these relationships is rooted in a form of emotional leverage and an influence of guilt or manipulation. This is most noticeable when you have a sense of "security" with them one day, and the next feel trapped by the relationship. For example, if you change the agreement and set a boundary, letting them know that you only want to participate in the solution, you may quickly be replaced, bashed, or shamed for not allowing them to continue with the same arrangement. In families, there's often an agreement that since you're family, you're automatically there for each other, no matter how you treat each other. Here's a helpful scenario:

DO YOU RELATE?

> Ray calls his sister Kris screaming about how terrible his day was, making sure that Kris feels just as awful as he does by the end of the call.
>
> Or, Ray calls Kris to complain about his wife while Kris sits back and justifies all the reasons he's right, even if she doesn't believe it.

These are both unconditional attention-seeking phone calls made to the person Ray knows he can "rely" on for the attention and validation he's seeking.

An unconditional attention relationship can feel like love because of the momentary high or chemical rush we get from these interactions. Some scenarios include: trying to get someone "on our side," telling someone the bad news, delivering gossip, or when we believe someone is hearing us when we don't feel heard somewhere else. We form a bond of mutual dissatisfaction and misery. It feels like "support" in the moment, but what is it really supporting? Our old trauma-influenced ways of being. It really becomes a habit, an addiction to seeking attention. Something we do over and over again as a pattern, and that back-and-forth energetic exchange, even if it's unpleasant, leaves us feeling "loved." This is really unconditional attention.

DEFINITION

> **UNCONDITIONAL LOVE:** the feeling, intention, and/or choice to love someone, regardless of level of trustworthiness, respectful treatment, or mutual interest.

There are some who would say this doesn't exist. There has to be a moment when we stop loving someone due to their behavior, right? I don't know the global answer to this. Perhaps a parent will feel anger, disbelief, and sadness if their child committed a horrible crime, and even separate from their life, but does that mean they stop loving them? Read these unconditional love statements. Imagine that someone close to you (e.g., your child, spouse, sibling, close friend, etc.) is saying it to you.

- "I seek your freedom and happiness."
- "I support you in doing the things you enjoy."
- "I encourage you to grow and follow your heart."
- "We listen to each other and behave kindly toward each other."
- "If we have a disagreement, we remain calm and attempt to remedy it with cooperation and understanding."
- "Our emotional health is our own responsibility."
- "Our health is important to each other."
- I consider both of our well-being within this relationship. If it becomes unhealthy for me, I'll set boundaries or remove myself from it. I'll understand if the same were to happen for you."
- I choose to feel love for you, regardless if we're together or apart."

When you hear these words said to you, or something like it, you may have a feeling wash through you. It won't be something you need to think about, rather your whole being will know it's unconditional love. Now go back through and read each statement a second time and imagine you're saying it to someone close to you (it may be back to the same person or someone else). If you don't believe it when you're saying it, or it isn't true regarding one of your relationships, then perhaps you're in an unconditional attention relationship.

Unconditional love can exist in your romantic partnerships, families, or friendships when you've worked on yourself and your relationships (and in the rare few that seem to have been graced with an easy time with this from the start!). You can sift through and remove past resentments. It's also a choice you can make during the many moments of your life when you may not be in a direct relationship with another, but you still choose to love them without giving or receiving attention. With unconditional love relationships, there's rarely ego-based desire to be correct or to win; instead, there's consideration of the other from both sides. There's vulnerability and honesty, as well as the relationship being focused on freedom and ease. The health of the relationship holds the priority of importance for you, not the mere existence of the relationship itself.

Let's explore unconditional love in relationships you have that don't carry as much pressure as these primary relationships. These may include ex-spouses, friends you don't see often, co-workers, cousins, and more. These relationships have less expectation and neediness. Resentments are often released more fully here, and there's a deepening of appreciation available in these relationships. These less-pressured spaces are a great place to practice unconditional love and personal integrity, which can then be brought into your more full-time relationships.

> *The health of the relationship holds the priority of importance for them, not the relationship's existence itself.*

If you're wondering why you don't have this as easily accessible in your close relationships, it's likely because there is residual irritability, expectation, and anxiety as a result of your intoxicated identification. For example, if you've felt the need to be someone else when with a certain person, you're not practicing integrity and you're not free.

Here's an example of an unconditional love point of view from someone who doesn't have an active relationship with his brother, yet still chooses to hold immense love for him.

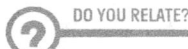

### DO YOU RELATE?

Rick shares that he cannot reason with, nor have a healthy relationship with his brother, Jamie. No matter what his brother does or says, or how his brother seems to despise him, Rick simply remains detached from the relationship, while still loving his brother. Rick recalls the multiple times Jamie beat him up in their family home when they were kids. Now, as adults, Jamie has patterns of demanding money from family members, attention for his problems with friends, and losing jobs. Rick won't give Jamie the money he wants, and Rick won't allow himself to be used in the ways Jamie expresses he needs. Rick smiles when he sees his brother at family events, and continues to offer the possibility of a future relationship if Jamie chooses to treat him differently someday. What he's demonstrating is that he won't offer unconditional <u>attention</u> to his brother, but he does continue to offer unconditional <u>love</u>.

Rich is using what I term a "spoken boundary" in EMSO Advanced Practices). There's no condition under which Rick will stop loving his brother; however, there are conditions under which Rick won't be in his brother's life.

Continuing to give attention to someone in an unhealthy dynamic (abusive, dishonest, manipulative) is an act of codependence, martyrdom, or self-deprecation, demonstrating that your filters and self-beliefs are at the helm of your life. You're most likely within the relationship contract of unconditional attention, not unconditional love.

Love is:
- care
- gratitude for the other
- humility in the face of disagreement
- seeking to understand
- offering support in seeking solutions

Love is not:
- continuously offering attention without solutions
- continuously offering support when the other isn't seeking solutions

Codependency is a misinterpretation of unconditional love. Unconditional in the context of a codependent relationship means: No matter what happens, how you behave, or how you treat me in this relationship, I will always be here for you and actively support you. I'll never leave you. I'll allow you to treat me as you like to—whatever makes you comfortable. My happiness, reputation, integrity, and personal growth are secondary. This isn't unconditional love. This is unconditional attention or codependency.

You can love others while not engaging in the behaviors you no longer find useful or resonant with the *you* you're choosing to be now. Understanding is an act of love, so bring this new tool along. With it, you won't be able to harbor anger or resentment; rather, you'll move forward and wish goodness for them. You may need to part ways with someone for a period of time. As I've shared, simply offering someone understanding and love doesn't necessarily entitle them to your attention. You can absolutely have unconditional love for someone that you choose not to see again.

*You can love others while not engaging in the behaviors you no longer find useful or resonant with the* you *you're choosing to be now.*

In this chapter, you learned that you can choose continued insobriety in the form of blame, PANE, punishment, and seeking or giving unconditional attention, or you can choose freedom. Use your new tools of self-responsibility, understanding, consequence, and unconditional love to begin stepping into freedom from PANE and unsober patterns. Remember, you're new to this, so be patient with yourself as you gain momentum over your cycles of PANE and ETBs, and the pattern of your brain, body, and ego pulling you back to what your Intoxicated Identity considers its "norm."

With each of these in your toolbox, let's move forward to the 4Rs.

# 31

## Review

*Our lack of healing from past trauma is evidenced by the intolerable, seemingly "unlearnable" lesson.*

I've depicted this healing process using a DNA strand, as I'm proposing the possibility that you're now able to make changes that will literally change your internal chemistry.

The scientific study hasn't yet taken place to prove that when we overcome our emotional addictions, that it also changes the way that our genes express and can then be passed down to future generations. For example, do you often hear yourself say: "I get my anger from my mother," or "My dad's afraid of everything... it's in my genes"? This is the field of epigenetics, or "the study of changes in organisms caused by modification of gene expression rather than alteration of the genetic code itself."[17]

My question is: If we can inherit insobriety from ancestral trauma, can we pass on sobriety from the work we do today?

I invite you to join the experiment that we're executing right here, right now. By continuing your EMSO Training with the 4Rs, you're a part of the next movement in human evolution! Now's the time to re-invoke your desire for your intention to be truly sober and take these next four clear actions.

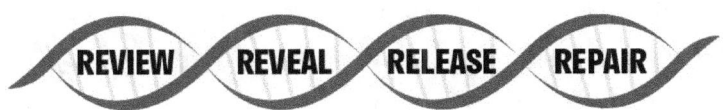

I can imagine that after the depth of investigation that you've now given your entire life, you may be seeing some similarities in the way you've been thinking, feeling, and behaving in various circumstances, with various people. Discovering your patterns will give you access to what's real about you. Mistakes are mistakes. Repeated mistakes are character flaws. Acknowledged mistakes are opportunities. It's for this reason that I've been putting "mistakes" in quotations throughout the book. Whatever you're feeling, I now reintroduce you to a powerful invitation: your choice to uncover the real you.

*Acknowledged mistakes are opportunities.*

Your first R: Review directly reinforces the teaching and practice of internal humility. At this point, you've discovered that you're the common denominator of your problems. Perhaps you still don't quite know how to fix them. This is where humility can continue to be used and help contribute to your relief. I like to define it as:

DEFINITION

**HUMILITY**: the ability to see who you've been in the past, and open to seeing that you're no better than anyone else.

During the EMSO Master Chart process, you outlined who you feel negatively about, if you're continuing to harbor blame, having any expectations, and by considering your rewind, uncovered what parts of the interaction were your responsibility. Your R.E.A.Life Investigation was a deep and thorough review of what specific aspects of your Anatomy of Emotional Insobriety were at play in each situation. I imagine this process was humbling for you, and for every single one of my students. You've now begun earning this humility.

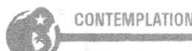 CONTEMPLATION

**REVIEW WITH HUMILITY**
Can you now contemplate and answer any of these questions more succinctly, with your earned humility? Do this internally now.

- Who have you hurt?
- What did you do?
- What were you hoping to accomplish?
- What were you thinking and feeling when you hurt them?
- What were the consequences of this?
- What could you have done instead?

Additional questions specifically for those in your intimate past:

- Who were you with and why? To feel desirable?
- What were you thinking and feeling when you did this?
- What was the consequence of this act?
- Were you harmed because of this? Were they?
- What would you choose to do now if you could do it again?

This is only a review. Look through your EMSO Master Chart for any remaining withholdings of complete facts or untruths. If you feel strange and withdrawn when you read them, seek to know if you're continuing to hide something from yourself. As the saying goes: "Where there's smoke, there's fire." If you sense that something is missing, it means that something *is* missing—a hidden abuse, a blocked memory, or a lie you've told or have been told. Recall the principle I shared: Whatever you bury will bury you. So, recommit to digging it up and putting it in plain sight, and then go do it. You're welcome to add details to your EMSO Master Chart at any time.

You may be asking: "Why do I have to look again?!" You're looking again to make sure you've been thorough and look for missed opportunities for deeper humility. Your ability to clearly see your part in your struggles is essential to overcome them. Make sure you aren't focusing on the negative attributes of others, comparing yourself to others, or "gossiping" to yourself about others.

*You're looking again to make sure you have been thorough and look for missed opportunities of humility.*

Again, any behavior that you'd change if you could <u>is</u> your part in it. No matter how small it may seem, you have a part in all of the events of your life, even if that part was that you didn't protect yourself, didn't pay attention, didn't listen to your intuition, or didn't ask for help.

*Behavior that you would change if you could <u>is</u> your part in it.*

For the situations that happened when you were a child, it can be difficult to find your part in it. Keep asking yourself questions such as: "Is there something I could have done differently as an adult to help myself or someone else after this event?" Be compassionate with yourself—especially around childhood trauma—yet also be honest and thorough.

For the students who've done their 4Rs directly with me, I say something to this effect when I can sense that they're struggling with finding humility: "Know that your ability to express these things to me is brave, but the ability to be honest with yourself about your part in them, is remarkable. If you can be honest about who you've actually been, and feel the consequences of being that way, you'll be able to change. You'll be inspired to become someone new. This is why humility is the secret to your healing."

*Humility is the secret to your healing.*

## Learn the Lesson

I was sitting in a waiting room one spring day, working on establishing a R.E.A.L. look at who I had been being. When I finished reviewing a particular area of my life, I realized there was a pattern. It was as obvious as a bright yellow line on a charcoal black road. I read through my discrepancies with both shock and embarrassment. I saw that the events and behaviors in one particular theme were identical! I knew in that moment of realization that I really only had to make this "mistake" one time to learn the lesson.

The problem is, I didn't make it only once. I did it countless times and didn't learn the lesson. Instead of learning the lesson, I ignored it.

It seems that not only do we not learn our lessons on the first round, most of the time we never learn our lessons at all. Why do we keep making the same problems? Why are we so angry? Why are we so selfish? I was so struck by this realization that I literally asked out loud, "What is it about us that hinders us from learning lessons from all of our mistakes?!"

The answer came quickly: We don't learn the lesson because we don't know <u>how</u> to learn the lesson, and we certainly can't learn the lesson that we can't see. This is why it's essential to make written and visual markings of who we've been being. When the state of our past and current lives isn't enough proof of our need for change, we clearly draw out our unlearned lessons. Then, our "lesson plan" is easily laid out for us.

*We don't learn the lesson because*
*we don't know <u>how</u> to learn the lesson.*

With obvious visual feedback of your patterns, you can't deny their existence. When they're displayed clearly in front of you, you may either feel overwhelmed, or in contrast, you may feel a surge of desperation to learn more. Some receive a glimpse of freedom simply by seeing their pattern one time! Personally, I was impressed by the fact that I could be surprised by a pattern of behavior that was happening in my own life, about me, by me, and because of me. If it was happening in me, how could I have not seen it all along? Patterns are great visual indicators that something needs to change within us. They're an obvious sign of our previous steps, and that who we've been will most likely be repeated if we don't observe and make new decisions.

---

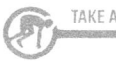
TAKE ACTION

### REVIEW: PAINT MY PATTERNS

This exercise will clearly reveal the tendencies you portrayed within the situations and with the people and groups on your EMSO MASTER CHART.

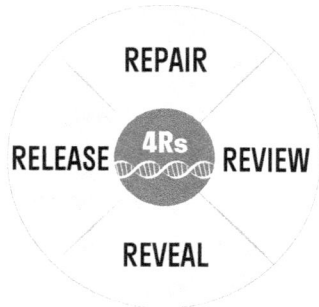

Use highlighters or colored pencils and color-code Columns C, D, & E on your EMSO MASTER CHART. Choose one color for each BELIEF/FILTER, one color for each PANE, and one color for each ETB. You may choose to use the same color palette for all three columns, because we're looking only for patterns within each column.

For example:

- in Column C – BELIEF/FILTER: "UW" could be blue, "L" red, and "IA" yellow
- in Column D – PANE: "F" could also be blue, "E" red, and "R" yellow
- in Column E – ETB: "DF" blue, "CH" red, and "JL" yellow

By clearly labelling each with a color, you'll be able to see a visual display of certain destructive patterns. For example, if you use "blue" for all your fears and you see a lot of blue in Column D, you'll have a clearer sense of just how much fear has been influencing your life.

Do you see any colorful patterns? Do these match your Anatomy of Emotional Insobriety?

**COACHING MOMENT**

In his book "E-Myth," author Michael Gerber writes, "The truth does set you free, but it can make you miserable at first." No matter what your pattern looks like, or how "miserable" it feels to look at it, know that no one does this kind of work without feeling this way at first. No one—no matter where they are on their path to Emotional Sobriety—is "better" than you. We're all in this together. You've made tremendous efforts toward changing your negative patterns already. Now's the time to notice the misery and keep moving forward anyway!

**TAKE ACTION**

**REVIEW: HIGHLIGHT WHAT NEEDS REPAIRING WITHIN ME**
Get a highlighter and review each person, group, and situation you wrote in Column A: NAME on your EMSO MASTER CHART, one by one.

Highlight the name for any that you feel the following when you review.

- PANE (resentment, anger, guilt, embarrassment, fear, or sadness)
- Body Signals (Do you feel uneasy when you think of them?)

That's it! You've now completed your first R and done some internal healing with humility. I'm happy to include you in our community of brave and humble students. The next R invites us to move outside of ourselves, while continuing to grow our internal humility.

Let's discover the next key to your healing...

## Reveal

*When you can look at yourself with perfect humility,
looking perfect to others won't matter to you.
And it won't matter to you when others are imperfect.*

The 2nd R: Reveal teaches <u>outward</u> humility. It requires readiness to be vulnerable and reveal (without resistance) your patterns of hurting yourself and others, exposing your "mistakes," and sharing your fears. Humility puts us in a position to heal through change, as it's a form of surrendering the ideals of our ego and Intoxicated Identity.

*Humility puts us in a position to heal through change,
as it's a form of surrendering the ideals of our ego.*

TAKE ACTION

**REVEAL: MY INTOXICATED IDENTITY**
Now that you've reviewed all of the components of your emotional insobriety that have created or are adding to the problems in your life, reveal them to yourself in a very direct and loving way. This is who you became because of Early-Age Trauma.

Read your entire EMSO MASTER CHART out loud to yourself.

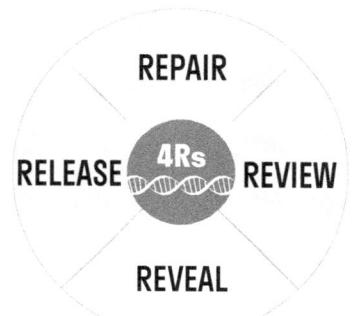

**Take the time to really acknowledge the things you've done, failed to do, or what happened to you in your childhood that formed your Intoxicated Identity.**

**Then respond to these prompts:**

1. I acknowledge my patterns of: _____

2. I could have saved myself and otheres from unnecessary pain by: _____

3. These Predominanty Accompanying Negative Emotions (PANEs), Trauma Filters, and Emotionally-Triggered Behaviors (ETBs) have been my biggest blocks: _____

Allow this to sink in and resonate with you. Look at how your past or current behaviors, filters, ways of thinking, and emotional triggers have contributed to your suffering. Give yourself permission to be outraged, sad, embarrassed, confused, shocked, and even remorseful. It's okay to have real pangs as the consequences of your choices or compulsive behaviors are revealed to you. Now you'll use these pangs as motivation to learn the lesson.

The lesson is learned through humility, vulnerability, and action. You'll use action to remedy these problems by illuminating your "mistakes" by placing them "outside of you" via "confession." As with some of your investigation, confession is inspired by ancient methods of spiritual and emotional clearing, and seen in many wisdom traditions. For example, methods of confession inspired the twelve-step programs, and now I'd like to introduce you to this freeing practice. Through this work, you've cornered your Intoxicated Identity and said, "I see you." Now how will you let others see it? This will bring you freedom from it.

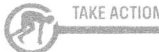
TAKE ACTION

**REVEAL: WHO I'VE REALLY BEEN BEING**
This is a unique opportunity and freeing exercise to reveal your biggest secrets, lies, and overall Intoxicated Identity to someone else.

OPTION 1: Reveal your Intoxicated Identity (what you uncovered on your EMSO MASTER CHART) to an EMSO Coach, to the EMSO Community (on the group page or in a meeting), or to your EMSO CO.

OPTION 2: Choose a truly trusted person to talk to—a rabbi, teacher, mentor, clergyman, therapist, counselor, or the like. Ask for a meeting to express what you found in your EMSO MASTER CHART and any revelations you've had about who you've been being.

Remind yourself that this exercise isn't about the therapy or advice that you'll receive from others; it's simply another human being that you can reveal these secret to. It's a place for you to humbly purge your past. Once you've finished revealing to them, don't engage in much discussion, unless you need support from a professional mental health practitioner.

*HINT: Some people have a hard time revealing due to fearing judgment. Remember, to whom you choose to confess is only an ear, not a judge. In the same way, you'll openly listen without judgment to another when they reveal to you.*

COACHING MOMENT

I've coached hundreds of people toward Emotional Sobriety and have sat for countless hours as they revealed their versions of intoxication to me. I've heard what some may think of as treacherous things. I've borne witness to their lies and affairs, their abusive behaviors, their hysteria, selfishness, and blatant childishness. When they finish this part of their revelation work with me, I remind them, as I'm sharing with you now, I don't judge you because we cannot condemn what we ourselves once were.

We're all the same.
You're not alone!

# 33

# Release

*Whatever your belief system is, to become emotionally sober, you must release your insobriety to a power greater than your insobriety.*

By learning to release with humility, you're learning to release your grip and give it over to your higher power, or your future self, and relying on them for help. At this point, you can <u>intellectually</u> understand how whole you already are, and maybe even are beginning to <u>feel</u> your wholeness. Releasing your past comes from the desire to release the old version of you. This requires faith in the power that you're made of.

At this point, you may have already felt its presence by doing some if this altering work. It may have snuck up beside you and "whispered in your ear" to give you support during the previous, difficult parts of this process. You may have felt a shifting within you when you dove into looking at your past with great focus and honesty.

This intentional work has a connecting effect—an effect that allows you to become more in line with this energy, humbled by it, and sensing your worth and lovability, perhaps for the first time. This is who you can be, with continued desire and intention, and more moment-to-moment action. This is only the beginning of the real you coming forward to transcend your Intoxicated Identity!

Now, we can understand that the energy that made us in the womb can recreate us by helping rid us of all the traits we no longer wish to carry. Then we can rely on it to help us build anew. This creative energy will be the power to which you release your lifetime of emotional insobriety. It will help you energetically remove your self-beliefs, filters and PANEs. You may already have a clear intention to be rid of them, yet because you'll always have an ego, you can't rely on intention alone. Along with your re-commitment and desire for Emotional Sobriety, you also need to learn to rely upon this egoless energy.

*This is only the beginning!*

Utilize your desire, intention, and action to obtain new behaviors in this next exercise. When it seems impossible to change, releasing shows us that we can move away from our faulty reliance on our old ways of thinking and behaving. If you regret what you've done in the past, don't be that same person today. If you haven't been able to change by yourself up to this point, maybe it's time to outsource this job to a great power, the power that was within you and around you all along.

*If you regret what you've done in the past,
don't be that same person today.*

CONTEMPLATION

**READY TO RELEASE?**
Ask yourself: Am I ready to replace the past and current self that I wrote about in my R.E.A.Life Investigation? Now that I've looked deeply into my past, am I inspired enough to release all of those behaviors and old patterns that have hurt me and others?

You've seen by now that your old way is not the way, otherwise you wouldn't be in the position you're attempting to change. I often say in my rehabilitation clinics that the road to health is going to look a lot different than you think;

otherwise, you'd already be there! Both humility and courage are required to hear that and take action in a new direction.

I recall the list of my "mistakes." I remember revealing them to myself and another person—seeing the patterns and the dysfunction. If you feel the way that I did back then, you're most likely ready to be rid of these things from your life. I want to enforce this condition—that this has to be your true desire.

I must say that of all the things I wish I could coach, I would coach desire. Yet, I don't know that it's coachable. I can't tell you how to make desire. Desire is a personal energetic state. It must be yours alone. I do know that when you have desire, nothing can get in your way—no one's opinion or fear, or an external event. Where there's desire, new opportunities will be in front of your face, and if you continue to feed it, change is imminent.

You learned in the beginning of this section that your desire must be sincere. You must have the absolute intention of being different, and you know that your intention cannot be turned into reality until you take action.

As Albert Einstein famously stated, "Nothing happens until something moves." So, let's take our next action!

 TAKE ACTION

**RELEASE: THE OLD TO MEET THE FUTURE**
Visit liftedacademy.com/tyynm and listen to the recording, "Release." Lie in a comfortable location, close your eyes, and listen deeply. Remove all distractions ahead of time.

Notice if your heart begins to swell as if you've just watched an inspiring or heartfelt movie. This is your energy touching you.

Once you feel confident that you're surrounded by it, declare your readiness and read the following statements.

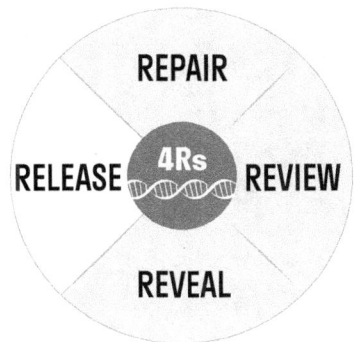

*"I'm ready for the energy that made and keeps me to help me remove and destroy my hurtful compulsions, my past pain, my anger, my guilt, and my belligerence.*

*I release this and ask that you remove every hurtful compulsion, my past pain, my anger, my guilt, and my belligerence. Remove everything that stands in the way of my usefulness and peace, and let me outgrow fear."*

**Visualize this actually happening in real time. Feel space freeing up inside of you. Feel yourself getting lighter, freer, and emptier as these things leave you.**

**Then say, "Thank you." Say it only when you mean it, and feel it with humility. Stay in this moment for as long as you can. Continue to feel the blocks from your old self getting removed as the real you begins to shine through.**

**When you come out of the visualization, take some time to free-write and/or draw how you feel and what you notice.**

# 34

# Repair

*Repairing your past in this way can feel like time travel or like we've actually altered the past, sometimes allowing for what feels like a do-over.*

Repairing with humility is a big part of the journey to Emotional Sobriety. Let's make some much-needed repairs. Here, you'll be practicing more honesty than you've even yet mustered up, in addition to using your EMSO Choices to invoke self-responsibility, understanding, consequence (what happens next), acceptance, and unconditional love.

As with some of our investigation and confession, repairing our "mistakes" is inspired by ancient methods of spiritual and emotional clearing, and is seen in many religions. A more modern (yet somewhat aged) example would be what twelve-step programs refer to as "making amends." In this context, let's think of them as "Repairs"—the final link in your EMSO Essentials. It means to communicate or demonstrate our understanding of what we've done and who we've been being and change it.

To repair is to attempt to literally mend the hurt you've caused. Whether in the past or present, you acknowledge where you've caused harm by being under the influence of your biochemical addiction, resulting in ETBs. Now, with your EMSO Training underway, you know exactly where you've been dishonest, defensive, childish, jealous, and more. You can rid yourself of the negative feelings created by their memory, or situational angst, by repairing them—within yourself and eventually either indirectly or directly with the other person, group, or situation.

Additionally, with your newly practiced skill of self-responsibility, you're much less likely to create any more "damage" that may need repairing in the future. This is an important part of your EMSO Training as it's the process by which you'll rid your life of the issues that cause chronic dis-ease, discontent, and pain. There's a large amount of correction that can be made for your past. I'll walk you through your Repairs using my broad personal experience as well as showing you the specific methods designed for this curriculum.

*You've begun a new chapter of your life where you won't rely on old behaviors to get what you want.*

If how you once thought, felt, and behaved created these experiences for you, how will your new understanding of cause and effect continue to shape the new you? How will you show the people around you what you've learned about yourself, and the effects that your behaviors have had on your life and theirs?

You've begun a new chapter of your life where you won't rely on old behaviors to get what you want. You recognize that they don't work, and they never will. You have suffered the consequences of your actions and inactions. You choose to no longer suffer or create suffering for others. You've looked deeply into your past, you're clear on the ways you could have behaved differently, and you've made a new promise for your future. You've acknowledged your faith in an intelligent energy that made and keeps you, and that you're connected to it at all times and can rely upon it for assistance.

You know that you're closer to being able to rely on the real you and your ever-growing maturity in <u>all</u> areas of your life.

The Repair process utilizes all of the work you've done in your training thus far. The good news is that you simply begin within. It's an extremely powerful experience and creates lasting change within us when we take it seriously. There are three ways to make repairs.

1. **Repairs from Within**—within you only. These are completed now in the EMSO Essentials.

2. **Indirect Repairs**—not in-person; to be completed in the EMSO Practicum curriculum.

3. **Direct Repairs**—in-person; to be completed later in EMSO AP (Advanced Practices).

COACHING MOMENT

You have new tools and are committed to using them going forward, but haven't yet had much experience practicing using them. To expect to be a master at levelheadedness at this point would be like someone considering themselves a master carpenter the first week or two that they were handed a hammer. This is why you don't necessarily jump right into indirect and direct repairs. However, the faster you complete your deep understanding of what you've done and find the courage to make your repairs, you expeditiously forge your growth with increased skills of clarity, honesty, and levelheadedness.

Making repairs in some form of contact with the people on your list is premature. This requires a stable footing in your Emotional Sobriety. Therefore, I won't invite you to make these repairs before you're ready to handle the potential pushback, disappointment, or rejection from the person with whom you're attempting to repair. We have great tools to make these repairs, but we have to do the prep work. Repairs begin with a clear plan, and they always start from within.

## Level 1: Repairs From Within

You now know that when you caused or experienced each of these hurts, you were filtering a perspective that caused negative emotions. This led you to react with Emotionally-Triggered Behaviors (ETBs). You may have had underlying motives such as a need for control, expectations of "promised" unconditional attention, or to prove that you're important to them. You've explored what you could've done differently, and now with more time and experience, could add to your "Rewind" Column with even greater clarity. You're working and committed to who you'll be in the future, starting now! Revisit your EMSO Master Chart now, and fill it out as much as you'd like. Then, continue your Repairs.

 TAKE ACTION

**REPAIR: WRITE REPAIR FROM WITHIN LETTERS**

Using the template on the following page, translate the contents of your EMSO MASTER CHART into one letter per person, group, or situation. Start by addressing each NAME you highlighted in a previous Take Action. These letters are for <u>you</u>, so don't write them as if someone will read it.

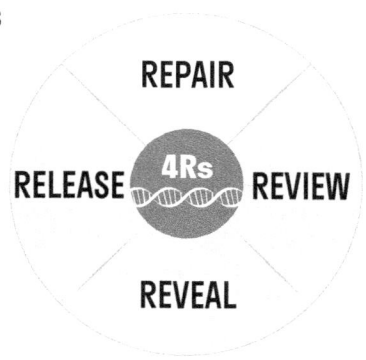

You can address each portion of your letter by looking at the respective columns on your EMSO MASTER CHART, indicated by the letter in the outline.

For example, [C] is found in the BELIEF/FILTER column, [E] is the ETB you displayed, etc.

Use this template as a guide to write your letters, yet make sure each one is written from your own voice, and that you truly mean it. Use your humility, modesty, and honesty. Ensure you're coming from a place of new maturity.

*HINTS:*

- *Use stationary or a dedicated notebook and find a quiet place without time pressure.*
- *Use the sample letter provided on the following page.*

- **Address the letter.** Dear [A:_____],

- **Begin the letter by stating your intention.** I intend to clarify what I've learned about myself and our relationship/the situation.

- **Share the situation.** At the time [B:_____] happened...

- **Indicate your belief and/or filter.** This situation was difficult for me because I believed it meant [C:_____] about me, and I recognize that I filtered this situation through this lens.

- **Share your PANE around the situation.** Due to this belief seemingly being validated during this situation with you, I felt [D:_____].

- **Write down your ETBs.** These feelings in me caused me to behave [E:_____]. I specifically behaved this way by_____.

- **If you had any blame and/or expectations,** communicate this next in the letter. [F/G]

- **Reveal your motive.** By behaving this way, I was hoping to accomplish [H:_____].

- **Share what happened next.** I recognize the natural consequence of this is/was [I:_____].

- **Rewind.** What I would now do differently is [J:_____].

*The last four parts of the letter aren't derived from your EMSO Master Chart, rather through The Real Me process and the skills you're developing with the EMSO Choices (understanding, acceptance, etc.)*

- **State your new intentions.** I've chosen to be [emotionally sober traits, new strengths, etc.]_____ from now on.

- **Communicate that there are no lingering expectations.** As I'm sharing this, I realize that I don't have any expectations of you.

- **Express your gratitude.** You added _____ to my life. This situation or discord brought to light _____, which I'm now thankful for.

- **Close the letter** respectfully and modestly, with no emotional leverage. With respect, _____.

Dear Tony,

I intend to clarify what I learned about myself by looking at our past situation. I was disrespectful toward you at dinner last year when I recognized you may not have considered our dinner to be a date (which I wanted it to be at the time). This recognition was difficult only because I allowed your disinterest in romance with me to mean something negative about me. I believed it meant I was unimportant, rejectable, and unlovable, and I filtered our whole interaction through these lenses.

Due to these beliefs seemingly being validated during this situation with you, I felt fearful, sad, and embarrassed. These feelings caused me to behave with defensiveness, childishness, judgmentalism, self-centeredness, and dishonesty, which may have confused or even hurt you.

I specifically behaved this way by rolling my eyes, huffing, holding expectations, thinking for you by interpreting what your actions meant, and being dishonest about my true feelings for you at the time. I realize I was blaming and punishing you for not choosing me, but now I see that my behavior must have made it challenging to even want to be near me.

My motive for behaving this way was to make you see that I was a "good catch," important, and lovable. I believed this would get your attention, make you see me, and make you want a relationship with me. I recognize the consequence of my behavior is that we didn't have a romantic relationship or even ongoing friendship. I now see that I could have been honest, vulnerable, open, and kind at our dinner together by telling you what was going on within me, even if that meant you might still choose to not have a romantic relationship. If I could do it differently, I'd be clear and communicative with you, instead of assuming the "date" should be what I thought it should be. I would be myself. I would've simply had fun and gotten to know you for who you are, not the attention and validation I compulsively believed I needed you to offer me.

I'm currently working and committed to being authentic in regard to my feelings and behaviors. I now intend to be honest, humble, more courageous, grateful, and strong.

I want you to know I don't expect anything from you, including a response to this letter. Although a response from you in any form is welcomed, my intention with this isn't to seek ongoing communication, but to clarify my understanding of what I've done and to show my respect by attempting to mend it.

I'm grateful for the time and energy you gave to read this letter from me. This situation really helped me grow, by looking at who I was really being back then.

All the best in your future,
Mary

As I've stated, at this stage in your EMSO Training, that's enough. Write one Repair From Within letter for every person on your EMSO Master Chart that you have lingering PANE around, and/or have a body signal with you think about them—the ones you highlighted. The next Take Action allows you to keep track of those with whom you've decided to Repair. Their name will go in the left column, as you're already doing your Level 1 Repairs by writing a letter addressed to them. This letter is, however, for you and you alone.

This process often inspires students to want to reach out and connect and heal with these people directly. I suggest you first get a bit more understanding of what that may entail, and then simply indicate their name in one of the subsequent columns. These next two levels of Repair are outlined in great detail in the follow-up curriculum, but I'll offer a brief overview here:

## Level 2: Indirect Repairs

Indirect Repairs means that you are not meeting with them face-to-face. There are three primary ways to make Indirect Repairs:

1. Action-based/Non-communication—this would be relevant with deceased persons, irreconcilable relationships, or anything you would consider unsolvable, and those where there may be more hurt created by reaching out (e.g., if you cheated with someone's partner and they still don't know)

2. Hand-written letters (usually based on your Repair from Within Letter)

3. Email

Most of the time, the scariest reparations are the most correcting for our lives—taking away the pain of years-long feuds, dysfunctional marriages, and shifting deep resentment to light-heartedness, connection, and even renewed friendships. This can prevent our minds and hearts from experiencing a lifetime of continued anger and fear. This allows us to conserve the creative energy that's normally drained from us due to the unnecessary tension of shame in holding onto these memories. It's powerful to know that you don't need forgiveness to mend your life; just change your life.

*It's powerful to know that you don't need forgiveness to mend your life, just change your life.*

## Level 3: Direct Repairs

I consider making Direct Repairs an Advanced Practice, and I don't suggest doing this form of repairs unless you already have experience with this process. The primary ways to make Direct Repairs are:

1. Phone call

2. Video call

3. In-person, face-to-face meeting

TAKE ACTION

**LEVELS OF REPAIRS**
After you've written your Repair from Within Letters, you may notice that you want to reach out and make additional efforts toward healing your relationships, using your newfound humility. For now, keep the letters to yourself and use this chart to write in the names of people you may eventually wish to repair with in other ways. This will aid you in preparing for the more advanced step of Indirect and Direct Repairs, which you will learn in future trainings.

## EMSO REPAIRS: HEALING WITH HUMILITY

| LEVEL 1: REPAIRS FROM WITHIN | LEVEL 2: INDIRECT REPAIRS | | | LEVEL 3: DIRECT REPAIRS | | |
|---|---|---|---|---|---|---|
| Write Letter (not sent) | Action-based | Hand-written letter | Email | Phone call | Video call | Meet in person |
| | | | | | | |

## 35

# Merciful Lessons

*Our mercy isn't only to bestow upon others.
It's also a gift to be used for ourselves.*

Understanding leads to mercy, and we can now begin to understand others' "mistakes" (and reasons for them) by first "knowing thyself." Just as you've been angry with others for their mistakes, you may feel shame or guilt because of a mistake you've made, and you may hate or resent yourself because someone was successful in getting you to believe you should feel that way. You've now begun to learn how to influence your resentments toward others by igniting them with understanding, self-responsibility, acceptance, and unconditional love, and by seeing the natural consequences (what happened next). Has this begun changing your anguish into peace? I consider forgiveness an EMSO Advanced Practice, so we won't cover that in this book, but mercy is a great middle ground.

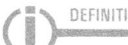 DEFINITION

**MERCY:** a power that when activated can shift us from hate/blame to understanding/ease, and when used in repetition (or when accessed at its most pure point) thrusts us into a state of ultimate and permanent forgiveness.

When you begin to learn mercy toward others, you become more free. But what do you do when <u>you're</u> the one who needs mercy? Find out where you're feeling guilt and shame. Guilt is often the consequence of making a "mistake," while shame is punishment—specifically a self-punishment.

DEFINITIONS

**GUILT:** self-resentment derived from past mistakes

**SHAME:** self-punishment derived from past trauma or current mistakes

Relief from self-resentment and self-punishment isn't between you and someone else. Even if the mistake you hate yourself for has hurt someone else, its resolution isn't dependent on them having mercy on you. Rarely when we as humans are "forgiven" for something, do we permanently feel absolved of the self-inflicted guilt and shame.

Having mercy for someone else may have an effect on their peace, but in the grand scheme of things, your mercy is for you. Mercy doesn't mean forgetting what you did or what has been done to you. You don't actually <u>want</u> to forget, because that would take away the valuable wisdom of the lesson.

The only way to truly change your way of being after you've made a "mistake" (or many!), is to actually be someone different. How? Learn the lesson. By gaining and stabilizing the wisdom from the experience, you save yourself from creating more pain for yourself and others. The best way to make up for your past mistakes is to stop making the same ones again, and the best way to steer clear of negative emotions is to have the wisdom to work through each situation.

There are cases when it really wasn't your doing. For example, a fight in self-defense with someone who was attacking you, a sudden accident, or being forced to do something you didn't want to do. In these cases, there was nothing you did that you could've done differently at the time, because you did everything the way you would do it today. You just <u>think</u> you should have or would have done something differently if you'd known what would happen.

Your ego wants you to stay committed to your filter—feeling like a failure, a worthless person, or a fraud. You may still carry guilt, thinking, "It's my fault that this happened." But that won't bring back your past and let you change it.

Your biochemical addiction is asking you to keep making shame; and you will, until you learn the lesson the training is lending you. Thus, the only option is to move forward, and the best way to move forward is to take responsibility for your behaviors, self-beliefs, and feelings. In this case especially, taking responsibility does <u>not</u> mean taking the blame; it means <u>releasing</u> the blame you placed on yourself by finally realizing the truth.

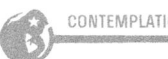

**CONTEMPLATION**

**MAYBE IT WASN'T MY FAULT**

Self-assigned guilt is often an attempt to go "back in time" to control something by taking blame for the outcome. I see this a lot in first responders and veterans who lose comrades or witness the darkest of the dark—in parents who lose children, or in friends, spouses, or relatives of those who commit suicide. If this is the case for you, please contemplate the following:

- Have I taken blame or shoved guilt and shame into myself for something that truly wasn't my doing?
- Am I holding onto the past pain, subconsciously thinking I should also suffer like another did?
- Did I really do it? Was it <u>really</u> my doing?

Pause and use your impeccable honesty skills right now. Catch your ego if it tries to talk you out of looking at what really happened. If you can finally see that you aren't to blame for something and yet you still feel the PANE of guilt, really ask yourself why:

- What is my motivation for holding this guilt or shame? Then ask it again.

It's important to search for this right now. If you can see the truth around it, turn your guilt into the necessary grief over what happened in reality, not the grief over what you <u>thought</u> you'd done. Work through the real grief you may have been avoiding—the grief that something truly difficult occurred, and do so without the guilt. You don't need a distractor to help you through it. You don't need drugs or alcohol, food, or destructive behaviors. You need access to the truth, the real healing, and the necessity of moving on.

Many people who undergo this training are able to easily step away from their secondary distractors and dependance on alcohol, food, painful relationships, and more, because they've now overcome their real, primary addiction—to their biochemistry.

## Your "Mistakes" Are Valuable, So Flaunt Your Failures!

The real you isn't just who you're revealing, it's who you've always been at your essence—otherwise, you wouldn't be working so hard! As these new traits become more and more embodied, and as you keep making repairs and advancing in EMSO Training, you may notice that your perspective of the past completely changes in relationship to both your traumas and mistakes.

The idea of mistakes being valuable is a difficult idea to grasp and understand when you're still sitting in a pool of them. I assure you that on the other side, with Emotional Sobriety, there are beautiful opportunities available because of or thanks to these mistakes. It's seeing with experienced eyes that these were actually gifts not only for your future evolution, but for your ability to one day share your learned lessons with others.

In the beginning of your transformation, it may have seemed unlikely or unbelievable that your mistakes could ever be positive or valuable. Now that you've been given a chance to imagine how your past could have been different, these exercises helped you identify where you were responsible—and we know that these were not actually mistakes, meaning "wrong" or "bad." If you could go back, would you do it all again to be where you are now—now that your observation and understanding of these mistakes has helped you actualize this truer version of yourself? This is the self-actualization that many teachers and preachers talk about!

When we feel the consequences of our past patterns and flaws, we choose more awareness. Once we're aware, we gain experience and knowledge. When we overcome them, we're handed a degree in transformative inspiration. We succumb to the depths of work that's entailed to produce a change within us.

We're diligent with our sanity, ridding our lives of the destructive behaviors we've relied on for many years, and we practice our new ways. Upon reaching our destination, we have a pass to Emotional Sobriety. We now have an opportunity to share this with others who are struggling as we once did—others who also can't imagine a way out of their problems and compulsions. We can now offer this gigantic, life-lightening gift to them, and if that calling arises for you, you'll be in awe of its power. You'll be grateful for having made the same "mistakes," and realize that it is <u>only</u> because of them that you now have the wisdom to guide others to a different choice. You'll see the value of your mistakes glaring you in the face when you can offer solutions to a suffering friend.

Before becoming a hero to others in this way, first become your own hero. When you can stand solidly on your own and offer your hand of help with genuine usefulness, your past mistakes not only become <u>your</u> experience and wisdom, they offer hope and courage to the person who's currently still making them. I now give thanks for all of my mistakes—they fashioned my growth through observation. They had an essential function in my life and many others' lives.

*Your past mistakes not only become your experience and wisdom, they offer hope and courage to the person who's currently still making them.*

When you've changed, the person you used to be must be remembered. Who you used to be can be described to those who may be in a similar position. They can witness the contrast of your old and new way of living. You can utilize the memories of your old self as an objective measurement of how far you've come into your new identity.

If you truly want to help others, flaunt your past failures, because your past mistakes now get to be a source of catalyst and hope for another in need. I told you that your mistakes would be worth something someday! By learning the lesson, your wisdom will grow, which will often move you to share this wisdom as inspiration and guidance for another. By exposing who you'd once been to someone who's struggling like you have, you're expressing (in real time) the opportunity for them to also change. Offer them a hand.

By being an aid to others, you learn more about yourself and are reminded of your past, reigniting the quest away from it. You are granted the gift of usefulness. When you're your best self, if you feel safe in their presence, even the person who may have hurt you the most in your life (who's now seeking guidance to change) will be able to ask you for help. Should they arrive at your doorstep and ask for help, you could supportively invite them in. You'd be able to deliver guidance and love to this person who's struggling in similar ways to you. As unlikely as that may sound to you right now, when you're demonstrating Emotional Sobriety, you won't even think twice about it. You'll be honored and eager to have the opportunity to help where you've been helped. You'll be thankful you know how to guide them. You'll thank <u>them</u> for asking you for help and trusting in you.

*An important component of helping someone change is to expose who you used to be, rather than who you are now.*

When you flaunt your past failures and can display the success of your present, you influence people to grow. In my personal experience as a coach, there are many opportunities to guide or help people in their change process. However, you don't have to be a coach to help others. We can help friends, relatives, children, spouses, and coworkers through their weaknesses and patterns if they are desirous, and if we have the skills.

An important component of helping someone change is to expose who you used to be, rather than who you are now. When I first meet with a student, I'm honest and transparent regarding how I used to think, feel, and behave. This brings a sense of comfort to the space by exposing the fact that I was sitting in the same place that they are. We now have this in common. They see that all of my problems have been solved, and they may choose that for themselves.

I've never helped anyone complete a transformation process without first being vulnerable myself. I have to show my past "ugliness" to give the other person an allowance to share theirs. I have to speak of my past compulsions, dishonesty, and fears for them to express what they're hiding. I happily flaunt my failures happily because I realize that all of the "mistakes" that used to cause my problems are now at the presupposition of being massively valuable to the person in front of me who's deeply scared.

My failures provide a jumping-off point, and invitation, for someone else's self-examination and vulnerability. They can see where I was once stuck and see themselves in me. When they can witness who I am today, with the contrast of reviewing my past, they are often filled with hope.

By showing those who are struggling your past flaws, the flaws now become inversely as powerful as they were once damaging. They're showing the other party that they're not alone in their "sickness," and that their troubling biochemical addiction is extinguishable.

If sicknesses can be caught by standing near someone, then sobriety can be contagious as well! Although you cannot impress your values or attitudes onto someone else, you can be an example in how you now choose to live. Be careful not to simply parrot EMSO information. Instead, be a beacon of self-honesty and integrity. Be a great inspiration of self-improvement through action and demonstration. Don't focus on appearing a certain way, rather be the way. Please don't only read books and take the classes. Take action! Do the work and embody the person you'd like to become—the person who prioritizes their EMSO Training. Be the person who's more aware of their own behaviors than they are concerned or attached to others'. Be the real you!

*If sicknesses can be caught by standing near someone, then sobriety can be contagious as well!*

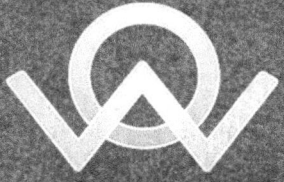

# THE *YOU* YOU'VE NEVER MET

## 36

# Fighting to Stay the Same

*What can derail us from our path to change?*

Even if you're feeling sadness, fatigue, or some residual resentment (even toward me!), let's take a look at the Emotional Sobriety scale and notice that you may have less severity in your tipping toward dysfunction. You may be in a careful balance between your emotional insobriety and sobriety. As you've become more aware and acknowledged so much, you may notice a difference already!

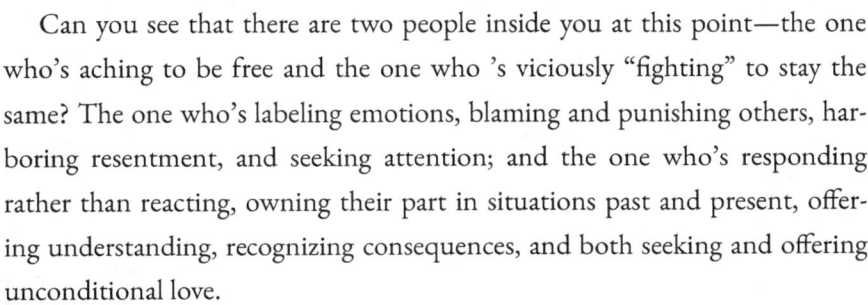

| NEGATIVE PATTERNS | PEACE |
| DESTRUCTIVE TRAITS | CLARITY |
| DYSFUNCTIONAL BEHAVIORS | LEVELHEADEDNESS |
| EMOTIONAL INSOBRIETY | EMOTIONAL SOBRIETY |

Can you see that there are two people inside you at this point—the one who's aching to be free and the one who's viciously "fighting" to stay the same? The one who's labeling emotions, blaming and punishing others, harboring resentment, and seeking attention; and the one who's responding rather than reacting, owning their part in situations past and present, offering understanding, recognizing consequences, and both seeking and offering unconditional love.

After a big upgrade, it's quite common to backslide a bit, and in this chapter and the next, we'll explore exactly why that is and the mechanics of how it most often occurs.

First, as we've learned, both your ego and your brain/biochemistry want to stay as they were. Because of our ego's "training" throughout your life, and our natural, survival-based addiction to our biochemistry, we often fight to keep that which we can change, even when it continues to hurt us. We can intellectually understand that the ego's job is to maintain our status quo—physically, emotionally/chemically, mentally, and energetically—in order to protect itself from the traumas that we once lived through. It keeps us ready for the potential of these same traumas happening again. This makes it seem as if we want to stay in disharmony, sadness, discontent, self-pity, or anxiety, so that we get to "keep" our behaviors. In this chapter, we check in and see if there are any areas in this process where you're unconsciously attempting to stay the same. I call these EMSO Barriers. They're the behaviors and tactics of the ego itself, which has been reliably acting on behalf of your Intoxicated Identity, not the real you. EMSO Training allows the ego to find its right relationship in your life as a support for your sobriety, rather than a stalwart for your insobriety.

*We often fight to keep that which we can change,
even when it continues to hurt us.*

When you meet resistance in your growth, I urge you to read and remind yourself of the following five EMSO Barriers to support you to continue moving forward.

### 1. Wall of Resistance

Everyone has a limit when growing—a wall of resistance. <u>Everyone</u> hits this wall at some point. My purpose—and the essence of EMSO Training—is to assist in getting you over that wall, to elicit lasting behavioral and biochemical change. Have you already experienced this wall during the first portions of your training? Maybe you even began to dislike me for asking you to do all this work because you didn't want to or thought you couldn't muster the energy needed to climb over it. It may feel wrong and painful, but when I push you, it doesn't mean I don't care about how you're feeling; rather, I push you because I both know how it feels to not want to climb it, and I know how it feels on the other side after pushing myself. It would be wasteful to commiserate over how hard it is when the solution is so close by. I made an agreement with you when you decided to walk on this journey with me. I won't give up on you, so don't *you* give up on you. Refocus!

*I won't give up on you, so don't you give up on you.*

## 2. Enemy of the Ego

Let me reiterate the significance of the ego! This ego has a big role thinking it's the most powerful thing about you, and when you allow it to be, it is. Your ego thinks it's the master of your life, the master of its life, and the master of everyone else's life, and you're attempting to challenge it. Did you think it was going to change quietly?

Prior to beginning EMSO Training, when you may have desired to make a change, you most likely asked for help in some way. You may have excitedly hired a coach, consulted with a teacher, read books, or even attended workshops. Now you've made a new plan and an "agreement" to become the *you* you've never met. You may feel an incredible high... the possibilities... the potential! You've decided you're going to have a blissful future devoid of all of your past suffering. You've thrown away the idea that you must remain in turmoil, complacency, or victimhood. You're willing to go to great lengths, and your courage and commitment in that moment are 100%.

When I come together with a student—no matter the subject at hand—and plan out their path to betterment, we often set a clear intention:
- Physical transformation: Intention of getting stronger, losing body fat, or rehabilitating an old injury to an area of reliability.
- Emotional metamorphosis: Intention of revealing the real you, eliminating old beliefs and filters, and committing to a new way.

Regardless of the object we're changing, we make an <u>agreement to reach a goal</u>. I bring this topic up here because this isn't the end of your path to remarkable change, and the ego doesn't like change. So let's make sure you know the tricks it will use to keep you the same. Even when you may think you're finished with your journey to Emotional Sobriety, the ego is still part of you.

Often after your decision to change is made, or after a big breakthrough, it is followed up with a <u>long</u> sleep. Most of my students tell me that when they get home from our initial visit or get halfway through this intensive work like you've just done, they fall asleep for several hours. You may have already experienced this within this work so far.

This sleep is due to the immediate and new relief from your current self, simply by making the agreement. Because you've made an agreement out loud with another person as a witness, your brain and body need to recalibrate and assimilate your new decision and all of this new information—especially the message it's received that the current version of your life will soon be gone. That's a lot to take in!

Since you've made an agreement, done some big work, and are getting ready to climb the next "rung of the ladder," a long sleep (or more than one!) may provide momentary ease in your situation as well. As you near the completion of your EMSO Essentials Training, this will be one of the most aggressive times the ego steps in, outside of when you first began. Because of some initial relief, it may say: "See, you feel fine, you don't need to change. You've got this! Plus, you're too tired to work more than you already have."

Initially, this can be met with standing up for yourself and saying, "No, I'm going forward with the plan!" You're now at battle with the ego, and if it wins over, there is a back-pedaling or complete turnaround in the opposite direction. It interprets the sleep as laziness and lack of motivation, when in reality it's simply your body's way of re-setting itself to ready you for the next step. So take a moment to know what the true function of the sleep is, and don't let your ego's interpretation win the battle!

Another trick the ego uses is to make an enemy out of your new support system. How? It will seek to find flaws in the methods and type of support you're receiving wherever possible—blaming the process for any of your setbacks, and mixing a lack of real desire with the genuine fatigue that this work produces.

The ego may create resentment within you about the people or person whom you've asked to help you transform. By making an issue of contention here, you now have a built-in excuse to <u>not</u> move forward. An alternative won't be sought because you've hit another area of temporary relief, as you did in the initial making of the agreement. This time, you may find your relief in the <u>breaking</u> of the agreement with yourself or someone else.

*The easiest way for the enemy to win is to make an enemy out of your new support system.*

It's a sneaky thing, your ego. The oldest parts of you will be threatened by the newness, and angry at the people who are helping guide you there. Your ego will attempt to convince you that anyone and anything that resembles change—even positive change—is actually the enemy. They <u>are</u> the enemy: The enemy of the ego.

Yet another trick up the ego's sleeve in to step is as your "enabler." As you may have experienced in other realms, the enabler support system is so pernicious and powerful in keeping us the same. The enabler is the one in your life who has "always loved and supported you" for "who you really are," and you now offer them a common enemy. This feels as if it reinforces the bond between you, and also reaffirms your belief of the ego's teachings and your old, familiar self. It toughens old patterns and creates a super-attachment to the old you. The enabler will be more than happy to appease your backslide.

This is especially true after you've recently made a big breakthrough toward a new version of you. In EMSO Training, I witness remarkable displays of the beginnings of transformation and then often a big regression afterward—making the student feel they're "never going to get it." Another common response is: "It's no use, this won't work for me." Similarly in strength coaching, I see this when someone makes a huge lift for the first time, or can do something in a conditioning modality in which they're now demonstrating as an athlete, when before it was "too hard." These people exclaim with joy and bliss that they're really starting to become someone new. Then after a day or two, this initial taste of what their future feels like becomes too surreal to comprehend and they don't continue right away. These successes and positive strides are all enemies of the ego. This concept is essential to recognize as you progress in your EMSO Training. When it comes up, once again... refocus!

### 3. Thoughts of Quitting

There may have been times during this process already, and in the future, when you may want to quit and remain as you are. Staying as you are will give you the exact same life. The same issues and the same disharmony. A decision to change, and the work to get there, is challenging to say the least. World-renowned strength coach and developer of ParaPhysical Training, Ted O'Neill, says, "If getting strong were easy, everyone would be strong. It goes beyond just showing up in the gym; you have to learn techniques, have a plan, and bring courage, understanding, and the humility that goes with knowing that you aren't already considered physically strong."[17] Similarly, if becoming emotionally sober were easy, everyone would already be emotionally sober! Therefore, many people unconsciously choose to remain within their norm of suffering or discontent because change is challenging.

In addition to the discomfort of change keeping you the same, you may have formed a belief that your particular "disorder" is special, and possibly one that's unsolvable. Whatever the case may be, recognize that you're on a path of healing, and healing can be perceived as pain.

As a Doctor of Chiropractic, I see many physical injuries. There's a time period directly after an initial trauma when the first high level of shock chemicals are flooding and then leaving the system. This is a particularly painful period. There's realization of the level of trauma, and the reality of what has happened. Then, as we begin the healing stage, the body deeply aches as it rebuilds. At times, this aching is an even deeper and more consistent pain than our initial injury.

The same goes for your emotional, mental, and energetic healing process. You <u>will</u> feel uncomfortable. You <u>will</u> ache. If you're suffering while you practice your changes and you choose to stick with it anyway, your outcomes will be exponentially as prominent as the discomfort you felt to achieve them. The more uncomfortable your body is with the change, the more deeply seated that habit is. Your habituated behaviors, beliefs, and feelings may be strong, so your desire to change must be stronger! The most successful people in EMSO Training are the ones who look for the moments when they want to quit and use them as signals to work harder. These people find inspiration even at their "lowest" points. Don't quit. Instead, <u>refocus</u>!

### 4. Regression & Doubt

"Regression"—moments of seemingly going backward—is an essential part of the process. You're shifting your biochemistry that's been habitually created since your Early-Age Trauma... these chemicals don't surrender easily. They put up a fight, and the tools I provide allow you to be ready to lovingly fight back! These regressions also allow you to see the contrast in your forward journey. You can see who you're still changing from being, and also use the "mistake" as a new jumping-off point, creating new momentum.

*If becoming emotionally sober were easy,
everyone would already be emotionally sober.*

For example, if you snap at your partner, yet immediately recognize what you've done and aim to practice the new way of being the next time, then you're headed in the right direction! Defensiveness may be the behavior you're focused on in your EMSO Training right now, and in this case you're able to "get over yourself" and see it from new eyes. As a new trainee, you're unlikely to be strong in all areas at once.

In addition to regressions, doubt may creep in. You may at times feel overcome by the fear that you cannot change, or your fear of what you'll experience as the real you may take the wheel and attempt to stop you from progressing. Remember that sneaky little ego that makes you feel fear and thrusts you into the Center of Self? It will want you to regress if you're moving forward with great strides. It will fill you with doubt.

Empower yourself with the knowledge that you might make mistakes, mess up, fall, or slide backward. You may feel all the old feelings flooding back to you, sometimes in small amounts or in landslides.

You may have days that you feel you've made no progress in your climb out of Emotional Belligerence. For some time, you're likely to struggle with the same anxieties and fears, the same anger and blame, and even the same temptation to manipulate and control others. When this inevitable regression and doubt come in, see them for what they are… a moment that you've allowed your Intoxicated Identity to take the reins. This work offers a moment of sobering up, emotionally speaking. Yet without day-to-day training, we easily return to our Intoxicated Identity. I offer ongoing support for this practical daily application of what you've learned about yourself in the curriculum thus far in the second-tier training: EMSO Practicum. This is required for growing and sustaining your Emotional Sobriety. It's earned. For now, when the regression and doubt creep in, remember that this is a natural part of this introductory process and… refocus

### 5. Hidden Motive for Doing This Work

We've discussed the role of your underlying motives behind your thoughts, feelings, and decisions. We've talked about the importance of knowing the motive behind your actions and communications. We've talked about finding your motive when demonstrating dishonesty, to keep you behaving in a R.E.A.L. way with yourself and others. Your motive is a very quick indicator of your level your sobriety. However, there may be an underlying motive lurking about that goes beyond your momentary behaviors, beliefs, and feelings. You may be staying in the training itself because you have a hidden motive for doing this work.

A hidden motive, in this context, is when you're doing the work and attempting to "better" yourself for reasons other than those you've outwardly stated. You keep these reasons to yourself—usually to establish or maintain some kind of control or to gain something other than your own clarity and peace. Hidden motive is a <u>conditional</u> means of "betterment." Some examples include:

- If I learn these things, I'll finally be better than my friends.
- I'll be able to make my spouse do what I want if I appear to be superior to them or act in a way that they'll find more attractive.
- My partner/parents/friend is doing EMSO Training and wanted me to do it too, so I'm doing it so I don't lose the relationship.
- I want the promotion (or to keep my job), and my organization is requiring that we do this.
- If I focus on the "inner work," I can therefore secretly keep my secondary dependence (sugar, alcohol, porn, etc.)

Hidden motive is an attempt to feign self-control in order to gain control over someone else. You put on a show after learning the right things to say and do, yet remain seething and resentful on the inside. You may worsen your sickness by demonstrating your compulsion to control and manipulate under the guise of getting emotionally sober. Not so surprisingly, this hidden motive is often not only hidden from others, but somewhat hidden from you! However, it's not all the way underground... you can feel its sneaky intention right now if this is true for you.

How, then, do you discover if you have a hidden motive? Here are the most common symptoms that there's a hidden motive at play:

- You've done all the work to this point in the training, and you're not feeling or noticing any significant changes within you.
- You aren't able to attain the outcome that's motivating your decision to engage in EMSO Training.
- You're moving in reverse and unable to retain the tools that will help you progress.

Think of hidden motives you have in other areas of your life. They're common in romantic relationships, namely when they're riddled with argumentative behavior or power-hungry partners. You may "learn new tricks" to appear more balanced and establish an emotional dominance over your partner. You'll be able to <u>act</u> a different part, but it's still not truly <u>you</u>. You'll play out this new role by saying things like, "I'm better now, so you have to take me back!" or, "I'm better now and we're still fighting, so obviously you're the problem." Over time, if you don't get what you want, there will be a display of significant Emotional Belligerence and ETBs. This is a desperate attempt at using the old ways once again as a means to "get the prize" when the "new tricks" don't work.

DO YOU RELATE?

Let's draw a parallel with someone who uses alcohol as a secondary addiction: In the back of her mind, and possibly not even recognized as a motive to get sober, Janet thought, "If I get sober and prove that I have myself under control, my family will see that it's okay for me to drink again." Her motive for improving herself and getting clean was to be able to continue to drink. Her intention was to learn to act the role of sober in order to continue to stay the same.

You now have another chance to uncover a potential EMSO Barrier—another way in which you may be holding yourself back. Discovering or knowing this is up to you.

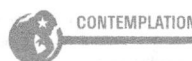

### CONTEMPLATION

**GO UNDERNEATH MY HIDDEN MOTIVE**
To rectify any possible hidden motive for beginning EMSO Training, and/or staying in it now, contemplate if any were present for you when you began doing this work.

Can you find a deeper desire and intention that truly drew you here? When you're stuck or regressing in any part of your life, ask yourself: Why am I <u>truly</u> doing this now? Use your self-honesty—a requirement in every part of EMSO Training.

This will allow you to continuously and lovingly keep tabs on yourself and your inner motive for staying connected to your Emotional Sobriety path. No one else can do that for you. No one else lives inside there... only *you* do.

The real motive that will propel you to true Emotional Sobriety is to be here for the betterment of yourself and the forward momentum of an honest life. If you're storing more secrets, telling more lies, attempting more manipulation, or increasing your level of gossip, you're continuing to live a life that sounds like a bad (or even sad) dramatic movie. I intend for this work to lead to you the opposite of this. If you're bitter that you didn't receive something from someone else that you wanted to gain from EMSO Training, <u>that</u> was your hidden motive.

*If you're bitter that you didn't receive something from someone else that you wanted to gain from EMSO Training, <u>that</u> was your hidden motive.*

## Closer Than You Think

There may be times that you think you haven't made any progress because you keep making "mistakes." Again, the fact that you're aware that you're making them simply means that you're catching yourself in old ETBs, and that's a good sign! Remember when you began and how hard it was to even <u>notice</u> when you were lying to someone else or to yourself, judging others, or behaving childishly? I imagine you're not only noticing these behaviors, but likely enacting them far less of the time.

*Catching yourself in old behaviors is a good sign.*

Recognizing the repeated pattern in the moment can feel like failure, but it's not. It's an opportunity to pause and be grateful that you now have the capacity to notice your behavior patterns. With additional training, you'll easily stop them in their tracks, or not even express them in the first place. In fact, you'll address the self-belief and addiction to PANE that created the need for this behavior and remove that biochemistry from your physical makeup altogether!

Too tired to work on yourself today? This is the day to put even <u>more</u> intention on being real. Resist coasting or "taking a break" on the days that you feel the strongest, bravest, and most centered. Instead, look for an opportunity to solidify your new way of being. The idea is to get so far ahead of your "problems" that you'll never fear falling back toward them. Even a small regression, when you have made it ten miles away from your past compulsions and chronic agitations, won't affect the quality of your life. Stay the course.

Allow yourself to be PANE-free by knowing you're worth saving!

*You're wanted in this movement of Emotional Sobriety.*
*Your advancements and insights will inspire the world.*

How long did it take you to develop these patterns of fear, anxiety, depression, anger, blame, frustration, impatience, and childishness? More than likely, this has required a lot of years. Give yourself patience as you work to resolve them. You've done extraordinarily hard work in discovering your Anatomy of Emotional Insobriety and matriculated through the full set of R.E.A.Life Investigation and Repair exercises. You've taken this seriously and honed in to become aware of and acknowledge your self-beliefs. You continue to take action to continue to grow in emotional health and sobriety.

Tell your transforming self that the habits and traits it had been using to get its way and survive are no longer usable traits. Invite your old self to move into a more powerful and useful version. Here, you become your own parent, your own teacher, and you coach yourself through your intoxication to make sure you're supported through your own efforts. Be patient with your ego and its childish fears, and lovingly invite it along on the journey with you. You're wanted in this movement of Emotional Sobriety. Your advancements and insights will inspire the world. What worked well for me was to say this to my old self:

 INTENTION-SETTING MOMENT

> "We aren't doing this anymore. Come with me over here, where all behaviors and attitudes that have caused harm will fall away. All the things you think you need will dissipate. Don't be afraid... you won't be left behind. I'll be strong enough for both of us. You'll be with me in wisdom."

It sounds as if the ego-mind is some conspiracy to keep you the same, but it's really there as a keeper of your habits and a seeker of homeostasis. It "thinks" it's doing what you've always asked it to, so to change (even if it's been several months) can feel sudden and threatening. To win a battle, you have to know what your "enemy" is planning. This is the ego's way of attempting to pull you back to who you used to be, to do what you've always done, and to urge you to quit doing the work you're doing to change.

## Landmarks

In my teaching over the years, I've seen common patterns in the moments and situations when the EMSO Barriers pop up. These are the landmarks that may delay or completely pause your new path soon after you reach them. Not only knowing these, but being hyper-aware of them will aid in your success. If you know what to look for, you can even use these setbacks to your advantage! When you complete each of these stages, be aware of what you hear from your inner egoic voice. Look for each of these landmarks as you continue your EMSO Training.

 CONTEMPLATION

### LANDMARKS

Look at the following set of landmarks and contemplate if you've already experienced them. If not, hold them in your awareness as possible future barriers to progress, and using the knowledge you've gained in this chapter, allow them to be springboards rather than setbacks.

**Time-Based Landmarks:**

- After your initial decision to change
- When you feel exhaustion or have excessive poor sleeping patterns (normal, but can be a cause of concern)
- When you have a big breakthrough and begin to demonstrate a new way of being
- When you feel you're coasting with new confidence, and it seems to be coming easily to you

The following can be the most difficult times. Remember that it's simply a sign that you're gaining ground on the mountain of change.

If your ego is fighting to stay the same, it means you're doing something to threaten it. Could the pushback from your ego be a good sign? Yes! It's showing that you're engaged in an active change process, or it wouldn't be fighting you to stop. Let these landmarks be signposts for your evolution!

**"Enemy of the Ego" Landmarks:**

- When you begin to resent the people whom you've asked for help
- When you're trying to talk yourself out of the next action step
- When you feel threatened by a new experience
- When your inner voice is telling you that your previous thoughts, self-beliefs, and behaviors were actually the right ones, or that you're okay now that you've made some progress

Though these may seem like setbacks, these are actually the transformative landmarks in your EMSO Essentials Training. These are the instances within which you prove your intention and commitment to uncovering the real you. You may have many battles surrounding these landmarks—with your fatigue, your familiar circles, and your thoughts. You may become sick, get injured, or experience some kind of new traumatic experience. You may break out in a rash or develop rushes of anxiety. Still... move forward, and of course... <u>refocus</u>! Continue to challenge your old self with love and motivation. Remind it who it's becoming. Show it who's in charge now.

Your success depends on each moment that you choose to stay committed—even when, and especially when, your ego doesn't want you to.

*Your success depends on each moment that you choose to stay committed.*

You may have been told you're not worthy, or contrastingly, you may have been told that you <u>are</u> worthy by certain teachers, counselors, friends, or a parent. Ultimately, neither makes a difference. *You* have to sit with *you*—alone in the darkness and feel what is true. You have to connect to that place that will remind you of the inherent worthiness that we all share. I cannot convince you of this. You cannot be told you're worthy. You have to find it and feel it, for yourself. When you know you're worthy to be and express as the real you, move forward.

## 37

# Familiar Energy Crisis

*It's okay to step away and heal.*

The most common place that our ego, brain, and biochemistry fights to keep us the same is in familiar settings.

You've probably been naturally sharing who you're becoming with those around you as you've been learning these EMSO Essentials—perhaps through direct sharing—"I'm in EMSO Training"—or simply through being who you are now around the same people with whom you used to act belligerently. Next, you'll learn why and with whom this will be the most challenging. Why does maintaining our change seem so difficult when we're around the people with whom we have had the longest-lasting relationships?

*When <u>you</u> change, by definition, the <u>relationship</u> is now changed.*

When engaging in a change process, the support you have around you is so important. I often say that there's a reason we aren't alone on this planet, and it's because we need community in order to evolve. What happens when your "support" is blocking you from your changes that you've chosen? Let's look at this topic calmly and see what solutions we can find to help you through this.

Long-term relationships can be the toughest for unhealthy individuals to grow within because they can be the most emotionally challenging. They expose our emotionally unsober ways. Depending on your current relationship maturity score, there may be many insecurities, expectations, old resentments, neediness, and assigned roles that make it almost impossible for a partner or family member to be supportive. When you change, your relationships change—all of them, whether they're romantic, familial, professional, or friendships.

Before your desire and decision to change, these relationships may have bombarded you with criticism and demanded that you change your behavior. The irony is that once you begin the process of real change and implement new behaviors into your life, these same people may express a desire that you revert back to the way you were. You may also feel that compulsion within yourself.

So why is that? In EMSO Training, it's the...

**DEFINITION**

**FAMILIAR ENERGY CRISIS:** compulsion to return to the person you've chosen to stop being by virtue of being near the energy of past familiar relationships.

Others may find you threatening to their own unique challenges because your energy, thoughts, feelings, and behaviors are now different than theirs. Maybe you're no longer arguing or impatient, and it doesn't match the way things have always been. It's new and unfamiliar to them, and it may be disorienting. They may subconsciously think, "What can I expect from this person now? What will it be like? I know how the arguing and fighting felt. I understand my role and necessary behaviors to maintain our previous relationship. What if we grow apart? What if I'm not good enough? What does this change mean about me?"

*Once you begin the process of real change and implement new behaviors into your life, these same people may express a desire that you revert back to the way you were.*

Whether you've mastered the EMSO Essentials or have only begun to live out your education through noticing your ETBs, when returning to the "norm"—your home or workplace—you will be faced with employing your new way of being within pre-sobriety relationships.

These are all the people whom you knew before you started sobering up, emotionally speaking—your friends, family members, romantic partners, co-workers, and acquaintances. Though you've worked on this process of change, your parents, friends, children, and bosses have most likely not experienced the same thing. You may feel great, yet the people you've known remain in old patterns of behavior. This leaves an obvious imbalance. Your transformation and dedication to making the healthiest choices in your life don't mean you're better than these people. This simply means you're different from what you once were.

Remember, when you change, by definition, the relationship is now changed. These relationships can be renewed and reconstructed, but they won't go forward without effort. This requires both a levelheaded and open discussion, along with an agreement of how the new relationship may look and feel.

New communication and action may be a challenge because the energy of these relationships is often so strong and bonded that they may pull you into the same habitual programming—behaviors, thoughts, and feelings—that you're in the process of changing. You may fall back into your old "normal." You may find compulsive urges of past actions, language, and feelings. If you remain new, calm, and humble within the conversation, you may even notice the other party attempting to get you emotionally "riled up" or feel ashamed of your desire to be calm. This is an unconscious reaction on their part to pull you energetically and chemically back to where they're comfortable.

This energetic pull to stay the same will be disguised as feeling familiar, natural, and normal. But just because it feels familiar doesn't mean it's healthy—it's only familiar. The power of the habit of the familiar is a threat to your change. The pull of judgment and resentment from learned racism, political stance, and even religious myopia can energetically become the custom of the family or the routine in a friendship. Hating the boss and gossiping at the office can be a strong "policy" of the social workplace.

This familiar energy has often caused people to regress into their Intoxicated Identity to the point that they stop their process of transformation and go back to who they were when they started. They return to lying and manipulating everyone by playing the role that they are expected to play. They then suffer with the same problems, think the same thoughts, and have the same conversations. They're experiencing the Familiar Energy Crisis.

When you change, the people around you must therefore adapt, and there may be resistance. It's so important to be 100 % committed to your process of change, no matter how many aspects of your life look differently than they did before.

In the educational space of EMSO Training, you may still be heavily embracing the use of your Emotional Intelligence, or awareness—asking yourself to pay attention to the details of your day, thoughts, emotions, and habits. You may need to be on highest alert within these familiar relationships.

Let's explore each type of relationship in your life, and how the real you can find greater ease and connection during your early development with EMSO Training.

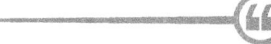

*Just because it feels familiar doesn't mean it's healthy.*

## Your Growing-up Family

If you continue to do what you've always done, your life will continue to express as it always has. Your Growing-up Family includes all the family members or people with whom you lived while growing up—the people whom you were surrounded by, learned from, and mimicked. They either witnessed or contributed to your experiences, your Early-Age Trauma, your triumphs, and more.

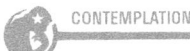
CONTEMPLATION

> Take a moment to feel compassion and gratitude for your Growing-up Family. No matter what it looked like, what are the pieces that you can really be thankful for? How were you loved? How were you taken care of? What can you respect and appreciate about your parents or caregivers? Your grandparents? Your siblings? Think about what they may have gone through in <u>their</u> childhoods. If they were adults when you were a child, what was their life experience? Do you know their pain or the issues they were dealing with? Were there other children in your home? What were their experiences? It's okay if you do not know the answers to these questions, they're here for you to question and sense into—to see that they're individuals like you. Take the time to think of this now before moving forward. No guilt or shame, judgment or anger... simply acknowledge them. All of them.

A healthy and open Growing-up Family can be one of the most supportive and safest places for you. It's important for you now to be the healthiest you can be while observing the habits of your family and deciding where there's unconditional attention, unnatural "obligation," expectations, punishment, shame, manipulation, etc. It's your duty now to discern where it's safest and supportive enough to continue your growth. If you have healthy relationships here, that's something to be truly grateful for; and if you don't, contemplate the reasons behind this (looking at yourself always) and see why and how the energy of the family may be blocking you (temporarily) from growth. Remember, it's nobody's fault—not even yours.

*In the childhood relationships that you've maintained into adulthood, you can easily fall into an inebriated state of habitual emotional reaction.*

More than any other group of people in your life, your Growing-up Family will have the most pre-established roles. Therefore, it can seem absolutely impossible to step outside of your role in these relationships, especially when you're in fairly constant connection with them. There are many ETBs within these relationships that aren't consciously developed. In the childhood relationships that you've maintained into adulthood, you can easily fall into an inebriated state of habitual emotional reaction. It is a challenge attempting to navigate and communicate within relationships that you entered into as a less sober version of you.

The Growing-up Family is often made up of the people with whom we feel "at home," yet there are often years and years of dysfunction. I've learned many things about family dynamics in my coaching practice—about the function of secrecy and lies, emotional leverage, distractors, and tactical defenses, and ways the dynamics protect members of the family feeling their fear, anger, sadness, or shame.

The intricacies of your family dynamics may feel like a complex maze to an outsider, but to you they're your native tongue... your tribe's way of doing things. You may not even have been aware of just how much energy it takes to maintain the maze. The maze of patterns is more easily established in families than anywhere else. Because your Early-Age Trauma occurs in childhood, you access your Center of Self and develop your filters and ETBs in the context of your family. You learned to "protect" yourself the way that they did. Maybe you hide away, drink alcohol excessively, or have compulsive attention-seeking behavior like one of your parents did. Maybe you find yourself yelling at your spouse and children, just like you witnessed someone in your family doing to their loved ones. There's so much energetic communication going on in your Growing-up Family—most obviously with what are commonly called "unspoken agreements."

*The intricacies of your family dynamics may feel like a complex maze to an outsider, but to you they're your native tongue... your tribe's way of doing things. You may not even have been aware of just how much energy it takes to maintain the maze.*

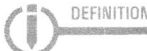
DEFINITION

**UNSPOKEN AGREEMENTS:** a system of one-sided imaginary contracts that are developed without a previous plan or discussion.

These are your family's ways of communicating via expectation and assumption. They are akin to expectations and showed up accordingly on your EMSO Master Chart. Unspoken agreements also have a way of advancing in expected understanding and translation over the years. If not met, or adhered to, they will cause great discomfort between members of your family. These could be facial expressions, body language, or reactions that are all designed to elicit a specific response, either emotionally or behaviorally. This response is what the other party has already "agreed to" without any actual indication. If you're part of a family that can "connect" based solely on imaginary contracts, past behaviors, punishments, and energetic coercion, think of the power that familiar energy has over you; and before you began your training, that <u>you</u> had over <u>them</u>! There may be unspoken insistence from your Growing-up Family that you remain in your previously agreed upon role. Do any of the following ring true?

- If I say _____, they'll think _____.
- If I give her _____ look, they'll know what I mean.
- If I do _____, they'll do _____.
- If they see me doing _____, I'll make them feel _____.

> *When you choose change and solution, you must surround yourself with supportive confidants, until you get your footing in sobriety, or be at peace with being alone for a while.*

When you go back to visit your Growing-up Family, it's quite common to suddenly feel all the same fears and anxieties that your family has been bathing in together. You may feel the same shame and embarrassment, or instantly shrink in the presence of your siblings. You may become angry and resentful and start to engage in various ETBs with them. In some cases, you may actually feel, speak, and even physically begin to look as you did before you began your change process. The sound of your voice can change back into what the family member is used to hearing,—both in tone and language. This is how strong the familiar energy can be in your Growing-up Family!

**DO YOU RELATE?**

> Jorge started a fat-loss program and he's two weeks in. He's lost eight pounds of body fat and is feeling really excited about it. Tonight is his mother's birthday gathering and everyone's meeting at his parents' house for dinner. He packs up a gift and puts on an outfit that he bought a couple years ago that didn't fit until today. He's feeling confident and accomplished.
>
> He enters the home of familiar surroundings. There's the smell of dad's famous home-cooked steak and potatoes, along with a giant birthday cake and ice cream for dessert, beer flowing alongside the wine, and a table with crackers and cheese, chips and salsa, and more. Jorge's other family members are watching the game and casually placing chip after chip into their mouths.
>
> He no longer wants to participate in most of these activities, as they don't match the statement of who he's now committed to becoming. He finds a seat next to his dad who hands him a beer.
>
> "Oh, I'm not drinking tonight, Pop," he says. Everyone looks over in disbelief and asks "Why?!"
>
> "I'm on a food plan to lose body fat," he responds.
>
> "A diet? But it's mom's birthday!"

More than likely, within a short time of arriving at the home of your Growing-up Family, you, like Jorge, will be drawn into the familiar behaviors. Food habits are a simple example to show how this is also true for habitual attitudes, language patterns, and emotions within the family. If you can be coaxed into eating the food you consciously went there <u>not</u> intending to eat, you'll also undoubtedly be pulled into the habitual emotional tornado—the anger, hysteria, gossip, or fear—of your Growing-up Family.

If you choose to eat the cake and drink the beer anyway, you're eating like the person who's overweight rather than the new person you're becoming.

With enough EMSO Training and integrity with your identity, nothing can take you off the path. No criticism, energetic pulling, or attempted guilt-trips would have swayed you into participating in any unhealthy habits of the family. When you choose change and solution, you must surround yourself with supportive confidants, until you get your footing in sobriety, or be at peace with being alone for a while.

If you choose to remain part of these relationships, it's now your responsibility to create a new agreement with each and every member of your family, You must be clear with everyone with whom you're currently co-existing that you're committed to a change process or training program (however you feel most comfortable wording it).

It can be challenging to do so amongst those who don't change alongside you, but I assure you that it <u>is</u> possible to change into the best version of yourself and still manage to have your family relationships.

How do you communicate your new intentions? This can be done only with acknowledgment of who you're being and why you're choosing to change. This requires demolishing the old "agreements" and creating new clearly spoken agreements. The new spoken agreements often start with getting real about two points of view: yours and theirs. You'll most likely discover that the unspoken agreements were interpreted differently by each person in the Growing-up Family. Anything not clearly communicated can be confusing and misinterpreted. In fact, all interpretation is a misinterpretation.

DO YOU RELATE?

> Veronica's dad has an unspoken agreement that he check her gas tank each time she visits to ensure she has an adequate amount of gas. When it's close to empty every time he checks it, he gets frustrated with her, and rather than voicing it, he gets in her car and goes to fill the tank. She interprets that her Dad derives enjoyment from having an act of service that he can offer her, so she purposefully comes to his house with an empty tank… it's a maze!

*All interpretation is a misinterpretation.*

In the EMSO Practicum curriculum, as well as in the EMSO Advanced Practices, you'll learn how to create precise, spoken agreements. For now, this will get you through the basics. I've provided three of the most common types of family members here to support you in practicing making clear, spoken agreements to replace the outdated, unspoken ones.

**The Neutral Parent:** Your parent loves you, is perhaps a kind person, but doesn't know how to effectively communicate and isn't yet emotionally sober. If it's been challenging to navigate a new relationship with them, especially now that you're changing, sit down and specifically state the things that would support you in having a relationship with them. Be sure to let them know that you're here to help create it with them.

**The Emotionally Belligerent Family Member**: This person may not have space for you to have a new kind of relationship, especially in the beginning. There may be someone in your family who's gossiping about you, or even being hateful toward you. You may be disappointed or hurt, especially in the beginning of your EMSO Training, when you don't yet have your "sea legs." You won't necessarily have a breakthrough with this person, and that's okay. The practice is releasing your need to have their attention. This looks more like having a boundary with them, which is spoken on your part. The new contract with them may even result in no contact for now—a new contract of no contact.

**The Ones Who Don't Know You're in Training**: Let them know that you're on a new path. It's okay to keep it vague and use language such as, "I'm going on a healing journey and may be calling you less often, but it's not personal to you. I'll be back."

Do you see how simple it can be to have clear communication about what's real? One of the initial responses I received from one of my students was, "But nobody talks that way!" I had to giggle and respond, "Yes, not many do... only <u>effective</u> communicators."

Like making your repairs, creating new agreements may yield disappointing results. If this is the case, it simply means you came into the conversation with expectations of a specific outcome; perhaps that they would magically know how to do all the things you're now learning in your training. Patience, understanding, and levelheadedness are imperative here. This group may be the most difficult to talk to.

When you're facing someone who's not supportive of your change from the beginning, discuss it gently by stating what's true for you. <u>You</u> can be understanding of <u>their</u> lack of understanding by taking time to reassure them. If that doesn't work, there may be too much resistance for you to grow. All you need to do is set your boundaries and create new spoken agreements. If it's met with resistance, you may simply need to create space. If/when they're ready to accept your change, they'll come to you. Judgment of others will block you from further growth and get in the way of your usefulness. Judgment is not benign; it's born from resentment. How helpful or destructive has resentment been for you before? Choosing the real you is to choose your sobriety, and this positively alters the energy you'll emit in and beyond these relationships, which impacts the world.

If you can't get along with someone or you have a lack of trust in them, then you can create a boundary, or physically separate from them. Remove your judgment and blame, and you can still love them. It doesn't make you wrong for continuing to love them. It's okay to love people whom you don't trust.

Can you imagine how beautiful your family relationships would look if you were levelheaded, genuine, and open? What could you contribute to their life?

*It's okay to love people whom you don't trust.*

### Your Children

Teach your children Emotional Sobriety and inspire through example, action, and consistency. The energy you emit around you is palpable. Think for a moment of the last time you knew someone was mad at you. If they didn't say anything at all, would you still have been able to feel it?

In the same way, your kids can <u>feel</u> you. In my experience as a mother, they can nearly read your mind. So to say we must be emotionally levelheaded and sober as parents is the bare minimum for our development. Our kids love us, rely on us, and depend on us to teach and protect them. In many ways our kids <u>become</u> us, so let's be the best we can be for them.

We must be consistent with our development as we can see the responsibility we have to bring up these children. We require the motivation to think good thoughts, maintain positive emotions of gratitude and love, and be compassionate when our kids act like... well, kids. The issue here is maintaining our composure in times of combustion. Learning EMSO, we not only become more aware of our anger, sadness, and frustration when dealing with our personal life, but also we acknowledge our impatience or anxieties and we reason within ourselves in a different and realistic way. We aren't shoving away our feelings or pretending to change our behaviors. We're working through our insobriety quickly with a clearer mind and actively choosing something more productive in their place. With mastery, we don't even receive the feedback of offense or frustration anymore, and our children notice!

*A great thing about self-control is that we get to decide what mood we'll be in moment to moment.*

Children may emulate both your strongest points and your weakest. Our children deserve to have parents who are in moods that they'll feel comfortable being around and talking with, and in which they can trust. Our children will go through different stages at different ages. As parents, we have to adapt, and that can be challenging! But as EMSO parents, we're steadfast and strong in our identity and therefore don't waiver from this strength.

In moments of "crisis," remember who you want to be. Instead of becoming the teenage girl who's yelling at you, be her levelheaded and reliable mother who can bring her into peace. In lieu of acting as the impatient toddler, choose to be the grown-up father who can be a steady hand of reason and example. Our reactions are particularly patterned as caretakers, so we must now declare who we are, and be a voice of reason with understanding, even in events as common as them needing our attention and not knowing how to ask for it.

We have to be forward-moving with our own development as adults, or our children may never learn to be adults. It's not our job to raise good little children. It's our job to raise content and contributory adults.

Think about what your intentions and motivations are, especially in the case of your children. These are the questions I asked myself regarding my daughter: "Who do I want to be that would most greatly influence and benefit her development? What would she be learning if she learned from me? How would she behave in relationships if she behaved like me? How would she suffer inside if she felt like me? What would she think about if she thought like me? Where might she get in trouble if she emulated me?"

I decided that the best version of me had internal clarity, less external neediness (wholeness), self-control, integrity in challenging situations, positive emotions as a default, an honest thought process, and a strong voice. I intended to be tolerant of where others were different than me, while at the same time be able to set boundaries where necessary. I chose to develop into a version of myself that could be trusted, and I could trust as well. My intention was to bestow my daughter with a familial tradition of realness and peacefulness.

*It's not our job to raise good little children.*
*It's our job to raise content and contributory adults.*

Can you imagine how beautiful your relationships with children would look if you're always levelheaded, genuine, and open? What could you contribute to their life as this new version of you? How will you inspire them, encourage them, and demonstrate Emotional Sobriety to them?

CONTEMPLATION

**UPGRADE YOUR ROLE-MODELING**
How would you like your children to be raised? If you currently have children, may one day, or have children in your life, contemplate your responses to these questions:

- What behaviors of your own do you want children to emulate?
- How would you like them to differ from you?
- Where can you make changes to your traits so that children in your life have an improved role model?
- Did you learn these ways of being in childhood?

## Your Friendships

A friend will support your growth, and you, theirs. Surround yourself with others who live life in the place you intend to advance to. Many of these people will most likely have undergone arduous work to develop into who they are. By not separating temporarily from our norm, we remain in the cycle of the same. Not because the people around us are to blame, but because <u>who we are</u> in those circles is what needs to change. We cannot do the same things and expect a different result.

As I've shared, staying in the same circles may confuse your decision to change and pull you right back under the wave of the status quo. You may find yourself caught in the looped undertow of coming up for sanity and drowning in unconscious insanity.

Some experiences that my students have shared when they're in the change process and run in their normal friend circles too soon include:

- Excessive complaining, gossip, slander, guilt, manipulation, and non-communicated management of others
- Worst-case-scenario thinking: anxiety, depression, fear, injury, and sickness (usually followed by colds/flus)
- Drug or alcohol use / too much "partying"
- General negativity
- Discouragement for their growth, hysteria, and other unhealthy habits that contributed to their regressing back to old patterns

But they happily participated in all of it because that's what they usually do in this setting. It's the habit of the circle. They found that continuing with the same friendships caused massive blocks to their evolving away from who they had been being. And the fastest way to begin and sustain change is to <u>actually</u> begin and sustain change! Meaning, you must start changing your life by changing your life.

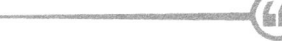

*They happily participated in all of it because it's what they usually do in this setting. It's the habit of the circle.*

We must separate from the areas where we can easily find these patterns or communicate effectively that this behavior is no longer what we intend to display or tolerate. We don't get sober by remaining in circles of addiction. We don't get levelheaded by being "allowed" to be hysterical. We don't get stronger by being enabled to act weak.

We become new by forming our life into the way we choose it to be. We don't find sobriety by talking about our problems, anger, or victimization. We don't find peace within the practice of gossiping, complaining, or discussing our current dramas in the same circle in which we personally perpetuated the drama. We don't continue to assign each of our friends to take on a role in perpetuating our problems.

Talking with an emotionally unsober friend about the problems in your life and expecting to change your problems is comparable to asking a drunk person to drive you home in a car with no headlights, in the middle of the night, with no map of where you need to go... and expecting to get home.

If your friends are constantly digesting your new life dramas, they're not gaining positively from their current relationship with you. Digesting their dramas won't show that you love them more. Your sadness won't bring joy, and their sympathy for your sadness won't bring you more joy.

During this process, seek out support that will resonate most with your newfound desire for growth. You can connect with fellow EMSO students, for example. There are plenty of options for support, but you must choose wisely. Look for those who encourage, but don't enable. Look for those who are seeking and maybe have gone further than you in their journey—then, you have immediate community and support from like-minded growth seekers.

*Talking with an emotionally unsober friend about the problems in your life and expecting to change your problems is comparable to asking a drunk person to drive you home in a car with no headlights, in the middle of the night, with no map of where you need to go... and expecting to get home.*

As a coach, I'm only interested in helping people transform. I'm not invested in maintaining people at their current level of circumstance, because I know that they're capable of more. I also choose friendships based on similar intentions and honesty. Where I spend my time and create my deepest connections is with those who want to do the "impossible." It's not only okay for you to be selective about whom you surround yourself with, it's imperative for your evolution. They will be great influencers on the path you take.

I want to be clear that this doesn't mean you have to change all the people in your life—you have to change only your relationship with them. I've recreated beautiful friendships with many of my pre-sobriety friends, and these relationships are healthier than ever! These friends were excited, encouraging, and even inspired by my process and progress of change, as I was by witnessing and supporting each of them on their own paths. When you change, communicate your change. At this point, you'll still have the history together, and now the opportunity to create new memories with new behaviors focused on cooperation, contribution, and creativity. Of course, be grateful, as true supportive friends are a real gift.

Can you imagine how beautiful your friendships might look if you're levelheaded, genuine, and open? What could you contribute to another person's life in this new form, as their friend?

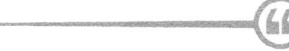

*Where I spend my time and create my deepest connections is with those who want to do the "impossible."*

### Your Workplace

Some find that leaving their job to change their lives is impossible. It's possible. I won't ask you to do that. That is for you to decide. We're surrounded by stressed-out people, and we've contributed to that stress within our workplace and circle of influentials—energetically and emotionally. We've been high-strung and bitter, and we entrain to the same tendencies of communication style, overreaction, underreaction, lies, oversharing, and abuse, all while avoiding rocking the boat.

When you become emotionally sober and begin a new way of being and living, you'll have to change your contribution to these circles. In the workplace, specifically, you'll go through "growing pains." You may be likely to give yourself away here, and lack integrity corresponding to your new identity, due to fear of creating discord. This is where you believe your financial security lies and sometimes you may be tempted to just be "normal" here, or not express boundaries that may cause disruption to your paycheck or initiate social pressures.

 **DO YOU RELATE?**

> One of my students, Angelina, had a lazy relationship with one of her male co-workers. She was attention-seeking and wanted to be validated, special, and attractive. They would flirt and go to lunch together. Once she completed her EMSO Training, she realized that she no longer desired that kind of relationship, as it didn't serve either of them.
>
> She told him that she was going to be changing her behavior, describing her reasoning for her past behavior, and initially he was a bit defensive. At the end of the talk, he admitted that he also struggled with needing attention, and because of that need—though he didn't genuinely have romantic feelings for her—their relationship had become flirtations instead of platonic.
>
> They committed to changing their behavior together, and now have a more relaxed and genuine friendship because it isn't buried under neediness or attention-seeking. It's now based on what's real in the moment.

This doesn't mean you have to walk into work one day and make a grand announcement to reveal the real you. You don't have to reveal this individually with each working relationship you have. But in cases like this one—the more unsober, compulsive relationships—you can step up and be confident in the new choices you're making and communicate them directly. This may even look like an apology to your boss or co-workers for some of your previous behaviors. If you're closely knit and seated near each other in your workplace, keep it simple and just do the next best thing. Modify and use any of the communication practices provided for families.

## Your Marriage or Romantic Relationships

Any healthy relationship mandates that all participants are healthy. Romantic relationships can be tricky on your journey to stabilize your Emotional Sobriety. As we spoke about when creating our EMSO Master Chart, our insobriety may be most obvious in these relationships, because they often easily expose our sickness. Many of us find we're the most needy, insecure, attention-seeking, dishonest, and we expose more parts of our Intoxicated Identity in these cases (though it may be a near tie with our Growing-up Family!).

In pre-sobriety, we often choose our partners to fill our deficits based on our Trauma-Influenced Self-Beliefs and Trauma Filters, as do our partners in their choice with us. One needs to be needed and one needs. One seeks attention and one over-gives. One wants to keep their addiction, and one will ignore the addiction as long as they aren't abandoned. One is constantly dissatisfied, and one is addicted to the discomfort of their partner nagging them. Our polarity of deficits can give the illusion of a perfect fit. It feels "good" and "right" to find someone who makes us "feel whole." Even if the relationship isn't necessarily healthy, it feels comfortable. In reality, it's each of our Intoxicated Identities finding a "match" so that our ego can sustain our insobriety and our body/brain can keep our biochemistry as it is.

So now that you've been able to get over yourself to see your own insobriety patterns, coming face-to-face with your pre-sobriety decisions can seem alarming. You may find that your romantic relationship is unhealthy. If you're in an unhealthy relationship, it means you are, or were, both unhealthy in some way. A healthy relationship cannot exist if one person is healthy and the other is unhealthy. With this realization, you may be tempted to stay the same so that your change doesn't rock the boat and alter your dynamic. This temptation will most likely be subconscious, like your other survival skills that try to keep you the same.

You may find yourself planning vacations and setting dates far in the future to keep the status quo at home. You may have the urge to have a child to keep your partner with you. You may buy a home together. If you aren't married, there may be discussion of it to create the "security" as you change, or stay the same. You may lack integrity in your new ways to appease the dysfunction of the relationship, being a newer version of yourself at work and with friends, and falling backward to the old you when returning home. This is why it's called the "familiar" energy crisis. You're tempted, manipulated, lulled, or even scared into being something you don't want to be anymore, due to familiar rank. At its worst, if your partner feels insecure due to your growth, you may even drop the idea of your continued training altogether to make sure your partner feels safe.

*Choosing to push down the deepest passion of your life to relieve or enable another's anxieties is not love. This is codependency.*

In most relationships, there's often some attachment of responsibility to someone else, and needs that must supposedly be fulfilled. This is compulsive behavior based on learned obligation of societal norms and upbringings. How can you make improvements on <u>you</u> when there's someone on the <u>outside of you</u> demanding you stay the same, creating obligation about when you should arrive and where you should be, what you should and shouldn't do, saying, "Stay exactly as you are, for me, even if you want to be and do more. That's how you can show me love."

Ignoring your own true desires in order to feed the insecurities of another is <u>not</u> an act of compromise. Denying your heart's truth to make someone feel more comfortable is <u>not</u> an act of compassion. Choosing to push down the deepest passion of your life to relieve or enable another's anxieties is <u>not</u> love. This is codependency.

Possible solutions include direct communication with your partner regarding what your intentions are, such as "I'm now committing to my healing process." The best option would be for you to take this journey together, which requires special vulnerability. If you can be accountable and help each other with your growth, it has the potential to be connecting instead of separating. Either way, gently invite them to do some kind of self-improvement practice to remind them of their wholeness. Otherwise, you'll always be the one who they'll look to to make them feel whole.

Make sure that you're aware that "filling" them isn't offering you any real security either. Heal together, and continually check your motive for creating a healthier partnership.

Once this is in place, you can make new spoken agreements and move forward together in individual and mutual growth. If there are negative emotional outbursts from them when you change, know that your changes may feel threatening to them. If their filter is distrust and you know this, the best things to offer are patience and support for their healing, and plenty of communication. Ask them what they would like the relationship to look and feel like. Ask yourself how you can help guide them to remember their own wholeness without giving any of yourself away. Then answer those questions for yourself as well.

That said, if you're fortunate enough to have a loving and supporting partner during this time, it can be a very beneficial addition to your process. As positive as this work will be in your life, this can still be difficult for everyone involved, so be kind to each other.

If you're single, I suggest refraining from dating until you have a solid proficiency in Emotional Sobriety and have cleaned out your past and overcome your Intoxicated Identity. If this isn't managed before entering into a new relationship, you'll likely experience significant backslide, mental overwhelm, and a revival of your past belligerence. Even though it's a new relationship promising new beginnings, it will bring up the same energetic tendencies of your past: The Familiar Energy Crisis.

## 38

# Choose the Real You

*Seeking perfection creates unending suffering.*
*Seeking betterment creates unending inspiration.*

You've cleaned up a lot of who you used to be by searching for the things that have held you back—the behaviors that didn't allow your life to flourish, and the ETBs that harmed you and others. You've begun to activate some essential practices toward experiencing truer freedom. To grow, you need a very clean foundation. Let's take a moment to delete some recognized Trauma-Influenced Self-Beliefs and perhaps even some of the really hidden ones. Dig a little deeper now.

When you're cleared of those additional blocks, you may feel a lightening, a spaciousness, or a sense of freedom. Some people actually see colors around the room they're in, or feel a warmth wash over them. They're experiencing a sense of the massive amount of energy that they're saving and receiving by releasing all of the things that have weighed them down. They're feeling it encircling them and within them, sometimes for the very first time. They've left their Center of Self and opened up to what's around them.

> *They're experiencing a sense of the massive amount of energy that they're saving and receiving by releasing all of the things that have weighed them down.*

On the other hand, the next rung on the ladder of transformation can feel a bit daunting. You're in the process of shedding your old self and are left with the opportunity to create a new self. You may feel raw as you're in uncharted territory, having not spent the majority of your life living as the real you. Use the following three contemplations to put yourself in touch with yourself in a new way. Recordings of each are available at **liftedacademy.com/tyynm**.

 CONTEMPLATION

**CHILD-SELF CONNECTING**
Imagine you're sitting next to yourself as a child. Notice what this child looks like, what they're wearing, how they act around you. Make sure you see this child as an individual, separate from your current grown self. Now imagine you were right there next to them when they were traumatized or emotionally overwhelmed. Find that child (perhaps sitting on a playground alone) and sit beside them. Make sure you're the current, more sober version of you as you sit beside them.

- Communicate to them who you are. What would you say?

- Show them how they will eventually grow up and can be anything they want to be.

- Tell them what's true.

- Tell them things like: "You aren't breakable. You're powerful. You're unconditionally loved."

- Flaunt to them who their future self becomes and is still becoming.

- Look into their eyes and feel all the love they have for you and you for them as you make them proud and inspired for their future.

- Remind that child how smart they are, how beautiful, how strong and honorable.

- Tell them all the things that they need to hear from you to allow them to flourish and ease their pain.

- Talk to them about courage.

- Remind them that if they ever hear their minds saying negative things about them, that it's a lie or they can change it if it's true.

- Love and care for them right now, like you're their parent. Maybe even hug them if you feel the pull to do so.

- Linger there for a while as you look into their eyes.
- Let them feel your love as you reach out your hand, inviting them to come along with you. You're reaching out to them to say, "Come with me. You can trust me. You can see we turn out great. Just keep going. I'll fully support you."

Let this child inspire you to become even more than you already are. Do it for them too! Remember you cannot take away anyone else's Trauma-Influenced Self-Beliefs, but this child <u>was</u> you! So, you're uniquely qualified.

Now that you've met, hopefully experienced love for your child self, and awarded them with relief of knowing how bright their future can be, it's time to move forward.

 CONTEMPLATION

**FUTURE-SELF CONNECTING**
As you are now, imagine the future *you* coming to visit. They've completed their full EMSO Training. They've already done the work, and they're here for you!

- First, admire their poise. What do they look like?
- Feel their confidence and the pride they have for you.
- Notice all of the new traits they resemble from the list of STRENGTHS you made. Acknowledge each of these strengths in them, and tell them thank you for embracing these new traits.
- Let them remind you how smart, beautiful, strong, and honorable you are.
- Let them tell you all the things that will allow you to continue to flourish and ease any residual pain.
- They'll talk to you about your courage.
- Let them remind you that if you ever hear yourself saying negative things about yourself, that it's either a lie, or if true, can easily be overcome.
- Let them love and care for you right now, like they're your parent. Maybe even hug them if you feel the pull to do so.
- Let them linger there for a while as they look into your eyes.

- Feel their beaming pride and love for you as they reach out their hand inviting you to come along with them. They're reaching out to you saying "Come with me. You can trust me. You can see we turn out great. Just keep going. I'll support you the whole way."

Take a moment to realize that you already are your future self somewhere in time. Become them now by building from here. Your previous thoughts, beliefs, and decisions have built your life to this point; now continue building.

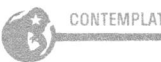
CONTEMPLATION

**BLANK CANVAS**
Read through the following visualization until you have it in your mind. Then find a comfortable place to sit and close your eyes.

Imagine you're completely alone and not in any specific location. There's no one around—no family, no friends, no pets, no relationships of any kind. (This won't last forever—just for a few moments!) Now, I want to imagine you've never had a relationship of any kind with anyone or anything (to the best of your ability). Once you have a clear enough idea of what that would be like, use this opportunity to start imagining a new you. Imagine what thoughts you have, how you feel, and what you notice in your body. Imagine the choices you make, the people you surround yourself with, and the places you go. Imagine anything.

Solitude can be important for certain aspects of your change or healing process—your inner remodeling. In moments of solitude, there's no external influence over who you should be. You can go within and connect with what you want for yourself, without anyone telling you what they think, urging you in a certain direction, or judging you for what you like, dislike, relate to, or believe. You're free in all aspects to make your own choices.

You now get to decide what your values are, your beliefs, your thoughts, your dreams, your desires, your sense of humor, your taste in music and food, and more. All of these are decisions that aren't based on anyone else's opinions, ideals, or influence over you. There's no one to please or disappoint. Only you.

You can choose from a menu of character traits and positive attributes. You can select the highest vibrating emotions. You can decide who you want to become.

# 39

# You Are Not Alone

*Even when it feels like it.*

Let's pause for a moment and acknowledge where you are now. You've completed a rare and brave undertaking—everything from uncovering your Anatomy of Emotional Insobriety, to completing your EMSO Master Chart process, and then the all-important 4Rs. Rest in this awareness for awhile.

You've embarked on a new path, and that often threatens people. It even threatens parts of you (namely your Intoxicated Identity!), so you can be understanding of their concerns. However, you can't let them obstruct your advancement on your path either.

As you learned about in Familiar Energy Crisis, if you aren't surrounded by supportive people, you may need to leave your immediate environment to get well—to separate from any and all unhealthy adult relationships. This may be necessary for you to carry on with your growth without backsliding every time you're near them. This separation doesn't need to be permanent.

EMSO students observe the unconscious ways that they engage in emotionally unsober relationships. This can include manipulation, codependence, dishonesty, insecurity, fear-based behaviors, high-anxiety thoughts and actions, worst-case-scenarios, violence, or shaming.

If, as motivational speaker Jim Rohn says, "you are the average of the five people with whom you spend most of your time," and you're not emotionally sober, then you can probably bet those five are also afflicted with some similar symptoms. You may even see examples of your negative behaviors in the people with whom you spend most of your time.

Being around the strife of anyone during a process of rigorous maturation can be counterproductive, especially if they're skilled in the habitual behaviors you're specifically attempting to overcome.

Even if you decide to step away for a long while, remember that one of the most valuable gifts you can give your loved ones is your clarity, levelheadedness, and peace. I'm not suggesting you're required to move to a remote island to get healthy! Yet due to the reality and possibilities of resistance in your process, it's up to you to come to the decisions of how and with whom you'll be going through this continued transformation. That said, experiencing this pushback can make you feel isolated. On the other hand, if you <u>are</u> supported, that's fantastic!

*Being around others' strife during a process of rigorous maturing can be counterproductive, especially if they're skilled with the habitual behaviors you're specifically attempting to overcome.*

Although it may sometimes seem that you're solo, I want you to know that you are truly not alone. All who are undertaking this journey alongside you, whether you know them or not, are in the same boat. They're having relationship tribulations as they maneuver through this, frustration with being able to see where they're responsible for their own "mistakes." They're feeling pity for themselves, and they sometimes think about quitting. Sound familiar?

Many times, students think that they're alone on this new path, so they may begin to "drag" their friends and relatives to their side of the street in an attempt to collect a new community—telling them that they "have to" do this work to change themselves too, instead of just living as and being an example.

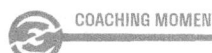
**COACHING MOMENT**

> Many people want their loved ones and colleagues to engage in EMSO Training once they've reached this point. It can be challenging when people in your life don't want for themselves what you've devoted so much of your time and attention to, or when they have a difficult time believing the new you is real. But think about what you're doing by expecting this... families, friends, co-workers... everyone has their own individual challenges, traumas, ETBs, filters, multitudes of unspoken agreements, perceived conclusions, resentments, dishonesty, and inability to reveal everything accurately in life (R.E.A.L.). They're all already juggling a lot, and now you may be asking them to take on even more.
>
> To invite them to look at all of it and undergo this immense task of EMSO Training isn't like asking everyone to get together to paint your house—it's asking for metamorphosis! It is an "all-in" proposition. This work is useful for everyone, but it's not something that everyone chooses. As you well know by now, it requires rare bravery and personal desire. Allow the timing for your loved ones and colleagues to come as it will.

Everyone has to come to EMSO Training by their own decision. You cannot force your newfound ways or opinions onto anyone else. If you wish to see others change for their own benefit, simply demonstrate your own upgrades. If they want what you have, they'll ask you what you've done to change, and maybe even ask for your support and guidance along a similar line. You don't have to shout your Emotional Sobriety from the rooftops. Instead, choose to be it! You'll share it because you'll "wear" it!

While you must know that you're indeed courageous and unique for what you've accomplished, it's also helpful to remember that you're not alone. You're now part of a community of people engaged in EMSO Training.

I'm here to say that if you don't yet know anyone who has begun EMSO Training, or you haven't yet connected with the community in some way, you can now make the choice to do so. Visit **liftedacademy.com/tyynm** or use this code to connect with the EMSO community, hear about upcoming events, revisit the recorded contemplations as often as you need, learn how to share EMSO with friends and family, and more.

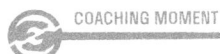
**COACHING MOMENT**

Imagine us all virtually holding your hand and assuring you that it's okay that you've made "mistakes." It's okay that you've made a fool of yourself. It's okay that there are people out there who don't like you or don't forgive you. It's okay if you haven't fully overcome all of your traumas or abuse. It's understandable that you're angry, sad, and resentful.

You're now changing all that. There isn't anyone on this planet who hasn't been handed a lifetime that contained challenges. Everyone has experienced some form of manipulation, control, or abuse.

Regardless of our circumstances, our empowerment is in deciding whether to remain victims, or be free of the chains of emotional intoxication. There's a version of you that will choose empowerment no matter what has happened to you, no matter what you've done, no matter how alone you may seem. Begin to believe that you're becoming a more resilient, new you.

Know that we're all the same, and you're not alone.

# 40

# The *You* You've Never Met

*Our same problems cannot exist when we've changed ourselves.*

No matter what you've left behind of your old self, find peace in knowing that no past traumas can persist within this new version of you. Any past trauma that occurred happened to a version of you that doesn't exist anymore.

After advancing in EMSO Training, your body will eventually stop making the biochemical that went along with your old beliefs and filters, and this is the next level of Emotional Sobriety. The traumas, of course, never go away. They happened. But you've now become the person that the traumas didn't happen to. They happened to the *you* you used to be. You now have wisdom from that trauma.

Give yourself a moment to recognize the work you did to achieve this. Realize you've reached a peak on this mountain. The long and arduous work to get here has begun to transform the *you* you were being. That version of you that has been dragged over rough terrain and starved of its usual "nutrition" of enabling and ignorance. It was dissolved in self-responsibility, courage, honesty, humility, vulnerability, and understanding. And with the wisdom your work has granted you, there will soon be effortless poise and integrity.

Now that you're at the peak of this mountain, look back on the trip you took to get here. You'll see the natural elements that surround you in a more profound way. You'll feel the powerful peace within you. These feelings of accomplishment may be the most intensely rewarding experience of your life up to this point. Having separated from your past behaviors, thoughts, self-beliefs, reactions, and resentments, you are now the real you—the *you* you'd never met. By now, you're more familiar than ever with the Anatomy of Emotional Insobriety, as you worked so hard to discover the details of your own. And though it may have felt like you were wrong or bad for having it, it's actually the most essential cog in the wheel of your Emotional Sobriety! Looking here, you can see that your insobriety is the "seed" that blossoms into your sobriety. Look at the Anatomy of Emotional Sobriety and all the components that make it possible at this point in your training. This will get larger as you advance beyond your EMSO Essentials Training through the next two phases:

- EMSO Practicum—second-tier EMSO Training to become the calm in the storm.
- EMSO AP—advanced practices for maintaining Emotional Sobriety, regardless of the circumstance.

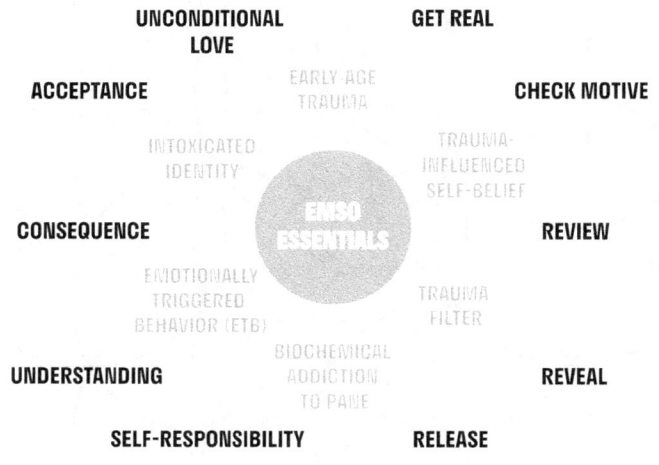

The real you won't be affected by pain like the old version was, yet they will retain the wisdom of what it's like to overcome suffering. And because of this wisdom—and with the practice of integrity—this new version of you can trust in itself completely.

The memory of your old self can now be introduced to your unburied—once trapped—real self. And think of how proud that version of you would be! You'll show your old self gratitude and acknowledge what it went through to get you here—how it sacrificed itself because of its love for you.

Feel immense love for the past version of yourself, because that person was brave enough to make the choice to change, even when it seemed impossible. Your past self-sacrificed the things that made it feel comfortable. It allowed its secrets and lies to be looked at, giving the child within you a new place to happily dwell.

*Feel immense love for the past version of yourself because that person was brave enough to make the choice to change, even when it seemed impossible.*

As our movement of Emotional Sobriety grows, our excitement for growth expands, and our love for ourselves and others braids us a new community. We're evolutionary creatures. We naturally seek growth and improvement. You may be eager for more growth, even while standing on the mountain after the journey of self-recreation. If you look, you'll always notice there are more mountains yet to climb. You won't be able to stop yourself from taking that next step toward becoming even freer, and to witness the greater sights of meeting the real you.

I consider this journey we've just taken together the primer for your advanced personal growth. It will allow numerous new teachings to come into your life, and even a return of some you've left behind (thinking they were ineffective). Without your blocks, fears, victimhood, trauma, ETBs, insecurities, attempted control of others, and dishonesty of your past, you're in a new life. You're ready to hear the lessons your teachers are speaking to you. You suddenly understand their language, feel their intention, and seek more and more information to apply directly to your own life.

We cannot learn or hear even the most articulate and talented teachers until we're in the right place to receive the information—until we're open in a different way to apply it to our lives.

EMSO Training contains your "prerequisite" teachings, meaning they're required as a prior condition for something else to happen or exist. As I've said before, this is only the beginning. Practicing these new intentions and ways of being to the point that they become your new default requires additional training, which is now waiting for you in the EMSO Practicum.

# Afterword: Evolution of Emotional Sobriety

*If you desire to see more miracles in the world, start performing them yourself.*

Humanity has evolved technologically by leaps and bounds over the last 100 years. However, we haven't really evolved in emotional wisdom or maturity as a group. If I were to sit down with any average person and their family and ask them what their problems are, they would most likely tell me the same things that their parents did. Continuing from there—grandparents and great-grandparents—the complaints, emotionally speaking, would all sound similar.

We've learned to become angry, depressed, sad, jealous, judgmental, and lack awareness around our manipulations and dishonesty. Our society tends to fight, cheat, and complain. We're often sick, we gossip, we're riddled with shame, and we sprinkle guilt over ourselves and others. In current times, we seem to continue to have these very basic emotional problems even alongside our masterful technological evolution.

*Can we ignite a massive revolution for our emotional evolution?*

Generation after generation, we find this drama, hysteria, and frantic demonstration. We find the same pain, the same depression, the same anxiety. Thus, I ask us all: Can we ignite a massive revolution for our emotional evolution? We can take the quality of our lives into our own hands and say, "I'm not doing it this way anymore!" There are far more useful ways for us to live—through love, service to others, honesty, connection, and even bliss.

Let's not settle for minor emotional evolution. Let's choose massive metamorphosis for our families, society, and the generations to come. If you didn't have an example of Emotional Sobriety in your life, and you wish you did, <u>be</u> the example. By becoming an example of Emotional Sobriety, you can help advance your community. Be the miracle that people look to emulate. Stand out, educate, and mercifully love those who will let you. When you're looking around for a leader and there is none, step up and be the leader.

---

*Our responsibility is to be self-responsible.*

---

Imagine what our workplaces, our families, and our world will look like when we're each committed to self-responsibility—when we blame no one, resent no one, and focus diligently on our own sanity, thoughts, feelings, and behaviors. Imagine a time when our eagerness to love others is so great that we can't feel hate, when our reactions come from the new norm of mercy and goodwill, and our communities work together peacefully and cooperatively. Imagine a culture filled with people who can see their flaws and work on their betterment for the good of all. When our focus and refocus are placed on making sure that we're having healthy and contributing thoughts and behaviors, all of the community around us has the opportunity to entrain to that.

Our mission: Emotional Sobriety—to enhance our capacity to give and receive love, and to find our personal integrity and develop to a new level each day. Our responsibility is to be self-responsible.

We are to be examples. That intention, when taken seriously, will lead us into the contagious nature of freedom—into massive change and a new age of self-responsibility.

When we do this, we'll be placed into our future. We don't think about <u>how</u> to get there, we live and demonstrate as the people who already belong there.

# Author's Notes

### Why Don't I Talk About Recovery?
I chose not to use the word "recovery" when referring to Emotional Sobriety, because to me, it indicates that we're aiming to return to a previously healthy state.

The overwhelming majority of people I've met—myself included—did not <u>first</u> experience sanity, balance, or levelheadedness before becoming "unsober." We didn't fall from grace and are now seeking to return there. We don't need to re-cover, or return to where we were, under cover of our shame, guilt, embarrassment, resentment, and more. If I'd been told that I would return to life as it was before my insobriety, I may have asked, "Return to what?" I'd been fearful, anxious, emotionally reactionary, and self-centered for as long as I could recall! If I were to return anywhere, I would be returning to actual childhood, and that would put me in the same position as an innocent, young being to develop the responses to my Early-Age Traumas that I already had.

So, for these reasons, <u>this isn't a book on recovery</u>. This isn't the work of getting you back to somewhere you've been already; it's the work that thrusts you face-to-face with the choice of being brand new.

### Chapter Symbol
This is the symbol that came to the artist as "the symbol for Emotional Sobriety." So we simply now call it the "EMSO symbol." It translates differently for each person and their unique journey. Some see it as "getting over the self," or a sun rising over a mountain representing an arduous climb, while others see the moon over an ocean wave.

Sometimes it's translated as the integration of our "stillness" (the whole circle) and "movement" (open-ended line) that Emotional Sobriety gifts each of us. When you look at it, what does it communicate to you?

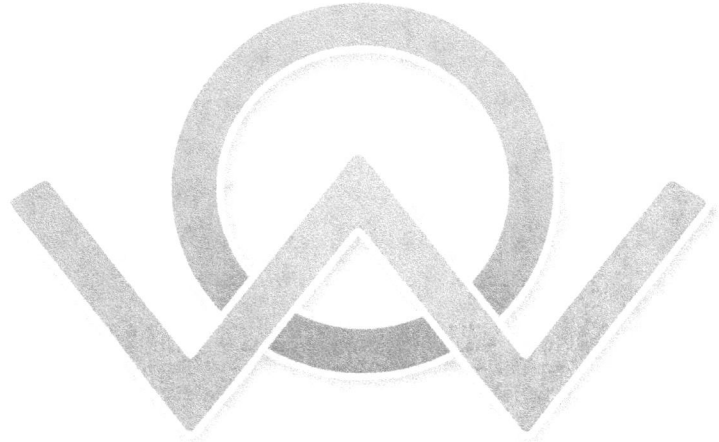

# Endnotes

**You're Here**

[1] Page 20 in "Ignorant, Not Innocent"–merriam-webster.com/dictionary/insanity

[2] Page 25 in "Ignorant, Not Innocent"–en.wikipedia.org/wiki/Ignorance

[3] Page 28 in "Common Misconceptions"– https://www.ncbi.nlm.nih.gov/pmc/articles/PMC4085815/

[4] Page 28 in "Common Misconceptions"–dictionary.cambridge.org/us/dictionary/english/emotional-intelligence

[5] Page 29 in "Common Misconceptions"–merriam-webster.com/dictionary/sober

[6] Page 30 in "Common Misconceptions"–merriam-webster.com/dictionary/sober

**EMSO Foundations: The *You* You've Been Being**

[7] Page 50 in "Early-Age Trauma"–Chapter 1, Healing Trauma, by Peter A. Levine

[8] Page 50 in "Early-Age Trauma"–childwelfare.gov/topics/preventing/preventionmonth/resources/ace/

[9] Page 67 in "Biochemical Addiction"–Paraphrased from Evolve Your Brain: The Science of Changing Your Mind, by Dr. Joe Dispenza

[10] Page 69 in "Biochemical Addiction"–Paraphrased from the work of Dr. Joe Dispenza, Breaking the Habit of Being Yourself & Becoming Supernatural

[11] Page 118 in "What Am I *Actually* Doing? Feeling? And Why?"–Paraphrased from the work of Bruce H. Lipton, Ph.D., The Biology of Belief

**EMSO Investigations: The *You* You've Never Noticed**

[12] Page 165 in "Outgrow Childishness"–learned from <u>Healing Trauma</u>, by Peter A. Levine

[13] Page 166 in "Outgrow Childishness"–Maslow's Hierarchy on simplypsychology.org/maslow.html

[14] Page 178 in "Free the Self"–Marcia K. Keating, Yale Unversity, "Memory & Reality"

**EMSO Repairs: The *You* You're Revealing**

[15] Page 262 in "R.E.A.Life Investigation"–<u>Transcending the Levels of Consciousness–The Stairway to Enlightenment</u> by David Hawkins, M.D.

[16] Page 278 in "R.E.A.Life Investigation"–<u>Illusions: The Adventures of a Reluctant Messiah</u>, by Richard Bach

**The *You* You've Never Met**

[17] Page 344 in "Fighting to Stay the Same"–Ted O'Neill, Strength and Conditioning Coach, Founder Diablo Barbell (diablo-barbell.com), Developer of the Paraphysical Training method (paraphysicaltraining.com), and co-founder of Lifted Academy (liftedacademy.com)

# Glossary of EMSO Terms

**Acceptance:** a premeditated, often spoken, peacefulness surrounding others' words, behaviors, and feelings.
**Action:** the doing part of life; the movement or work to achieve your desired intention.
**Advanced Practices (APs):** practices for the emotionally sober to advance them beyond their initial sobriety.
**Anger:** an immense "burning" of pain, directed at someone who was believed to have caused it.
**Avoidant Ignorance:** (lack of desire to know); an intentional closing of the eyes.
**Biochemical Addiction to PANE:** addiction to chemicals created within our body that can intoxicate our thinking and behaviors, which our body becomes chronically addicted to making.
**Confrontation:** (con-front); to bring to the front—to pick up a topic and set it down on the "table" for discussion.
**Consequence:** simply what happens next—after something.
**Courage:** to go "all in."
**Criticism:**
>**Exclusionary Criticism:** any 'ism or social phobia; to deny opportunity to someone based on race or color, religion or creed, gender or lifestyle preference, judgments that exclude other people due to different beliefs, statuses, cultures, or being born the "wrong kinds of person."
>**Loud Criticism:** an outward declaration of your judgments.
>**Vacuum Criticism:** this form of judgment appears as attemping to control your environment by continuously and disrespectfully pointing out flaws in it.

**Desire:** a strong, energetic drive for something to occur.

**Early-Age Trauma:** <u>any</u> event that creates a hard change in your emotional status... a stark contrast to the feelings you had before the event; a moment that changes or influences what you believe to be true about yourself and the world around you in a negative way.

> **Delivered Trauma:** trauma that you inflict upon someone or something.
> **Inflicted Trauma:** trauma inflicted upon you by someone or something.
> **Observed Trauma:** witnessing an impactful or dissonant event.
> **Perceived Trauma:** judging the intention of someone else's action.

**Ego:** the security guard of the status quo.

**Embarrassment:** strong feeling of shame; feeling exposed, overly-observed, objectified, or made a joke.

**Empowerment:** the experience of having once been a victim and now choosing to become victorious; to remember your power.

**Emotional Addiction:** see Biochemical Addiction to PANE.

**Emotional Belligerence:** to become overrun with harsh biochemicals, emotionally "drunk," losing the power of choice regarding behavior, along with the inability to be corrected until the chemistry changes on its own.

**Emotional Insobriety:** the chronic state of biochemical addiction stemming from Early-Age Trauma, demonstrated via dysfunctional behavior, negative patterns, or destructive traits.

**Emotional Intelligence:** awareness of your emotions.

**Emotionally-Triggered Behaviors (ETBs):** habituatl reactions stemming from biochemical intoxication, demonstrated under stress or threat.

**Emotional Sobriety:** to be rid of the filters, beliefs, and subsequent emotions that cause emotional overwhelm; to no longer feel the offendable biochemistry that promotes our triggered behaviors; to be able to experience all of life with levelheadedness, clarity, and peace.

**Endogenous Addiction:** addiction to the chemicals made within the body.

**Exogenous Addiction:** addiction to chemicals made outside the body.

**Expectations:** a premeditated, often unspoken, standard for how someone should speak, behave, or feel.

**Familiar Energy Crisis:** compulsion to return to the person you've chosen to stop being by virtue of being near the energy of past familiar relationships.
**Fear:** a feeling of helplessness.
**Growing-up Family:** all the family members or people with whom you lived while growing up.
**Guilt:** self-resentment; the feeling of having done something wrong; failed obligation.
**Humility:** the ability to see who you've been in the past, and open to see that you're no better than anyone else.
**Identity:**
>   **Chosen Identity:** how we present ourselves to the world based on who we have chosen to be—our values, beliefs, thoughts, feelings, behaviors, personality traits, how we speak, our level of energy, and our capacity to transform our energy depending on the situation.
>   **Intoxicated Identity:** becoming someone you didn't choose as a result of your Early-Age Traumas and the re̲actions and confusion from these experiences; to lack a chosen identity due to emotional insobriety; to take on a role in life rather than living as your chosen self.

**Ignorance:** unawareness; deliberately ignoring important information or facts about the self, including behaviors, beliefs, and treatment of the self and others.
**Integrity:** the state of knowing you're whole, entire, and complete, regardless of the circumstance.
**Intention:** the planning and aim toward your desired outcome.
**Mercy:** a power that when activated can shift us from hate/blame to understanding/ease, and when used in repetition (or when accessed at its most pure point), thrusts us into a state of ultimate and permanent forgiveness.
**Motive:** the honest "why" behind feelings, thoughts, and behaviors.
**Punishment:** a chosen sentencing, with the intention of promoting shame or balancing the suffering that you've experienced; making someone else feel the pain that you feel.
**Re-act:** behaving compulsively, seemingly without choice—a pre-programmed act or behavior.

**R.E.A.L.:** reveal everything accurately in life.

**Real You:** the innermost you, before you experienced any trauma; the original *you* that you were created to be; the *you* that you consciously create; the *you* you've never met.

**Resentment:** continued bitterness regarding having been seemingly treated unfairly.

**Respond:** behaving by choice or intentionally.

**Sadness:** a feeling of hopelessness.

**Sanity:** a comprehensive understanding of the self, the training and maintaining of the self, and the ability to have self-control...including control over our thoughts, emotions, and the way we respond to our inner and outer world.

**Self-centeredness:** believing that most things are <u>about</u> you.

**Selfishness:** believing that most things are <u>for</u> you.

**Self-responsibility:** the responsibility of a problem lies on the person whose life it belongs to.

**Shame:** self-punishment.

**Trauma Filter:** an unconscious barrier put in place after an Early-Age Trauma to validate our Trauma-Influenced Self-Beliefs by collecting events that are familiar to our past and adapting the picture of everything, allowing for repetition of our memorized feelings of trauma.

**Trauma-Influenced Self-Belief:** belief adopted about ourselves that becomes part of our identity as a remnant snapshot of our Early-Age Trauma; with unresolved trauma, these self-beliefs become the internalized "story" of who we are and what we expect the outside world believe about us as well.

**Unconditional Attention:** the compulsion to give or receive continued attention, regardless of level of trustworthiness, respectful treatment, or mutual interest.

**Unconditional Love:** the feeling, intention, and choice to love someone energetically, regardless of level of trustworthiness, respectful treatment, or mutual interest, not necessarily followed up with attention.

**Unspoken Agreements:** a system of one-sided imaginary contracts that are developed without a previous plan or discussion.

# Acknowledgments

This work was a calling, an order, and a non-negotiable to me. And this calling came to me alongside a full-time job, two businesses, and a family. Thankfully the people who make up my family encouraged me during the whole process. I spent most of my time writing during late nights or when my daughter was otherwise engaged so I was sure not to miss much more time with her.

In terms of acknowledgment, I want to clearly declare my love and appreciation to you, my daughter. Your unyielding enthusiasm during the composition of this book motivated me again and again. The happy tears in your eyes when I handed you a first run manuscript was one of the proudest moments of my life. Witnessing your inspiration in your own writing, and your fearless belief in me, enchanted me into believing I could also be a writer. Your precision and commitment to your internship at Levelheaded Doc helped bring the EMSO Training curriculum into new life in a more meaningful way. I promise to always continue to be a better me and make sure our relationship remains healthy and free.

Deep gratitude to Ted O'Neill for his remarkable support both in my writing this book and during my own personal Emotional Sobriety voyage. I cannot be descriptive enough in declaring how you've saved my life. Thank you for being so eager for this to be written, and fully supporting and advocating this from when it was only a glimmer on the horizon. I've been granted so much wisdom just by virtue of knowing you. I've collected so much self-confidence via achievement through your teachings. You're a master teacher in all four planes of our existence (mental, physical, emotional, and energetic).

You may say I owe you nothing, yet I'm indebted to you for one million lifetimes simply for helping me heal so profoundly in this lifetime, and putting me in the position to help thousands of others heal as I did. Thank you for showing me what it means to be loved.

Thank you to my parents for bringing me to Earth, for convincing me I was smart when I didn't always believe it, and for showing me how to work hard. If I didn't have all of that, this book would not exist. I carry the best parts of each of you within me everyday.

To Mark, for being a massive point of inspiration for me to take on this mission to ask people to go deeper and work harder to master Emotional Sobriety, so that no outside influence can derail their intentions. I know that even though you never met The Real Me—the emotionally sober me—you helped create her, and this EMSO movement, in spirit.

Thank you to my teachers, for breathing life into so many concepts and ideas which allowed me to articulate these teachings in a clearer way. Thank you for doing the work and research, for spending countless hours to become the teachers you've become, and for making sacrifices to teach what you know to the students who are ready to receive it.

Additionally, a sincere thank you to my outstanding friends, teammates, and patients. A list of loving and generous souls that are so numerous I couldn't list them all. You're a true demonstration of my fortune of friendship. We don't need a list because you know who you are. You've loved and encouraged me daily. Your eagerness for me to share this book was one of the biggest reasons I was able to complete it, and your interest in reading it re-validated the importance of its being written. I'm so blessed with so many wonderful people in my life.

To all my EMSO students that have come before, know that the process of teaching you taught me so much! I have loads of love for each and every one of you. I will always remember your first moments of vulnerability, honesty, and humility. That moment is an event that we'll always share and will connect us forever.

To the one who got me to the finish line, my editor and soul friend, Amanda Kay Creighton. There's absolutely no one on this planet who could have done this with me the way that you did. You've been such a supporter and influencer of this mission, and you're integral in its growth. Your value goes far beyond editing, attention to detail, and precision. You brought this book and curriculum to life with me. I will forever remember your example.

Thank you to Dustin Brunson and A.C. Gelicame for adding your clarity and art to this project's graphics and layout with such professionalism, gratitude, and excitement.

Lastly, thank you from the depths of my heart to the creators of the Twelve-Step Program. I believe that work will stand the test of time as an anchor and starting point for a reality-based life that always comes back to our own personal power and responsibility. I'm eternally grateful for its teachings and their impact on my life and the lives of others. EMSO Training comes next!

# About the Author

Dr. Andrea Vitz is founder and CEO of Levelheaded Doc, LLC, an educational platform committed to a global Emotional Sobriety movement, and the primary developer of EMSO Training. She is also the co-founder and one of the primary faculty at Lifted Academy. She leads others to their own healing by attacking the cause of suffering, opening the door for reinvention, and being an example of the power to welcome drastic correction and control of their lives. Along with being an Emotional Sobriety Educator, she's a Doctor of Chiropractic, Life & Relationship Coach, and Strength & Rehabilitation Expert.

Attaining her doctorate at age 23, becoming a mother at 25, and becoming a business owner soon after, Dr. Vitz hoped her successes were an indicator of certain maturity. It wasn't until someone she trusted expressed their concern that who she was *being* did not match her statement of what she intended. This remains one of the most influential messages that was ever spoken to her. Here, she began her work of self-investigation, self-reliance, and self-metamorphosis.

Her efforts as an educator and coach have provided her with countless hours of experience to draw from. As a result of her intense passion for Emotional Sobriety, she was coined the name "Levelheaded Doc" as it applies to both her intention individually and what she encourages in her students.

Alongside her process to levelheadedness, she was experiencing a major spinal injury. Refusing surgery, with her dogged determination she overcame all of her ails, via her desire and practice of the new. Her injury rehabilitation led her from disability to finding strength and earning an elite status as well as becoming a National Champion in the sport of powerlifting.

Dr. Vitz attempts to excel in many different areas in an effort to better serve her students, clients, and patients. Her belief is that she's never done growing and improving, choosing to be an example of inspiration to her clients and colleagues. She lives in California with her family while delivering chiropractic care in her busy, established practice, teaching strength and rehabilitation, and providing high-level coaching and EMSO Training to thousands of students and clients.

*Not only can you overcome your traumas, weaknesses, and pain, you can transform them into your strongest attributes.*

~Dr. Andrea Vitz

www.ingramcontent.com/pod-product-compliance
Lightning Source LLC
Chambersburg PA
CBHW071227070526
44583CB00017B/2083